Social Psychology for Nurses

Social Psychology for Nurses

Understanding interaction in health care

Charles Abraham BA(Hons), DPhil, AFBPsS, CPsychol
Department of Epidemiology and Public Health,
University of Dundee

and

Eamon Shanley BA(Hons), MSc, PhD, RNMH,
RMN, CPN, RNT
Department of Nursing Studies,
University of Glasgow

Edward Arnold
A division of Hodder & Stoughton
LONDON   MELBOURNE   AUCKLAND

© 1992 Charles Abraham and Eamon Shanley

First published in Great Britain 1992

British Library Cataloguing in Publication Data

Abrahams. C.
  Social Psychology for Nurses:
  Understanding Interactions in Health
  Care
  I. Title II. Shanley, Eamon
  302

  ISBN 0–7131–4577–3

Whilst the advice and information in this book is believed to
be true and accurate at the date of going to press, neither the
author nor the publisher can accept any legal responsibility or
liability for any errors or omissions that may be made.

Typeset in 10/12 pt. Palatino by Anneset, Weston-super-Mare,
Avon
Printed and bound in Great Britain for Edward Arnold, a divi-
sion of Hodder and Stoughton Limited, Mill Road, Dunton
Green, Sevenoaks, Kent TN13 2YA by Biddles Ltd., Guildford
and King's Lynn.

Preface

The idea behind this book developed in 1987 when Eamon was course leader of the full-time nursing degree at Dundee Institute of Technology and I was teaching a range of psychology courses on the nursing diploma and degree courses taught there. However, the history of this idea can be traced back to the mid 1970s. when both Eamon and I had studied for the specialized undergraduate degree in social psychology offered by Sussex University. Following different paths, as a psychiatric nurse and a psychology lecturer we had each become interested in applying social psychological ideas to nursing.

Many psychological concepts and research findings outside the domain of social psychology are relevant to nursing. However, given our backgrounds we are especially aware of the way in which social psychology is related to developments in nursing. Most nursing care involves joint action with a patient directed towards a health-related objective. Assessment, planning, implementation and evaluation are all dependent on nurse–patient interaction. Thus the management of interaction lies at the heart of nursing and interaction is the special focus of social psychology.

We hope that the book will help nurses develop a psychological insight into the social interaction involved in nursing care. It is written for those who have no previous knowledge of psychology and attempts to foster a cumulative understanding of social psychology through its chapter sequence. The book would be suitable for nurses beginning to study psychology at different levels of professional development (for example, both diploma and degree level). Sections and chapters may be read when relevant and readers are referred back to more basic ideas when this is foundational to material covered in later chapters. Although the book is suitable for the novice it attempts to provide a challenging excursion into the territory of social psychologists.

The aim of the book is to introduce nurses to the theory and research which social psychologists have used to illuminate the intricacies of interaction. We hope it will provide nurses with the tools social psychologists have used to analyse and explain everyday interaction so that nurses can apply these to developing ever more effective nursing interaction – most importantly nurse–patient interaction, but also nurse–nurse and nurse–doctor interaction. The book tries to take the reader gradually through social psychologists' exploration of interaction, constantly relating this to the health and care orientated tasks which constitute nursing.

Nursing intervention is often directed towards encouraging change, usually an improvement in a patient's well-being or health status. We have therefore been especially interested in the way in which social psychological research can help us encourage and predict change. Many chapters explore the way in which relationships or social context shape our behaviour and show that when social aspects of our everyday world are changed we too may develop and change. Understanding the social determinants of people's behaviour is the key to understanding how social forces can be employed to foster personal development. The book therefore focuses on the social foundations of routine and change in our lives and explores how a knowledge of these processes can enable nurses to facilitate social and individual change.

The book is written primarily for nurses but many of the social psychological issues it considers are equally important to those working with nurses. We feel that the book may therefore be of interest to a range of health-care workers who are concerned with the interaction of nurses and patients.

Charles Abraham
Dundee, 1992

Acknowledgements

We would like to thank Jenny Cross, Terri Shanley and Adam Shanley for their support and tolerance. We would also like to thank Jenny for her helpful comments on a number of chapters. Pat Sawers for her help with typing some of the chapters and Margaret Ross for her artistic help with figures and diagrams.

Dedication

To our teachers who took time to explain, to our students who brought enthusiasm to learning, and to patients who have shared their experience with us.

Contents

1

What is social psyschology?

1 Introduction to Social Psychology

The subject matter of social psychology

Social psychology is about understanding people and what they do. It is the study of how people behave in everyday social settings. It focuses upon what happens between people, that is how they *interact*. It attempts to discover patterns in this interaction and thereby poses questions about the kind of beings we are; questions about what controls and regulates our everyday activity.

Students new to the subject often adopt one of two views about social psychology. They think that studying it will enable them to 'analyze' other people (that is, understand their private thoughts by watching their behaviour) or, alternatively, that it will be a waste of time because we all already know about such things (that is, that social psychology is merely a restatement of common-sense). Neither is true but each contains some insight into the nature of social psychology.

The first view assumes that people's behaviour is controlled by private thoughts and feelings which we cannot easily understand. This is partially true in that individual beliefs, intentions and aspirations do shape behaviour. However, as we shall see throughout this book social psychologists have demonstrated that much of our behaviour can be understood in terms of beliefs and meanings common to all those brought up within a particular culture or belonging to a particular group. We can gain some insight into this by noticing how similar people's behaviour is in similar social settings, for example, in lectures or when meeting someone in a position of authority. Indeed social psychologists have suggested that the roots of our everyday behaviour are much more *public* and *social* than we generally think. Of course this does not mean than social psychology will not help the student understand others' behaviour. On the contrary, we believe that it provides important insights into everyday conduct. However, these insights concern *social* rather than personal processes, that is, beliefs and behaviours which are created by the interaction *between* people. This idea that social determinants shape our individual behaviour will be our underlying theme.

What can social psychology offer nurses?

The relevance of social psychology to nursing lies in the *interpersonal* nature of nursing itself. Much of what a nurse achieves in her work happens in the course of her interaction with patients[1]. Consider some key elements in the nursing role, for example, assessment, treatment-evaluation, health education and counselling. Each of these depends upon nurse and patient understanding one another, being able to communicate effectively and trying to modify their behaviour to accommodate the views and responses of the other. *Relationship management* then, lies at the core of effective nursing. Studying social psychology offers the nurse an opportunity to understand in greater depth the processes which regulate her[2] and her patients' everyday experiences, interactions and relationships.

Each of us has our own insights into such processes. Social psychological theory can substantiate or challenge, such insights by revealing the way in which our everyday experiences are related to the social situations in which they occur. The connections between our experiences and our social relationships can remain hidden in the 'cut and thrust' of moment-to-moment interaction but can be revealed by adopting a more detached, social psychological perspective. It may be obvious, for example, that a nurse needs to monitor her prejudices and ensure that they do not undermine her ability to care for and work with others. Social psychological theory can, however, provide a wider understanding of what we mean by 'prejudice'. It can help us understand how we form impressions of others and how prejudices are based on these impressions. It can explain why we are sometimes prejudiced and sometimes not. It can show how such prejudices unconsciously change the way in which we communicate with another person once we begin to think of her as belonging to a particular social group and what effect this has on any developing relationship. Examining such underlying social processes can help us explain why people act as they do and why we feel about others as we do.

Our intention then, is to offer the nurse a set of theoretical models and theories which will provide insights into her everyday experiences, her patients' behaviour and the nature of nurse–patient interaction. This will give her a better basis for assessing what can and cannot be achieved within the nurse–patient relationship in any particular setting and, we hope, enhance her ability to relate to patients.

The kind of questions we shall explore include: how can we promote health behaviour; why do we worry about what others are thinking about us; why do we often feel an acute need to 'fit in' and how does this affect nursing practice; why do we divide people up into 'us and them' and treat 'them' with less respect than 'us'; how can such prejudice be reduced; how can we improve our communication with others; how do we form and maintain personal relationships; how does becoming a patient affect our feelings and behaviour; why do we sometimes not help people in emergencies; why is it hard to say, 'No', to those in authority even when we think they are wrong; what is involved in good leadership; how can we help others change their thoughts, feelings and behaviour; what motivates and satisfies us at work?

Social psychology and the obvious

'But isn't this all just common-sense?', our second respondent is still asking. Certainly our language includes a great variety of common-sense understandings of peoples' behaviour. We might, for example, explain a person's conduct by saying, 'She's racist' or 'She very extrovert', and such comments could play an important part in decision-making processes, for example in student nurse assessment. Everyday interaction then is *embedded in*, and *directed by*, 'common-sense' psychological explanations. In a job interview, for example, the candidates attempt to live up to the expectations they imagine interviewers have concerning suitable applicants. In other words, they behave in accordance with their theory about the interviewers' theories about the ideal employee.

This relationship between everyday behaviour and common-sense psychology was explored by Heider (1958) who argued that, as social psychologists, we must regard 'common-sense psychology' as an important part of our subject matter. This means that as social psychologists we must reflect on our immediate, everyday psychological judgements in a critical manner. Thus we might ask; what assumptions are involved in categorizing a person as 'racist' do these assumptions provide us with a good explanation of when people do and do not make 'racist' remarks and what do these categorizations tell us about the way in which we regularly make judgements about others? Alternatively, we might ask why one person with chest pains explains these as the result of worries about work and does not seek professional help while another person becomes concerned about their heart function and goes to see their general practitioner. By asking questions of this kind we adopt the perspective of the social psychologist and begin to explore the very 'obviousness' such common sense judgements and their impact on everyday, social interaction. Heider (1958) summarized the aim of such social psychological investigation as an attempt to pierce 'the veil of obviousness'.

Schutz (1953) discussed this theoretical perspective on common-sense in some detail and distinguished between *first-order* and *second-order* theories. First-order theories are the 'obvious' psychological explanations we use in everyday common-sense, while second-order theories are those of social psychology. These second-order theories use first-order theories as part of their subject matter. In other words social psychological theory must explain *common-sense* psychological theories. Thus instead of restating common-sense social psychology attempts to analyse its effects on our behaviour. Throughout the book we shall be inviting the reader to adopt this critical, second-order perspective on her own everyday judgements of people and their actions.

We shall argue that, to a large extent, people are as they are because they collectively believe in particular common-sense psychological theories. In other words aspects of ourselves which we regard as 'natural', and describe as 'just the way people are', are in fact sustained by a general acceptance of particular theories about how we should be. Since most of us believe these theories, most of the time, and therefore act in accordance with them, it appears as if these theories are quite simply true. By adapting a second-order stance we shall see that common-sense theories are a shared construction of how the social world should operate. An example of such a theory is the idea that our behaviour is largely the result of our various personalities. In everyday conversation the notion of 'personality' is very useful for making sense of people's behaviour. We shall argue, however, that when we examine the assumptions upon which this notion is based and consider the ways in which our behaviour changes across situations, we discover that it is, in many ways, misleading; misleading, that is, as a general, second-order theory of how people think and act.

This does not mean that common-sense is generally flawed and mistaken but that it contains many different and sometimes contradictory psychological theories which we switch between as we move from one social setting to another. These are adequate as everyday explanations of particular experiences but, not as overarching, second-order analyses of behaviour in general.

2   Two Important Source Models for Social Psychology

The importance of models in theory building

In order to develop second-order theories social psychologists use models of interaction and people. By 'model' we mean a comparison, a simulation or an analogy. By examining a similar or simplified structure to the one we are studying we may develop a new way of thinking about some aspect of the thing we are really interested in. In trying to understand the human body, for example, we might use an anatomical model in which the organs are represented by plastic pieces of different sizes, shapes and colours. Studying such a model will help us understand the size and positioning of our organs but other models will be required if we are to understand their functioning. In order to understand the operation of the heart, for example, we might compare it to a mechanical pump. We already understand what a pump does and at least roughly how it works so by imagining the heart as a pump we gain an insight into its operation. Indeed Miller (1978) argues that our understanding of pumps led to our modern conception of the heart. He points out that the evidence on which Harvey based his theory of cardiac functioning, in the early seventeenth century, had been available 1500 years before to the Greek physiologist Galen but, because he did not have an appropriate model Galen could not 'see' the evidence in the same way as Harvey. As Miller puts it;

> There were no better analogies than those of the lamp or the smelter's furnace . . . Galen's inability to see the heart as a pump was due to the fact that such machines did not become a significant part of the cultural scene until long after his death. The heart could be seen as a pump only when such engines began to be widely exploited in sixteenth-century mining, fire-fighting and civil engineering.'(p.187)

This demonstrates two important points, first, that theories are based on models and secondly, that without appropriate models we may, like Galen, be unable to appreciate the significance of even very familiar experiences, that is, we may fail to 'see the evidence'. Harré (1983) refers to the models on which our theories are based as 'source models' and in this section we shall introduce two important source models for social psychology. These are the *person as computer* and *person as actress* models. At the end of this chapter we shall return to the relationship between 'evidence' and available models.

The computational model

Just as pumps helped us understand the heart so computers have helped us understand the relationship between mind and brain (Fodor, 1976). Computers manipulate information, that is they are information processors. Unlike other machines, such as pumps or watches, their functioning can be altered by changing the programs (that is, the instructions) they use. This is because the information-processing capacity of computers enables them to store descriptions of parts of the world as well as rules about how they should respond to certain features of this world. A computer can, for example, be programmed to play chess; to do this it must 'know about' the different pieces, the lay-out of the board and, of course, the rules. The computer 'knows about' chess in the sense that it's programs embody a representation of the game. This representation can be thought of as an internal description which (like it's human opponents) the computer uses to examine the moves it can legally make, anticipate it's opponent's moves and select the move which will give it the best position. Acknowledging that computers have this ability to represent the world and, after consulting their internal representations, to act according to stored rules, we can begin to think of our own behaviour as directed in the same way. We can ask, what kind of representations and rules do we need to be able to act as we do, and how do we use these to direct our behaviour? In other words what kinds of programs are our beliefs about the world embedded in and how do these programs enable us to anticipate everyday social interaction.

Of course, just as there are differences between a mechanical pump and a heart, so there are important differences between a computer and a person. One of these is that *people form complex representations of themselves*. A person can consider what kind of person she is, and can even think about the way she uses this representation of self. This kind of awareness of self-representation is referred to when we make statement such as, 'I thought I knew it all when I first qualified'. This is, as we shall see throughout the book, a crucial aspect of what it is to be a person and to be able to change by 'reprogramming' ourselves. Another important difference between persons and computers is that we gradually build up our 'programs' through belonging to groups of people who share whole sets of beliefs or 'programs'. In other words, our representations of the world, and even of ourselves, are very similar to those of other members of our culture. Again this is a crucial aspect of our social psychology. Finally, as Harré (1983) notes, while the programs used by computers are written in programming languages our 'programs' are likely to be based on our shared languages, such as English, Welsh, or Urdu. These differences remind us that we must remember the limitations of our source models.

The dramaturgical model

Our second source model, known as the dramaturgical model, draws a comparison between the performances of an actress and our real, everyday interaction. The model has been used very effectively by Goffman and others to reveal the underlying structure of social interaction (Goffman, 1969, 1974; Harré, 1979).

An actress must be able to convey to her audience that she is (meant to be) experiencing particular feelings, for example, sadness, excitement or enthusiasm and that she is following particular intentions, for example, warning or persuading another character. The audience's understanding of the scene or story depends on this ability to 'bring off' the performance. She must also be able to convey a sense of past experiences affecting present ones, that is, a sense of self-conscious consistency or character. This is done so successfully in many television soap operas that we begin to relate to these characters as if they were real, gossiping about what they will do next, reading newspaper articles about them and so on.

In our everyday lives we like the actress, must put together convincing performances so that we can convey how we are feeling and what our intentions are. If we do not we will be misunderstood, disliked and even feared by others. If we want to communicate that we would appreciate sympathy and support we must behave appropriately, otherwise those around us will assume that we are feeling something different, perhaps anger of irritation. Like an actress we need to be able to play our parts convincingly if our audience is to understand us. Thus, although we are not acting (in the sense of consciously putting on a performance) we are unconsciously using the same kind of skills as the actress. The importance of these taken-for-granted social skills is sometimes emphasized for us when we find ourselves in a different cultural setting where we are misunderstood because the people around us express their feelings and intentions differently. In this case we are running the wrong expressive programs; wrong in the sense that they differ from those around us, so that their interpretations of our behaviour does not match our intentions. Everyday interaction depends upon the automatic matching of our expressive intentions to others' interpretations and we may be quite startled by someone whose feelings and intentions remain unclear.

Of course, we also deliberately try to convince others that we feel or want something which we do not. In this case we are self-consciously using our expressive skills in the same way as the actress. As social psychologists, critically reflecting on everyday interaction we shall find it useful to regard both consciously and unconsciously 'directed' behaviour as dramatic performances. This model allows us to ask, *how are the participants 'bringing off' their performances, what 'lines', movements, expressions and props make them convincing* and how could they improve them.

So far we have used the dramaturgical model to focus on individual performances but actresses do not usually work in isolation. They cooperate with other actors and actresses who follow a *script* which is written so that they respond to one another in meaningful ways. Thus, if one character is upset another may try to cheer her up, and so on. The whole performance depends on meshing together the actions of a number of actresses and actors according to a shared script. This is also true of everyday interaction, bringing off our own performances means matching them to the social context and to those of others. Thus, using the dramaturgical model, social psychologists, may ask what kind of rules, roles and scripts are shaping the behaviour of groups of people. In this way we can see individual behaviour as part of a joint social achievement (see Chapter 4, Section 1).

The dramaturgical and computational models can be regarded as complementary. In order to bring off complex, scripted performances without, as Langer (1978) argues, even having to think about it, we must have ready-made guidelines or scripts stored away. This is analogous to the programs stored in a computer. However, unlike the computer the person must attend to others' behaviour and ensure that what she does will fit into others' representations of the shared situation. In this sense we are more like the actress ensuring that her performance corresponds to those of her fellow actors and actresses.

3   Interaction Through Shared Meanings

A symbolic interactionist perspective

The idea of a script, enabling actresses and actors to coordinate their performances into meaningful productions, highlights the way in which everyday interaction is dependent on, and directed by, a framework of shared understandings. We can appreciate the importance of these shared understandings by taking a detached look at a familiar setting and asking how we could enter into the interaction without these understandings. Imagine you have never heard of 'hospitals' and find yourself on a surgical ward. From this socially isolated perspective most of the activities of staff and patients would be incomprehensible. The uniforms, the instrumentation, the report, the filling-in of forms, the drug rounds, the doctor's rounds, indeed the ward activity as a whole would seem puzzling and bizarre. Even the act of taking someone's temperature is incomprehensible unless you understand what a thermometer tells you and how 'normal' and 'abnormal' temperatures are interpreted; to the uninitiated it might appear to be a religious or bonding ceremony (like exchanging rings or smoking a peace pipe!). Yet, to the ward staff, all these activities make sense and can be carried out, without puzzlement, in a fairly routine manner. Indeed, every morning nurses, doctors, psychologists, dieticians, domestics, and so on, come to work understanding their respective jobs, knowing how to perform them and having some awareness of how they relate to overall hospital functioning. Collectively then, they are able to take over the running of the hospital. This is because they have built up and stored sets of overlapping programmes which enable them to make sense of hospital activities in similar and complementary ways. Each of them has, as Berger and Luckman (1966) put it, *internalized* their social reality. This dependence of hospital functioning upon shared understandings is no exception. All our social activities depend on such shared, common-sense understandings.

This social psychological perspective on emphasizing the *shared nature of meaning* is known as *symbolic interactionism*. The work of Schutz (1953, 1967), Mead (1934) and Goffman (1969, 1972a) has been especially important in developing this perspective and it will contribute substantially to our exploration of everyday interaction. As social psychologists our task is to reveal the shared understandings which sustain the meaningfulness of social activities for the people involved. This is an example of how our second-order theories must look behind the obviousness of common-sense. The dependence of our everyday social performances on shared, taken-for-granted understandings is referred to by social psychologists as *intersubjectivity*, that is, understandings *between* people. This shared sense of what things mean and what should be done next, is the foundation for our individual plans and actions, without this assumed understanding we would, like our uninformed visitor to the ward, be left frozen, unsure as to what to do next.

Socialization – learning shared meanings

Of course, being 'dislocated' from shared understandings and failing to understand the meaning of social activity, is not an extraordinary experience. The feeling of bewilderment in a hospital ward is familiar to the first-time patient or the student nurse on her first ward. Such people have not yet learnt the meanings which sustain the obviousness of the ward routine. The actions of others around them do not make sense and consequently they do not know what should be done next. They are, as Peters (1958) and Berger and Luckman (1966) point out, in the same position as the non Christian at a Catholic mass, they do not know the pattern of conventions which make sense of the actions they observe. They have not yet built up the required store of programs they need to understand the social situations they find themselves in. This is an anxiety provoking and disabling state in which the individual does not know what behaviour is appropriate or how others' are going to judge her actions. The priority for a person in this position is to enter quickly into the world of shared meanings around them. Others are usually keen to help because they fear potentially embarrassing deviations from the shared script and because they want to increase the social usefulness of the individual. This is the rationale for introducing new, and even prospective patients to ward personnel and procedures. They are being introduced to a set of shared meanings which the staff take for granted. This enables them to move from a state of bewilderment, in which it is difficult for them to undertake independent action because of their uncertainties, to one of 'cultural competence', in which they can plan their own actions and make independent judgements about what is going on around them. Later these 'old hands' may be able to introduce new patients or nurses to ward routines.

This process of being introduced to a set of shared understandings which render a set of activities meaningful is known as *socialization*. This is of course the essence of 'bringing up' our children, they must be introduced to the vast range of shared understandings which constitute our culture. This is primary socialization while the introduction of adults to a new sphere of meanings is known as secondary socialization (Berger and Luckman, 1966). Thus we can speak of the whole process of nurse training as 'nurse socialization' (see Chapter 4, Section 2). As we progress through any socialization process we become members of the culture (for example, the 'ward culture') from which we were previously isolated, that is, we become party to the shared set of understandings which constitute that culture.

Socialization usually proceeds through various types of conversation with culture members, for example, lectures, gossip, individual instruction, reprimands, commands, and so on. This is because *language* provides the best medium for communicating and storing the shared understandings necessary to bring off our cooperative performances. There are, of course, other ways of 'storing' such understandings, for example, clothes can convey much about who people are and what they are supposed to be doing. Uniforms in nursing provide a good example of how clothes themselves embody a shared set of understandings, in this case understandings about the way people should relate to one another (see Chapter 5, Section 5). Language, however, remains the primary store for such understandings so that, socialization consists initially of learning new ways of talking about ourselves and others. Learning the meaning of the title 'ward sister', for example, involves at least a basic understanding of the way hospitals are organized into wards, the nature of hierarchical, authority relationships and the ratio of women to men in nursing. As we become culture members we internalize these new ways of talking about our experiences. Thus *new ways of talking gradually become new ways of thinking*. Progressing from candidate-for-nurse-training to staff-nurse to charge-nurse, for example, involves socialization into a new culture which means learning to think about ourselves and others in new ways. This in turn changes our experience of social situations so that, for example, concern about charge nurses' approval may be an important feature of student–nurses' experience while anxieties over leadership responsibility may be common amongst new charge-nurses.

Self awareness – representing our own psychology

This capacity to change ourselves by engaging with others in new ways of thinking about ourselves is a fundamental feature of what it is to be a person. It relies on our ability to represent ourselves, that is, to reflect upon who and what we are. Mead (1934) has argued that this ability to think about, or represent, ourselves comes about through social contact as an infant. It develops as a result of others speaking about us, and treating us as separate, named, 'objects'. Gradually we begin to recognize that we are indeed 'objects' which can be seen, described and responded to. Parents may say, 'How's Chris today then? You're in a good mood aren't you, and so on. In response, Chris begins begins to realize that 'Chris' is a particular 'object' which can be talked about. This is the first stage of self-representation and indeed the first stage in becoming a person. Following Mead, Luria (1981) has highlighted the role of language in early socialization, arguing that, initially, representations of ourselves exist only in adults' conversation but that over time we are able to internalize these and so think about, or represent, ourselves without necessarily speaking. Thus, as adults, we can reflect on what and who we are. We can engage in self reflection such as, 'I'm Chris. I'm a staff nurse on an intensive care unit. I'm feeling happy today' and so on. Figure 1 summarizes how the processes of primary and secondary socialization can affect self-representation and thereby determine the social roles we choose to adopt (see Chapter 4, Section 1).

To be a person then, is to be involved in a continual process of building up representations of oneself in cooperation with other people. As Harré (1983) notes: 'A person is a being who has learnt a theory, in terms of which his or her experience is ordered' (p. 20). This view of personhood is central to a social psychological perspective and is also very useful when it comes to understanding how people are able to change themselves. The issue of change is of obvious relevance to nursing and it is one we shall return to throughout the book. We shall see that, whether we are considering how a person takes on the identity of 'nurse' or gives up using a drug or changes

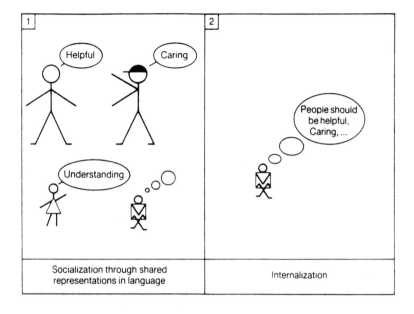

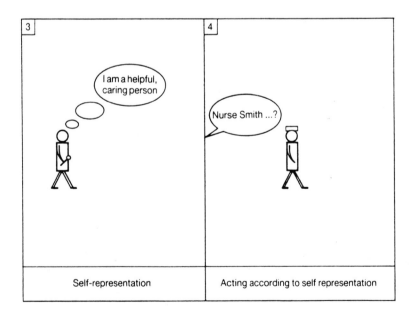

Figure 1   Socialization, self representation and social behaviour.

her sexual practices, we need to look at how they represent themselves and how these representations relate to those of others around them. Indeed, we shall see that this process of constructing, or more precisely reconstructing, oneself is the basis of many forms of therapy (see Chapter 7, Sections 2 and 4).

A socially constructed reality

We have argued then, that our experiences and behaviour depend upon our self-representations, that is, how we think of ourselves, and that these in turn, depend upon primary and secondary socialization, that is, the process through which we internalize ways of thinking shared by other culture members. We can see then that everyday reality is, as Berger and Luckman have it, 'socially constructed' and intersubjective. Since each of us has the capacity to change our representations, and since others' influence our representations through interaction, there is substantial opportunity for us to change the way we see ourselves, others and social situations. Thus a person who we think is friendly and helpful may later be thought of as manipulating and uncaring, or vice versa. Using the dramaturgical model we might say that everyday interaction is rather like a play in which there is a lot of adlibbing. This means that each performance is a bit different from the last and that, over time, as new lines are added and the characters change, the whole play may evolve into something quite different from the opening night show.

This potential for change has two implications for our thinking about everyday interaction. First, although some aspects of our shared representations may be fairly stable, for example, the meaning of 'cardiac arrest' and how it should be dealt with, others may be change quite rapidly, for example our view of sister Smith's assessments of nursing students. In such matters we may influence and be influenced by others' opinion of a person or their understanding of an event. This is not, however, simply a matter of establishing 'the facts'. Genuinely different understandings may be arrived at by people who have heard the same argument or conversation. In the case of our fictitious sister, some people may have little respect for her judgment and others may regard it as entirely reliable. To make things even more complex, people may change their positions as the social situation and personal interests change. Thus, interaction can be regarded as involving a great deal of negotiation and persuasion concerning which, of various alternative understandings, we should adopt. We may try to persuade others that we are a particular kind of person or that our job is a particularly important one or that something of which we are accused is not really our fault. We may be successful with some but not others. Those we persuade may change their minds and others will try to persuade us to adopt a different view. In other words, social reality is made and remade as we act out our parts in different ways across different day-to-day situations.

This daily variability and uncertainty is poeticly captured in T. S. Elliot's The Lovesong of J. Alfred Prufrock. Prufrock seems sensitively aware of the fragility of everyday intersubjectivity. Thinking of how we try to present a particular image of ourselves to others he muses that;

> There will be time. . .
> To prepare a face to meet the faces that you meet

then, recognizing the possibility of reconstruction, he reflects that;

> In a minute there is time
> For decisions and revisions which a minute will
> reverse

He is also aware that others will negotiate their representations of him;

> They will say: 'How his hair is growing thin!'
> They will say: 'But how his arms and legs are thin!'

We shall see later how these indecisions and revisions mean that the maintenance of one's social reputation is a crucial, ongoing aspect of everyday interaction (see Chapter 3, Section 2).

The second implication of this potential for social change is that in the long-term the whole background culture into which we are socialised can undergo revision. Over time, our shared representations of people in general may change. Thus different cultures develop different under-standings of what kind of beings people are and what place they have in the universe. Snell (1960), for example, argues that the ancient Greeks thought about themselves very differently to modern Europeans because of their belief in the everyday influence of hundreds of different gods who interacted with them; they did not, he proposes, see themselves as having the same power to shape their own everyday activity and long term destiny. Consequently their experience of life was, in our terms, very fatalistic. If Snell is correct then these people inhabited a different social reality because they shared different beliefs about how things happened on a moment-to-moment basis. Cultural diversity means that nurses must be aware that the same medical techniques may have very different meanings for people belonging to different cultures. The decision to pursue a particular medical procedure, for example, a blood transfusion or an abortion, will be very different for patients with different beliefs. In fact they will be involved in making *different decisions* regardless of similarities in their physical circumstances. Such potential for variation and change amongst people makes everyday interaction exciting and sometimes stressful. It also ensures that social psychology will remain a challenging field of study.

4   Social Psychology as Science

What is science?

We have begun to explore the subject matter of social psychology. Our next step is to consider its methods. This is important because it will help us understand and evaluate social psychological research. We shall begin by asking if social psychology is a science. In other words, is it similar to the natural sciences such as chemistry and biology? This question obliges us to ask 'what is science?', that is, 'what is it about chemistry which makes it a science'? Such questions could divert us into the interesting but complex area of philosophy of science. We shall, however, only pause to consider these issues in a superficial way here and interested readers wishing to explore further are referred to Chalmers (1978), *What is this thing called Science?*

In general, we might say that science involves the use of models to develop theories, which give us a better understanding of our everyday experience and help us to anticipate what will happen next in any given situation. Thus the 'theory' that air contains a vital substance which we consume through breathing, (that is, 'oxygen') helps us understand why being cut off from a fresh, air (or oxygen) supply will be fatal. Scientific work can therefore be divided into two stages:

1. developing new models or theories and,
2. deciding which of these theories are most useful for understanding our experience.

As new theories are developed scientists must decide which of two, or more, competing theories is the most useful. Our need for oxygen, for example, is explained by biochemical theories of respiration which, presently, appear to provide a very useful explanation of gaseous exchange during breathing. Included in this explanation is a theory of oxidation which today's students of biochemistry take for granted. However, prior to Lavoisier's work in the late eighteenth century a very different view of these chemical reactions prevailed. Focusing on combustion, the 'phlogiston theory' stated that substances *gave out* phlogiston when burnt. Lavoisier was able to demonstrate that certain substances, such as mercury, actually *take* in something (in fact, oxygen) when heated. These demonstrations did much to discredit the phlogiston theory and paved the way for further theory-building leading, eventually, to our currently accepted model of respiration (Bronowski, 1973).

The question of how scientists decide on one theory, rather than another, is a controversial one. However, in general, science is characterized by the 'testing' of theories through careful examination of those aspects of our experience to which they refer. Lavoisier, for example, made careful measurements of weights and volumes before and after burning. A century earlier Mayow had laid the foundations for Lavoisier's insight by demonstrating that part of the air is used by a burning candle and that this same part is also that used during breathing. He too relied on careful observation of what happened as circumstances changed, for example, how placing a burning candle in the same, sealed air-space as a mouse would affect the speed with which the mouse got into breathing difficulties (see Miller, 1978). This kind of careful observation is referred to as 'data-collection'. Data-collection can help us to test our theories but as we noted above in relation to Galen we may only know what 'data', or evidence to collect after we have formulated our theory (with the help of an appropriate source model). Thus the relationship between data and theory is complex and reciprocal.

Scientific observation – reliability, validity and experimental method

The work of scientists like Mayow and Lavoisier and philosophers of science, such as Mill (1872), has led to a particular form of data collection which is sometimes regarded as the hallmark of science, namely, *the experiment*. In an experiment the scientist changes, or manipulates, one aspect of what she is studying and takes various measurements of another to discover whether, or not, the first affects the second. At the same time she holds other aspects constant so that if her measurements of the second aspect do show changes she will know that the first aspect is responsible for these. The aspect which is manipulated is usually known as the 'independent variable' while the one which is measured is known as the 'dependent variable'. In Mayow's experiment, for example, the presence or absence of the burning candle was manipulated while the time it took for the mouse to get into difficulties in a closed air-space was measured. In this case the the presence or absence of the burning candle is the 'independent variable' and the time the mouse took to get into breathing difficulties is the 'dependent variable'. Mayow also took care to keep the size of the air-space and the mouse the same. This meant that when he found that the mouse got into difficulties more quickly, in the presence of the burning candle, he could rule out these other aspects of the situation as possible explanations, because they had remained the same, whether the candle was present or not. We could also use an experimental design to evaluate some new idea in nurse training. In this case the delivery of the new training package or its absence would constitute our independent variable and the competence of nurses who did or did not receive this training would be our dependent variable. Again we could control for other factors by, for example, ensuring that the ability of groups who did or did not receive the training was equal before training began (for further details on experimental design see, for example, Greene and D'Oliveira, 1982).

Two important concepts in the measurement of independent and dependent variables are *reliability* and *validity*. A reliable measure will give us the same result on different occasions when our variable is not changing. If, for example, we wish to assess student nurses' abilities to carry out nursing procedures then we require reliable measures of nursing competence. Such a measure must give the same result on different assessments if the nurse's ability remains the same. This is called test–retest reliability. The measure must also give the same result when it is used by different assessors. Otherwise we may be measuring some aspect of the assessor's perception rather then the nurse's competence. This is called inter-rater reliability. Both types of reliability are crucial to scientific measurement.

However, even reliable measures can be misleading. The now discredited practice of phrenology was based on the assumption that the brain was made up of distinct organs which controlled different types of behaviour. Phrenologists developed maps of the scull which allowed them to relate bumps and hollows on people's sculls to supposed brain structures beneath. They then interpreted such bumps and hollows as if they were measures of brain structure and therefore of personality type. These maps were fairly reliable in that one could receive the same interpretations at different times and from different phrenologists. However, the underlying theory seems absurd to us and illustrates how reliable measures may be misleading if they are not really measuring what we are interested in. Measures must not only be reliable but also valid, that is they must measure what our theory is concerned with. The best way to check the validity of a measure is to investigate whether it predicts some future event. In the case of student nurse assessment our measure should accurately predict whether the nurse will be able to effectively carry out a procedure so that it will lead to the desired health outcome in future practice. This is called *predictive validity*. Phrenology measures fail to meet this criteria because the bumps on our head do not allow accurate prediction of our behaviour.

We have said that scientists use observations (checked for their reliability and validity) to assess the usefulness of their theories but we have not explained how they assess these theories. We might suppose that if the theory makes good predictions then it must be accepted as true. For example we might say that Mayow proved that the candle and mouse used the same substance in air. This not quite correct because it is always possible that something has been overlooked and our data is somehow misleading. This is the point Popper (1959) made when he distinguished between 'verifying' or proving theories and 'falsifying' them. Using one of

Popper's examples, it does not matter how many white swans we observe we can never 'verify' or prove the theory that all swans are white because a black one may always turn up tomorrow. It is always possible that a counter example (such as a a black swan) will be found in the future and such counter examples can 'falsify' our theories by showing that they are inadequate. Thus we cannot prove our theories, but we can test their usefulness by collecting data which could lead to their falsification. In this way misleading theories such as 'air contains two separate elements, one used in burning and another used in breathing' or 'all swans are red' can be falsified. A theory which is not falsified by data collection can be accepted as a useful, working theory which we know may be falsified in the future. It is not necessary for us to discuss Popper's position, or those of his critics in detail (see, e.g. Chalmers, 1978; Magee, 1973). However, it is important to note that while data collection methods may help us develop theories, test them and discard inadequate ones *they do not prove* these theories.

Social sciences and natural sciences

Science then is the practice of developing and testing theories which will give us a better understanding of our experience. Given this general definition, and our discussion of testing through data collection we can conclude that *social psychology* is a *science*. However, this does not mean that it is the same sort of science as the natural sciences. The question of whether, or not, there are fundamental differences between the social and natural sciences is a much debated one with important implications for social psychological research. Our position is that *social psychology is fundamentally different to the natural sciences*.

This difference is due to a difference in subject matter. The social psychologist studies people in interaction while the natural scientist studies the behaviour of animals or inanimate matter. Our behaviour is different to that of animals or chemicals because it is directed by our internalized representations of shared understandings about ourselves and the world we live in. Thus, the social psychologist, unlike the natural scientist, must always be aware of the understandings of those she studies. The natural scientist does not have to wonder how the chemicals, or for that matter the mice, would explain their current situation to themselves; she does not have to worry about participants in her studies looking back at her and asking themselves, 'What's she up to now?' or about whether their answer to this question will change their behaviour while she is taking measurements. Such concerns are, however, an inescapable part of data-collection in social psychology.

Data-collection is therefore more problematic in social psychology than in the natural sciences. Carrying out controlled experiments, like those of Mayow, becomes much more difficult because, just as people change their behaviour in interviews, they may change their behaviour in experiments. Experiments may be special social situations in which behaviour is directed by particular understandings which do not apply elsewhere. If this is the case behaviour observed in a social psychology experiment may not be a very good guide to how people behave in their everyday social environments. In other words we may not be able to *generalize* from our experimental data to the everyday social situations we are really interested in (Tajfel, 1972). In response some researchers such as Shotter (1980), have advised social psychologists to abandon data-collection altogether while others have tested their theories using data-collection methods other than the experiment (Mixon, 1972; Potter and Wetherell, 1987). In general, however, social psychologists have retained the experiment and attempted to overcome the complexities of observing self-representing beings. Some have tried 'candid-camera-like', *field experiments* in which the participants do not know they are involved in an experiment (Latane and Darley, 1970, see Chapter 4, Section 4) while others have deceived participants as to what their experiments are about (Milgram, 1974, see Chapter 4, Section 3). The idea of deception is that if people we are studying believe we are investigating one aspect of their behaviour (for example, learning) but we are actually observing another (for example, obedience) then their understandings of the experimental situation will not affect the behaviour we are interested in. The deceived experimental participant will focus on what they (mistakenly) think the experiment is about and so will not try to consciously change the behaviour we are really concerned with.

Of course deception raises important ethical questions concerning the trade off between dishonesty and the need for research. There is no simple resolution of these methodological problems and we shall consider how they affect social psychological research into particular topics in later chapters. Our intention at this stage is merely to alert the reader to the difficulties inherent in carrying out social psychological research and to encourage a critical perspective on the way in which scientific research in general is conducted. We should continue to ask whether social psychological theories fit her own experience (and, if not, why not?) and whether the research they are based on has demonstrated that they can be generally applied.

People change as cultures develop and therefore the nature of the social psychologist's subject matter changes over time. We may assume that the basic laws of the natural world are unchanging and the same everywhere across the globe. However no such assumption can be made about social psychological processes. We have already noted how our representations of ourselves and our behaviour is culture-bound and subject to historical change. Thus our second order theories always refer to a particular culture at a particular point in time. Indeed Snell has called 'the belief in the 'existence of a universal and uniform human mind' a 'rationalist prejudice' and Gergen (1974) has posed the challenging question of whether social psychology is really a special branch of history! None of this means that it is impossible to study social psychology. It means that we have to be sensitive to cultural changes and differences. We must be careful not to overlook such differences when comparing groups of people and we must not assume that because one group of people behaves in a particular fashion another will automatically behave in the same way.

This is especially important because data collection relies on observing using small groups or *samples* when we really want to develop theories which apply to larger groups or *populations*. Such generalization from the behaviour of samples of people observed in social psychological studies to behaviour in wider cultural contexts must be very carefully considered.

Since our representation of ourselves are subject to change over time the social psychologist must consider the possibility that her own theories might influence changes in the way people represent themselves. Moscovici (1961), for example, has demonstrated that present day, common-sense French explanations include concepts such as 'complex' and 'unconscious motivation' which were originally parts of Freud's psychoanalytic theory. It is possible therefore that the theoretical concepts of today's social psychology will be incorporated into the everyday, common-sense understandings of twenty-first-century people! It would seem then that the relationship between social psychology and common-sense is two-way. If social psychological theories are absorbed into common-sense they can shape the way future generations think then about themselves and therefore how they experience reality. Accepting this gives social psychologists a momentous responsibility; a responsibility to consider how any particular theory might influence the way we think about who we are.

Shotter (1974) makes this responsibility very clear in outlining the goals of social psychology:

> It's main theoretical goal is to make the experience of being a self among other similar selves intelligible, to understand the idea of what it is to be human. In practice it's goal will be to develop and expand the human self, to seek ways of expanding the sphere of genuine human action, to increase what people as individual personalities can do for themselves at the expense of what they just find happening to them whether they wish it or not (p. 57).

Shotter's point is that psychological theory should be seen as serving the social function of helping people to make the most of their lives by promoting greater understanding of our experiences and behaviour. He has called upon social psychologists to recognize their social responsibilities and accept that their work must be based on a particular set of values. Arguing the same radical position Taylor (1971) concluded that the social sciences are fundamentally distinct from the natural sciences because they are *moral* or value-based sciences. Characterizing social psychology in this way draws our attention to the correspondence of values underpinning social psychology and nursing; both aiming to optimize peoples' independence and sense of well being. Indeed Shotter's last sentence above might well have been taken from a statement of nursing goals.

CORE IDEAS IN CHAPTER 1

- Social psychology studies how people understand their social worlds and interact with one another. This necessitates an analysis of common-sense psychology.

- Effective nursing depends upon properly managed interaction and an understanding of others. Social psychological theory can provide insights into how we understand others and manage relationships.

- People use internal representations of themselves, others and their social worlds to direct their behaviour.

- These representations are learnt through interaction with members of particular cultures. By internalizing the language and common-sense theories of a culture one becomes a culture member. This is known as socialization.

- The meaningfulness of individual judgements and actions depends upon these shared, taken-for-granted understandings. This is known as intersubjectivity. Being out of touch with shared understandings is therefore a disabling and anxiety-provoking experience.

- People can learn new representations of themselves and situations. This allows for personal change and means that social reality is open to reconstruction and negotiation.

- Social psychology is a science in the sense that it generates and tests theories. It is , however, fundamentally different to the natural sciences in the sense that its theories are second-order theories concerning self-representing beings.

- Since the theories of social psychology may be absorbed into our first-order, common-sense theories it may be regarded as a moral science.

Notes

1. Throughout the book we follow the widespread convention of referring to those who are nursed as 'patients'. Of course not all those receiving nursing care are ill and the passivity connoted by 'patient' may be inappropriate even for those who are physically ill. These issues and the consequent problems with the term 'patient' are discussed in Chapter 4 Section 2.
2. Throughout the book we use the feminine pronouns to refer to persons in general. This highlights the implicit sexism of unquestioningly using 'he' and thereby presenting masculinity as social normality (see Chapter 4, Section 5). It also seems more appropriate in a book written for nurses at a time when the majority of nurses are women.

2

Modelling our understandings of health and illness

1   Modelling Representations to Predict Health Behaviour

Beliefs, representations and behaviour

We noted in Chapter 1 that a computer's move in a game of chess depends upon the representation of the game embodied in its programmes. Similarly our beliefs about ourselves and our health and illness determine how we respond to perceived symptoms or health education campaigns. If we believe rhinoceros horn reduces fever then we may buy it and having consumed it we will assume that any reduction in the fever was caused by it. If later we lose faith in its effectiveness we will stop buying it as a medicine and identify other causes for our previous recovery.

In order to understand health behaviour we must consider how people's beliefs affect the way they see the world and how their memory of past experiences affects their anticipation of the future. Our environment affects our behaviour (see Figure 2a) but it does so indirectly through our beliefs and understandings (see Figure 2b). We shall later consider an alternative view when discussing how environmental changes can support personal change (see Chapter 7, Section 3). However, throughout the book we shall be emphasizing how individual representations of reality direct behaviour.

Many of our individual understandings are shared with others allowing communication about joint reality. This is essential to our anticipation of others' expectations and the coordination of everyday social actions (see Figure 2c). If, for example, we ask someone to 'monitor Mr. Smith's heart-rate' we are assuming that they already know the significance of heart-rates (in general and for this particular patient), how to use the monitoring equipment, how to interpret its output and what to do if dangerous heart-rate readings are observed. Without this knowledge (embodied in representations, built up through secondary socialization) the person will be unable to respond as we expect them to. Dislocated from the intersubjective world we take for granted they are, like the naive visitor to a hospital ward we met in Chapter 1, unable to formulate intentions, or plan meaningful action.

Predicting Health Behaviour

Social psychologists have developed second order theories which model the representations underlying our everyday behaviour. These theories highlight key beliefs and understandings which we can measure and relate to actual behaviour. In many studies measures of people's beliefs form the independent variable while measures of their behaviour provide the dependent variable. Such studies can show whether the beliefs and understandings highlighted in our models are in fact important determinants of behaviour. In other words they can attempt to falsify our second order models and thereby prompt further model development.

Modelling how people understand their circumstances allows us to see the sense (that is, *their sense*) underlying their actions. Without this *psychological understanding of common sense understanding* others' actions, such as not following prescribed treatments may seem bizarre, random and unchangeable. If, however, we can identify the key beliefs which guide such actions (for example, the belief that prescribed treatment is ineffective) then we can try to change such beliefs and thereby promote behaviour change. This is the essence of health education.

Such second order models may be important to nurses both because psychological care presupposes an understanding of those cared for and because health education and behavioural change are increasingly central to the work of all health-care workers (for example, Stachnik, 1980; Eiser, 1982; Christie and Mellett, 1986; Feuerstein et al., 1986). We are becoming more aware that illness cannot be successfully combated at a purely biological level because its incidence and form are inextricably linked to lifestyle at both economic and personal levels. This means that understanding what people 'do' to themselves and others on a daily basis is crucial to understanding patterns of health breakdown and promoting better health (see, for example, DHSS, 1976; Doyal and Pennell, 1979; Inglis, 1983; Rowland and Cooper, 1983). Thus, whether we

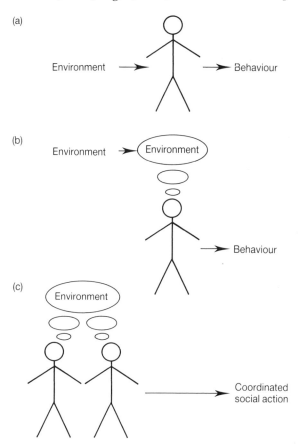

Figure 2 Behaviour depends upon our representations of our environment.

are confronting heart disease, lung cancer or AIDS we must be concerned with the behavioural bases of health maintenance and illness prevention. This leads inevitably to an examination of the psychological determinants of such behaviour, that is, to an examination of how people represent their worlds and plan actions within them.

An important aspect of illness behaviour is the degree to which people follow the advice offered to them by health-care workers. Indeed the effectiveness of any health service depends upon *compliance*. However, research evidence suggests that some patients do not intend to follow medical advice (Davis, 1968) and between 40% and 50% do not follow advice on taking medication or other health-related matters (see Ley, 1977; 1979a; 1982; 1988). Indeed, in 1984 King estimated that £100 million worth of prescribed medication was being discarded every year! This is particularly serious when one realizes that failure to comply with recommended health-care behaviours is a major cause of premature death and disability (Stachnik, 1980). The reasons for *non compliance* are complex. Ley, (1979b; 1982) reports evidence indicating that it is *not* affected by patients' economic background, their scores on personality tests, the duration or seriousness of their illness, or their doctor's characteristics. However, the number of medicines prescribed and time spent waiting reduces compliance while patient satisfaction with consultations appears to increase it. One important barrier to compliance may be the way such advice is given. Hauser (1981) reviews a range of relevant studies and concludes that 'doctor-dominated' consultations in which the doctor is unresponsive to patient needs and engages in only limited information exchange may lead to non-compliance (see Chapter 5, Section 4). While, in the field of media health education Hastings and Scott (1987) find that although recent UK AIDS-publicity succeeded in giving people a basic knowledge about the risks of human immunodeficiency virus infection it left them unsure about what to do, on a day-to-day basis, to reduce their own risk. It seems then that satisfaction and compliance can be increased simultaneously by ensuring that advice and health education communications relate directly to the beliefs underlying everyday health and illness behaviour.

2   From Attitudes to Health Beliefs

Attitude theory

Social psychologists have developed a set of terms which refer to our common sense representations. Many of these like *attitude* and *belief* have been borrowed from our everyday vocabulary. However, even when these terms are familiar it is important to remember that psychologists have defined them in specific ways so that their theoretical meaning may differ from the meanings they have in everyday conversation.

Attitudes are social in that we share them with others and they seems to guide our behaviour in that we act in accordance with the attitudes we express. Social psychologists have therefore tried to identify and measure people's attitudes in order to understand and predict their behaviour. Indeed much research has been devoted to discovering the structure of our attitudes and devising ways of measuring them (see Jaspers, 1978 for an introductory review). Unfortunately it has proved extremely difficult to define 'attitude' as a theoretical term (McGuire, 1985) and moreover measures of people's expressed attitudes have not corresponded as closely to their behaviour as social psychologists had hoped (Wicker, 1969).

One fairly widely accepted model of attitudes suggests that they are made up of three parts: *an emotional part*, involving our evaluation of, or feelings towards, the attitude-object, for example, we might value smoking cigarettes and feel the experience was a very positive one; *a belief part*, for example, we might believe that smoking less than 20 a day does not damage our health and is good for us because it reduces stress, and finally, a *behavioural or intentional component*, for example, we might intend to buy cigarettes each time we visit the supermarket. An attractive feature of this model is that, by assuming that the three components remain *consistent* with one another we should be able to predict peoples' intentions and therefore their behaviour by measuring the strength of their evaluations and beliefs. We should, for example, be able to predict who will give up smoking, or who will take suggested medicines, by asking them what they feel and believe about these subjects. Prediction of this kind would clearly be very useful to those responsible for health care delivery.

Unfortunately our representations of the world are complex and knowing people's general feelings and beliefs about something do not provide a very good guide to their behaviour in any particular situation. As early as 1934 LaPiere found a discrepancy between stated prejudice and actual discrimination. LaPiere and a Chinese couple were served in a sample of hotels and restaurants in the USA. However, when LaPiere wrote to these establishments 92% of the 128 who replied claimed they would not serve Chinese people! Clearly, the general policy of these institutions was not a good guide to the actual practice of their staff. Of course the reader will realize that the social situation the staff found themselves in when LaPiere and his friends arrived was more complex than LaPiere's written request suggested. After all LaPiere himself was European and the hotels were presumably happy to cater for Europeans. This is exactly the problem with general attitude measurement. The representation of the topic used to answer questions about attitudes is unlikely to be complex enough to include all the aspects of the situation in which the attitude-relevant behaviour is observed. It is easy to say 'I believe X' and 'I would have done Y' but when we find ourselves in a situation where we can live up to these claims we may not want to because there are other aspects of the situation we wish to respond to (such as what other might think of us).

The doubt LaPiere cast on general attitude measurement was confirmed by Wicker's (1969) review of studies examining the link between attitude measurement and behaviour. Wicker concluded that this 'link' was at best weak and, at worst non-existent. This might be taken to mean that attitude theory has been falsified and should be abandoned. Certainly simple attitude theory has been expanded and revised. It failed to take account of the complexity and detail of the everyday representations we use to organize our behaviour. Models which refer to the *multiple, specific beliefs* people hold about particular situations, or decision points, have been developed. Such models suggest that aspects of attitude theory may still be useful in understanding and predicting people's behaviour. Indeed Bentler and Speckart (1981) assert that when our models and measurement techniques are appropriate we can show that attitudes do indeed direct behaviour. However such models must take account of the complexity of our common sense understandings of specific situations. Wicker, for example, noted that in any given situation people's behaviour depends upon their beliefs about; acceptable behaviour in that situation, alternative action plans, the expected consequences of their action and their own abilities.

The theory of planned behaviour

Ajzen and Fishbein's (1980) *theory of reasoned action* attempts to provide a more appropriate model. They argue that we must look initially at the persons' intention to behave in a particular manner. Thus if we want to predict whether a person will take a prescribed medicine we should ask them first whether or not they intend to take it. This fairly straightforward idea could have important implications for understanding why some people follow their health-related advice while others do not. Davis (1968) found that 44% of patients who did not follow doctors' advice admitted that they had not intended to comply with suggested treatment and that only 8% of those who did not intend to follow advice actually did so! This suggests that formulating the intention to act in a certain manner is a crucial prerequisite to actually carrying out that action.

Ajzen and Fishbein propose that certain background values and desires determine our *behavioural intentions* and therefore, our behaviour. In particular:

1. *beliefs about the likely outcome of a particular behaviour* (for example, the belief that suggested treatment will provide symptom relief);
2. *the value the actor places on these presumed outcomes* (for example, the importance of symptom relief for that person).

These two elements correspond to the belief and evaluative components of the simple three-part attitude model discussed above. In this new model what was previously called the behavioural component has been separated in order to emphasize the importance of intentions as predictors of behaviour. Ajzen and Fishbeins' model also highlights how our perceptions of other people's views and our desire for their approval affects our behaviour. These two aspects of our representation of socially appropriate behaviour are referred to as our *subjective norm*. They are the second and third determinants of our behavioural intentions considered by the model:

3. *beliefs about others' approval or disapproval of our behaviour* (for example, beliefs about what friends, relations, or certain authority figures would think if we complied with a suggested procedure);
4. *the strength of our desire to please people who we presume will approve or disapprove of the behaviour*.

In a recent reformulation of the theory Ajzen and Madden (1986) rename it the *theory of planned behaviour* and include beliefs about the 'control' an actor thinks she has over a particular behaviour (see Figure 3). This adds a fifth determinant of intention:-

5. *beliefs about abilities, recourses, opportunities and obstacles relevant to the behaviour*, for example, beliefs about our ability to use medical equipment or about times in the day when we will be able to take a suggested medicine.

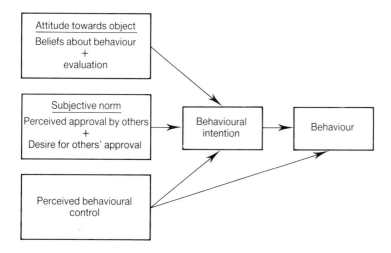

Figure 3   The theory of planned behaviour.

The theory of planned behaviour is a general model of how our representations of the world shape our behaviour. It takes account of many of the
factors mentioned by Wicker and is obviously more comprehensive than
the three-part attitude model. It has proved useful in predicting a range of
behaviours including students' attendance and study behaviour, adolescent contraceptive use and breast self-examination behaviour (Jorgensen
and Sonstegard, 1984; Lierman et al., 1990).

The health belief model

A similar model which has been used to understand common sense
beliefs which influence health behaviour is the *health belief model* (HBM).
The model was based on investigations of into the reasons why some
people adopt recommended health behaviours while others do not (see
e.g. Rosenstock, 1960; Rosenstock, 1966; Rosenstock, 1974; Becker et
al., 1977). It was initially applied to the problem of public response to
preventive health programmes (for example, cancer screening and anti-
smoking programmes). However, its use has been extended to investigate
non-compliance. The four central beliefs which the health belief model
identifies as important to health behaviour are:

1. *beliefs about how susceptible we are to the illness* in question, that is, whether
    we think that we are likely to contract the illness or, in the case of
    a health problem we already have, whether we think we are likely to
    suffer from recurring problems;
2. *beliefs about the seriousness or severity of the illness* if we do contract it (for
    example, how painful or life-threatening it is);
3. *beliefs about the potential costs* (for example, physical, psychological,
    and economic) involved in undertaking the suggested preventive or
    curative action;
4. *beliefs about the effectiveness of this action in relation to possible alternatives.*
    Unless we believe that a suggested programme will actually relieve or
    remove symptoms we will be unlikely to follow it. If we think less costly
    alternatives are just as effective we are likely to adopt them.

In addition to these measures the model takes account of people's exposure to *cues or triggers* to health behaviour. It proposes that when a
person already holds the beliefs outlined above they may be prompted
to engage in the appropriate health behaviour by bodily or environmental
triggers. The appearance of a symptom, a health education poster or a
conversation with a friend may emphasize the importance of the recommended behaviour and so trigger our adoption of it. Finally, a number
of studies (Becker and Maiman, 1975) have suggested that the model
should incorporate a measure of *health motivation*. In other words we
need to understand the extent to which the person believes it is valuable

to maintain their health. This is related to the theory of planned behaviour's measure of behavioural intentions but is somewhat less specific, referring to the broader motivation underpinning particular intentions. Overall then HBM comprises six separate psychological measures which it proposes are useful in predicting health behaviour (see Figure 4).

Including beliefs about severity, costs and effectiveness can be seen as adding specific detail to the theory of planned behaviour's focus on beliefs about outcome. However, HBM differs from the theory of planned behaviour in that it does not identify beliefs about others' approval or our own abilities as being important determinants of compliance. We shall examine the importance of other beliefs below and see that combining these with HBM and the theory of planned behaviour may enable us to make even more accurate predictions about which patients will comply.

Becker, et al., (1977) and Janz and Becker (1984) review research into the usefulness of HBM and conclude that the model has been effective in accounting for differences between people's health-related behaviour across a number of different contexts and conditions. A number of studies have demonstrated that in general people who say they hold the beliefs identified by the model tend to follow health advice while those who do not express these beliefs tend not to. In particular beliefs about susceptibility and severity seem to be very important determinants of preventive behaviour and treatment compliance. Becker, et al., (1972), for example, found that mothers who believed that their child was susceptible to illness, that the illness was severe and that the recommended penicillin

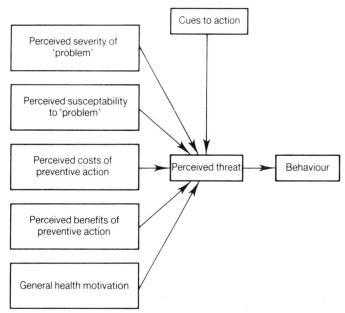

Figure 4 Simplified version of the health belief model.

regimen would be effective were much more likely to comply with the suggested treatment. Haefner and Kirscht (1970) used the model to set up an experiment in health education. They showed one group of people films about their susceptibility to and the seriousness of certain health problems (including cancer and heart disease) and then compared their behaviour with that of another group who had not received such education. Interviewing participants eight months later they found that (despite having no symptoms) the 'educated' group were much more likely both to see themselves as susceptible and to have had a check-up than the control group. Overall, the evidence suggests that the beliefs identified by HBM are important predictors of patient compliance. Thus, as Ley (1988) suggests compliance might be increased if nurses and doctors focused on these beliefs during interviews and consultations.

Psychological models and health education

Marsh and Mathensons' (1983) study of the health beliefs of 2700 British smokers' also provides useful insights into the application of HBM. They found that while almost half did not accept that smoking increased their susceptibility to health problems (for example, 33% believed that smokers were no more susceptible to lung cancer while 45% believed they were no more susceptible to heart disease) the majority (85%) believed that if they did get ill smoking would be at least partly to blame. These smokers seemed prepared to accept their increased susceptibility only if they become ill. This is, as Marsh (1985) notes, a gambler's mentality, denial of risk before losing and admission of risk after losing. Even those smokers who accepted increased susceptibility tended to believe that the danger level was above their own daily consumption, that is 20-a-day smokers thought susceptibility to health problems began at 30-a-day and so on. These results demonstrate that our health beliefs can be complex and somewhat inconsistent. This further emphasizes the point that psychological models simplify the nature of our everyday beliefs. In doing so they help us gain insight into people's decisions and behaviour but we should not assume that people's beliefs are always neatly consistent with one another or that our models provide more than a rough map of the representations used in everyday decision-making.

This complexity should not, however, discourage the health educator. Indeed Marsh and Matheson's results demonstrate the power of health beliefs to induce behaviour change. Marsh (1985) reports that those who believed in the *health benefits* of giving up intended to give up and were much more likely to do so. This illustrates a general point about susceptibility, namely that by itself it may not be enough to induce behaviour change, patients must also believe that their actions will result in health benefits. Marsh and Matheson found that smokers were generally unconvinced that giving up would bring health benefits; even those who accepted increased susceptibility seemed to believe that whatever damage they might suffer had already occurred. Marsh concludes that future health education concerning smoking must do more than emphasize susceptibility. They must make it clear that increased susceptibility begins at less than 20 a day and is decreased by giving up thus making good health more likely. Marsh highlights this point by suggesting the slogan *Stop smoking and stay well*.

The implications for health education are clear. Providing 'information' is not enough. Effective health education must be linked directly to the beliefs of those we hope to educate. Recent AIDS-related, educational material in the United Kingdom implored people not to 'die of ignorance' but this is rarely the problem; it is not ignorance but mistaken beliefs which prevent us from taking health-preserving measures. Marsh and Mathensons' participants were not ignorant, they just did not believe they were susceptible. Similar self-protective, 'not-me' beliefs may be developed in relation to any health threat. Abrams, et al., (1990) and Abraham, et al., (1991), for example, report on low perceived susceptibility in relation to the threat of human immunodeficiency virus or 'AIDS-invulnerability' amongst teenagers in Scotland. Combating such low perceived susceptibility means designing health education campaigns which are based on a knowledge of the beliefs of the target group. Messages can then be tailored to relate to widespread beliefs concerning the causes of ill health, the likelihood of disease transmission in everyday settings, the effectiveness of suggested health behaviours and so on. HBM and the theory of planned behaviour collectively provide us with a useful framework in which to model shared representations regulating everyday health and illness behaviour. However, we may need to 'fine tune' this framework to take account of beliefs relevant to a particular group of people or a particular health problem. Bradley, et al., (1984), for example, have used HBM to construct groups of questions capable of measuring beliefs relevant to those with diabetes while Abraham, et al., (1991) point to differences between groups of young people's beliefs about human immunodeficiency virus. In other words common-sense health beliefs may only be common to particular groups. Thus as Becker, et al., (1977) note we may need to emphasize susceptibility to some, severity to others and peer approval for health behaviours to others. This means that mass media campaigns which broadcast the same health education messages to different groups may be limited in their effectiveness.

Our discussion so far has focused upon preventive behaviour and treatment compliance but differences between health beliefs across groups may also affect the perception of illness and therefore the use made of available health services. Zola (1975), drawing upon the work of Koos (1954) and others, notes that what are regarded as 'symptoms' in one culture may be seen as quite normal in another. If coughing, backache or conversing with absent persons are regarded as a normal part of everyday life then such experiences will not be classed as illness and will not prompt help-seeking behaviour. Indeed Zola reports on a group in which a condition we would think of as a skin disease was so common that culture-members regarded its absence as a pathological condition which made men unfit for marriage! Zola also studied the perception of ear, eye nose and throat problems amongst Americans of Irish and Italian decent. He found that even when participants of the same sex and similar age received the the same diagnosis and had the complaint for approximately the same period there were systematic differences in how 'Irish' and 'Italian' participants described their problems. Irish people tended to report fewer symptoms and to see the problem as specific to a certain part of the body while Italians tended to report more, and more diffuse, difficulties. The general point here is that illness cannot be separated from culture; while biological processes may underpin illness, illness itself is a social construction. To identify 'symptoms' and define oneself as ill one draws upon shared beliefs concerning the nature of health and illness. Thus when we speak of internal and external 'cues' prompting compliance we must be aware that what counts as a cue may differ from one sub-culture to another.

A model of help-seeking

Mechanic (1978) has developed a model of help-seeking behaviour which takes account of the cultural context of illness and has the advantage of incorporating a number HBM components. We shall conclude this Section with a brief consideration of his model. The model consists of ten factors which may affect whether or not a person will respond to a bodily cue (for example, chest pains) by seeking help. However two of these factors concern the general understanding of the person and those around her. This includes their knowledge of bodily functioning and awareness of the different interpretations of a particular sign (for example, being aware that chest pains may be due to heart disease or anxiety). These factors refer to the general representations of health and illness available to the person at the time. The other eight factors are listed below:

1. *the visibility and recognizability of signs or symptoms.* Obviously the more noticeable a problem is the more likely the person is to acknowledge it and seek help. However, 'visibility' is culturally determined. It may, for example, be affected by acceptable mode of dress and body display.
2. *beliefs about the severity of the illness* once the problem is acknowledged. Mechanic points out that this HBM component can also affect help seeking.

3. *disruption to everyday life* caused by the signs. The greater the disruption the more likely we are to seek help. Again this will depend upon the relationship between the signs and the person's lifestyle; what is disruptive to one person may hardly impinge upon another.
4. *the frequency with which the signs appear*. When a condition appears persistently we and those around us are more likely to see help-seeking as appropriate.
5. *the tolerance threshold of both the person themselves and those around them*. Low tolerance levels promote prompt help-seeking.
6. *needs that lead to denial*. If the person or those around her see the signs as representing a serious threat to them or their lifestyles they may protect themselves by failing to recognize the presence or meaning of symptoms and thereby avoiding help seeking behaviour (see Chapter 7, Section 2).
7. *availability of treatment resources*. This factor corresponds to beliefs concerning 'costs' in HBM. Seeking help may be seen to involve travel, money, time as well as psychological costs such as humiliation or embarrassment.
8. *competing needs and intentions*. This factor could be viewed as a special type of cost, that is the 'opportunity cost' of seeking help. Help seeking may involve delays in acting upon other intentions. Thus the more daily demands a person feels they must meet the less likely help-seeking becomes. Some people feel themselves to be so busy they do not have time to be ill!

By adding Mechanic's model to our conceptual framework, we can model help-seeking, preventive and treatment-compliance behaviour. Such modelling can help the practicing nurse make sense of a variety of health and illness behaviour and acknowledge that what seems bizarre and irrational to her may appear quite sensible given a different set of health beliefs.

3   Beliefs about Causes and Control

Attribution theory

In this Section we shall examine models of our beliefs about *what causes what* and discuss how such beliefs influence health-related behaviour. Beliefs about the cause of a bodily sensation may affect how we respond to it. Mechanic (1978) notes that one of Koos' (1954) participants observed that if he knew his backache was due to lifting a bucket of coal he might not consult a doctor as quickly as if he could not explain why he had backache. Thus beliefs about susceptibility and severity and therefore help-seeking may depend upon causal beliefs.

Heider (1958) was one of the first psychologists to model our common sense notions of causation. He noted that when we identify a person or thing as the cause of an event we describe them in terms of some quality they possess which enables them to cause such events. We say that the needle is sharp and can therefore cut us or that Mary is allergic to pollen and therefore gets hayfever. Heider referred to this process of understanding causation as *attributing* causal power to a *disposition* of the person or thing. We understand the event, for example Mary's streaming eyes, in terms of the kind of person Mary is, that is in terms of her allergic disposition. This disposition then becomes part of our understanding of Mary and we will not be surprised if she shows the same reaction again when the pollen count is high. Of course if we know some noxious substance has been released into the air then we may form quite a different understanding of the event. In this case we may attribute Mary's problem to a dispositional property of this substance and having understood the event in this way we will not expect Mary to continue to suffer in the future because we have not attributed her suffering to a disposition characterizing *her*. Instead we will expect other people exposed to this 'noxious' substance to suffer in the same way as Mary. Representation of the causes underlying events depends upon such dispositional attributions which in turn shape our expectations regarding future events.

Of course different people may form different understandings of the same event by making different attributions, in which case they will disagree about the nature of the event. Thus one person might say that Mary has hayfever while another might argue that the air contained something which upset everyone. As social psychologists we are not primarily concerned with the truth or accuracy of these understandings but with the effect they have on people's intentions and behaviour. If Mary believes she is allergic she may buy drugs or see a faith healer (depending on how she attributes the power to alleviate her condition). It is *her* causal beliefs about symptoms and remedies (regardless of her doctor's views) which determine her behaviour. This connection between causal attributions and intentions corresponds to the theory of planned behaviour's identification of beliefs about control as determinants of our behaviour.

Kelley (1967) used Heider's analysis to create a simplified 'attributional' model which distinguished between internal attributions characterizing people (Mary is allergic) and external attributions which characterizing environmental features (the air contains a noxious substance). Weiner (1974) elaborated on Kelley's model by adding a stable-unstable dimension. This allows to distinguish between four broad categories of attribution. Namely:

1. *internal-stable*, involving a lasting disposition within the person, for example, being allergic or having some ability. This type of attribution leads to expectations of similar events involving this person in the future, for example Mary will get hayfever again.
2. *internal-unstable*, involving a temporary state the person may experience, for example, Mary being upset or 'run-down'. This type of attribution does not necessarily lead us to expect recurrence of the event for this person. We will only expect symptoms to reappear if Mary becomes run-down again.
3. *external-stable*, involving the identification of a lasting disposition in the environment, for example, the difficulty of a task or the presence of long-lasting radioactive contamination. This type of attribution will lead us to expect the event to happen to or affect other people in the same environment.
4. *External-unstable*, involving a temporary, environmental state, such as the presence of smoky air which will be dispersed by the wind. This is the type of attribution we make when we put things down to luck. Such attributions lead us to expect a recurrence of the event only when particular, unstable conditions are present.

Weiner's reworking of Kelley's model enables us to put peoples' causal understandings into rough categories and thereby anticipate the type of expectations they will have regarding the future occurrence of similar events. These attributions incorporate our understanding of the different causal processes which may be involved in different events. We distinguish between deliberate actions, involuntary reactions (such as emotional responses) and physical occurrences which do not involve a thinking or feeling being (Abraham, 1988).

Locus of control and health beliefs

Rotter's (1966) work on 'locus of control' is closely related to that of Kelley and Weiner. Rotter proposed that we could categorize people according to whether they typically attributed control over events to themselves (that is, internally) or to the outside world (that is, externally). Those who typically attributed internally (internals) would have a strong sense of control over events whereas those who typically attributed externally (externals) would have a more fatalistic view of their lives. Levenson (1974) divided Rotter's single dimension into three; the tendency to attribute control over events *internally*, the tendency to attribute control over events to *powerful others* and the tendency to attribute control over events to *luck or chance*. Wallston, et al., (1978) adapted Levenson's dimensions to deal specifically with perceived control of health issues and so developed the 'multidimensional health locus of control scales'. These sets of questions or 'scales' allow us to assess the extent to which an individual attributes control over her health to the three sources identified by Levenson. Thus a person might, for example, tend to attribute control over her health both internally and to powerful others but not to chance. Wallston and Wallston (1982) note that this particular attributional pattern may engender good relationships between the person and health-care workers and may therefore be particularly beneficial to people with chronic conditions who are in continual contact with health-care systems.

Wallston and Wallston provide a useful review of studies investigating the relationships between locus of control and health-related behaviour. Quoting Strickland (1978) they note that early work on Rotter's simple scale suggested that internals were more likely both to engage in preventive health behaviour and to comply with treatment advice. However, they also point out that since three-dimensional scales have been used to measure locus of control the evidence has been less conclusive. A number of studies on reducing smoking have shown a relationship between a tendency to attribute control over health internally and being able to reduce cigarette smoking (for example, Kaplan and Cowles, 1978). These support Eiser's (1982) finding that smokers who retained faith in their control over the habit were more likely to intend to give up, try to give up and be successful at giving up than those who saw themselves as 'hooked'. Some studies also suggest that those who attribute control internally or to powerful others are more likely to comply with treatment advice and report symptoms earlier. Wallston and Wallston argue that the evidence is not conclusive because locus of control cannot be studied in isolation from other health beliefs. They are an important component of the representations which determine our health and illness behaviour but they also interact with the beliefs we have considered above.

King's (1983) work is of interest here. She found that participants suffering from heart disease were more likely to believe themselves to be susceptible to further heart problems if they attributed their problems to uncontrollable factors such as an inborn predisposition, a change of lifestyle, bad luck or stress due to family illness. King also found that, after behavioural intentions (emphasized by the theory of planned behaviour) causal attributions were the most important influence on attendance at clinics screening for high blood pressure. Specifically, those attributing high blood pressure to stress and worry were more likely to attend than those who attributed it to too much exercise, a lack of vitamins or bad luck. This work reaffirms the importance of understanding patients' causal attributions by demonstrating that they have an important influence on beliefs about susceptibility and preventive behaviour. It also illustrates the value of using and models such as attribution theory, HBM and the theory of planned behaviour *in combination* (Cummings et al., 1980). Using social psychological models in this way we can consider multiple health beliefs and are more likely to capture the sophistication of our patients' representations of their situations. King (1983), Blaxter (1979) and Taylor (1983) also point out it is useful to examine patients' own spontaneously generated causal explanations. While broad categorizations (such as 'internal' and 'external') can help us make generalizations they can also obscure the sophistication of the individual's common-sense explanations. Again we are reminded that modelling peoples' representations of reality is not simple because these representations are themselves complex.

Perceived self-efficacy

Common sense causal attribution is closely linked to *perceived self-efficacy*, that is our perception of our own ability to handle events. Seligman (1975), Abramson, et al., (1978) and Seligman, et al., (1979) have argued that people prone to depression tend to attribute uncontrollable failures (that is, failures which the person could not have prevented) to internal, stable factors such as lack of ability. This means that where others would blame external factors (such as the difficulty of the task undertaken) these people blame themselves. Seligman has argued that this pattern of attributions teaches people that they cannot control their own destinies and leads to a state of *learned helplessness*. Thus such attributions lower their self-esteem, remove feelings of self-efficacy and lead us to anticipate failure. Indeed studies suggest that challenging such attributions and other self-defeating beliefs can be more effective than antidepressant drugs in alleviating depression in the short and medium term (Beck, 1976; Rush and Giles, 1982 – see Chapter 7, Section 4).

Bandura (1977; 1986; 1989) has probably done most to emphasize the importance of perceived self-efficacy on everyday performance and behaviour change. He presents evidence suggesting that high perceived self-efficacy allows people to perform better than those with equal ability but less faith in their ability. High perceived self-efficacy leads people to persevere with difficult problems, to discard ineffective problem-solving strategies more quickly, to reexamine their work for errors, to set themselves more demanding goals and to spend less time worrying about the consequences of failure. These psychological implications mean that perceived self-efficacy is likely to become a self-fulfilling prophecy; those who believe themselves to have the ability to perform well are more likely to succeed. Bandura (1989) discusses studies which show that performance on tests of strength, pain tolerance, susceptibility to headaches and the operation of the immune system can all be influenced by changes in perceived self-efficacy (Litt, 1988; Holroyd, et al., 1984; Wiedenfeld, et al.,, 1989). Thus modelling people's beliefs concerning their own abilities should be be a crucial part of understanding their success and failure. This may be vital when recommending a self-care procedure or preventive measure. Patients who are less confident in their ability to comply will be less likely to do so (Kaplan et al., 1984; Alagna and Reddy, 1984).

4   Challenge, Control and Coronary Heart Disease
Stress – in the eye of the beholder?

Each of us has our own everyday challenges (such as trying to understand social psychological research and its relevance to nursing). These give our lives structure and when we meet them successfully make us more self-confident (especially if we attribute our success to internal-stable dispositions). It is only when we doubt our ability to cope that such challenges become stressful (see Chapter 9, Section 1). In other words lowered perceived self-efficacy generates stress. Of course events which involve the loss of some well-known and important aspect of our lives are bound to make us unsure about our ability to cope. We build up sophisticated representations of the people and places in our lives and expect to be able to use such 'knowledge' to meet our personal goals (see Chapter 3, Sections 1 and 2). Losing key elements of the world we know leaves us unsure about how to plan and proceed with everyday life. Change and loss are therefore stressful to some extent for everyone because they require us to readjust, that is create new representations of ourselves and our world and to establish new relationships and routines.

In order to compare the readjustment demanded by some of life's more serious losses and changes Holmes and Rahe (1967) developed 'the social readjustment rating scale' which indicates the relative stressfulness of various events. At the top of the scale is the death of one's spouse scoring 100, lower down comes marital separation scoring 65, personal illness or injury 53, losing one's job 47, retirement 45, changing jobs 36 and moving house 20. This helps us appreciate the support people need as they experience such upheavals and warns us against generating too much change in our lives at any one time.

Holmes and Rahes' generalizations about stressful life events are based upon our understanding of the intersubjective nature of our social representations. We know that close relationships and jobs are crucial to most peoples' representations of themselves. Losing relationships or work-related activities will create stress and if no alternatives are available may lead eventually to depression (see Jahoda, 1982; Oatley, 1988). However, the stressfulness of any particular event depends upon the individual's representation of it so that one person's stress may be another's excitement! An experiment by Glass and Singer (1972) illustrates this point. They exposed two groups of participants to a loud and unpleasant noise. One group were told they could stop the noise by pressing a button but were asked not to while the other were given no control over the noise. None of the 'stop-button' group actually used the button so all participants experienced the same noise. However the 'stop-button' group did better than the 'no-control' on problem-solving tasks presented immediately after this experience. This suggests that the noise was *less disturbing* for the 'stop-button' group simply because they believed they were in control (see Figure 2b). Thus perceived self-efficacy appears to reduce the psychological disturbance that unpleasant experiences can produce (Bandura, 1989). This result underlines the destructiveness of a depressive attributional style. It seems that if we make internal, stable attributions when we fail and so regard ourselves as lacking in ability, we will not only feel discouraged but also be more disturbed by unpleasant experiences (such as failure). The destructive tendency to become annoyed at one's own lack of ability even in the face of impossible or uncontrollable events has been identified as one facet of what has become to be known as 'type A' behaviour (Brunson and Matthews, 1981).

Type A; type B

In 1974 two cardiologists, Friedman and Rosenman published *Type A Behaviour and Your Heart*. The book reported evidence for a theory they had been investigating since the 1950s. They proposed that some people were more prone to coronary heart disease (CHD) because of the way they represented and responded to the world. These people who exhibit what they called 'type A' behaviour are highly competitive and feel themselves to be involved in an incessant struggle to achieve more and more in less and less time. They are hard driving, aggressive, prone to hostile reactions and have a strong sense of time urgency. 'Type B' people are the opposite; uncompetitive, 'laid back', relatively unconcerned about time and slow to show hostility. Friedman and Rosenman developed a series of questions which, through interviews, allowed them to distinguish between these two types. This technique was used in the *Western Collaborative Group Study* (Rosenman, Friedman and Strauss, 1966) to divide a group of 3154 employed, Californian men aged 39 and 59 into 1589 type A's and 1565 type Bs. The mens' health was then monitored over the next eight and a half years. The study showed that quite apart from standard risk-factors associated with CHD (such as smoking and high cholesterol levels) those initially categorized as type A had twice as much chance of having heart disease as those categorized as type B.

Numerous research projects have investigated Friedman and Rosenmans' ideas and although some methodological problems remain unresolved the evidence generally supports their proposal that type A's are more prone to CHD (see Feuerstein, et al., 1986 for a useful review). It is worth noting, however, that some studies suggest that a subset of type A's are particularly at risk, namely, those who regularly display anger and hostility in response to everyday frustrations. A number of explanations of the type A-CHD link have been developed (see Carver and Humphries, 1982 for a review). Glass (1977) for example, has argued that type A people have an exaggerated need for control over their environment and therefore respond to events which challenge this control by doubling and redoubling their attempts to retain control. If, however, after this intense struggle they still lose control they tend to make negative, internal attributions and lapse into learned helplessness. The physiological damage that makes CHD more likely may be caused both by increased activity of the sympathetic nervous system during the struggle for control (including increased heart rate) and by the sudden shift to parasympathetic nervous control (including decreased heart rate) when type A's give up and retreat into helplessness (see Chapter 9, Section 1). Carver and Humphries point out that this struggle for control includes ignoring signs and symptoms of physical exhaustion, so that type A's will push themselves to and beyond normal limits more often than type B's. This also means they will delay acknowledging and reporting physical problems. Remembering Mechanic's model of help-seeking behaviour we can see that type As are indeed people who do not have time to be ill. Overall then type A behaviour appears to sacrifice physical needs to achieve psychological control against all odds.

Powell and Friedman (1986) have proposed that *low self-esteem* underlies the high need for control characterizing type As. The urgent need to keep things under control is a product of low perceived self-efficacy. The type A coping style is a vicious and self-destructive cycle; lack of faith in one's abilities leads to a chronic struggle for control which in the face of uncontrollable challenges leads to self-blame and helplessness. This prompts further reductions in perceived self-efficacy which heighten the need for control. Meanwhile the physiological processes sustaining this cycle result in cumulative damage and make CHD more likely.

The question raised by this body of research is whether the incidence of CHD, a major cause of premature death, could be reduced by inducing psychological change in those identified as type As. The results of Powell and Friedmans' (1986) *Recurrent Coronary Prevention Project* suggests that it could. They undertook a 54-month experiment with 1012 post-myocardial infarction patients. Ninety-five per cent of these showed some degree of type A behaviour. One group received cardiologic counselling (that is, advice about heart function, diet, exercise and so on) while another group received cardiologic counselling and type A behavioural counselling (that is, advice, materials and therapy designed to help them reduce their type A behaviour). The second group showed a reduction in type A behaviour after one year and a higher incidence of survival without cardiac recurrence over three years (94% of this group survived the three years without cardiac recurrence as compared to 87% in the first group). This suggests that, at least for people who have experienced a cardiac episode, (who may have stronger intentions to cooperate with preventive advice) we can intervene to decrease type A behaviour and thereby reduce premature death due to CHD (see Chapter 7, Section 4).

We have seen that representations of the world affect our health in two ways. First, through our *behavioural responses* to symptoms. These include help-seeking behaviour and responses to advice about health that is compliance with treatment and preventive programmes. Secondly, by means of *physiological changes which accompany changes in our our psychological state*. The recognition that psychology has a crucial impact on health in through both these routes has led to the development of a psychosomatic or holistic approach to many health problems including CHD pain-management and cancer. Christie and Melletts' (1986) collection provides a useful overview of this developing field including an interesting Chapter by Stoll on the way mood and stress may affect cancer growth through associated hormonal activity. Thus a healthy body may be dependent on a healthy mind in the sense that constructive beliefs about oneself and the world preserve good health through their affect on underlying physiological processes and health-enhancing behaviour. In particular it seems that high self-esteem and perceived self-efficacy helps us feel good and stay healthy. Thus therapies designed to change such underlying representations such as Powell and Friedmans' recurrent coronary prevention project or Beck's cognitive therapy have an important role in health care provision.

5 Using Psychological Models in Health Care

Understanding patients' understandings

Since health and health-related behaviour depend upon our beliefs and intentions, health-care workers, who want to understand and change their patients' behaviour, must be able to model these beliefs and intentions. We have outlined a series of social psychological models and theories which can be drawn upon in this endeavour. We have noted how important it is to understand peoples' beliefs about; the causes of events, the likely outcome of an action (including various costs and benefits), their own ability in relation to any proposed action, others approval of such action, their susceptibility to illness, the severity of any given illness and their current intentions. These psychological measures can provide a rough map of the representations which direct health-relevant behaviour. Such a map can enable health educators and those interested in personal change to target their explanations, recommendations and recourses so that they are likely to affect the particular beliefs that are maintaining destructive behaviour or blocking compliance (see Chapter 5, Section 2).

One area of application is the structuring of assessment interviews and health care consultations. Open questioning and appropriate recording formats could allow us to track patients' health beliefs over time. Such records could provide a basis for focused discussions about the relationships between individuals' beliefs and desired behaviour change. They could be jointly updated by staff and patients and provide a basis for subsequent consultations. Such cognitive assessment might be particularly beneficial to nurses who are engaged in day-to-day communication with patients and may act as intermediaries between the patient and other health-care workers. It would ensure that health-education discussions focused upon individual health beliefs and highlighted the patient's responsibility for evaluating her health situation and acting accordingly. Issues of non-compliance could then be addressed as psychological problems. If for example, a patient felt threatened by breast self-examination the risk of finding a lump could be discussed in relation to the potential losses involved in leaving a lump undetected (see Meyerowitz and Chaiken, 1987). Cues for forgetful patients could be arranged, for example friends or relatives could be given responsibility for prompting the patient (see Chapter 6, Section 4). This might be particularly useful for patients who attribute control to powerful others and may also benefit friends or relatives by giving them a sense of control over some aspect of the patient's condition. Causal beliefs affecting the patients' sense of self-efficacy could be identified, and aetiology and prognosis related to the patient's current health beliefs. In this way the patient would be involved in a self-reflective relationship directed towards establishing health-enhancing beliefs and intentions. This kind of psychological assessment and intervention could be accommodated within a number of nursing models such as Rogers' (1980) unitary model of nursing care or Riehl's (1980) interactionist model. Both these models acknowledge the importance of monitoring and facilitating change in patient's representations.

When health-care workers do not model their patients' representations they are likely to misunderstand them. Feuerstein, et al., (1986) for example, note that doctors tend to underestimate non-compliance, are inaccurate at identifying non-compliant patients and may attribute non-compliance to internal, stable factors, such as 'personality' or 'laziness'. Mechanic (1978) notes that patients' have particular expectations of their encounters with health-care workers and if these are not fulfilled then communication and cooperation break down (see Chapter 5, Section 5). Jones (1982) argues that doctors' failure to allow patients' to introduce material into consultations and their adherence to questions based solely inferences about the patients' initial statement of symptoms may (given the fallibility of patients' memory and the ambiguity of descriptions of bodily states) lead consultations away from the real problem and result in confirmation of erroneous inferences. Thus failure to understand problems from the patients' point of view may result in ineffective service delivery because of patient dissatisfaction, uninvestigated non-compliance, perception of patients as 'lost causes' and an increased likelihood of mistaken diagnosis and treatment recommendations.

Implications for health care practice

Using psychological models to enhance health-care delivery may necessitate changes in everyday working practices. King (1983), citing Stimson and Webb (1975), notes that taking account of the patient' beliefs means that the consultation process must become a negotiation between patient and health-care worker in which each becomes aware of the others' views and any diagnosis or recommendation is acceptable to both. After all, if it is not acceptable to the patient they are unlikely to comply. Wallston and Wallston (1982) point out that such 'democratic' consultations are also likely to enhance patients' perceived self-efficacy. This may, however, require redefining the role relationship between patients, nurses and doctors (see Chapter 4, Sections 1 and 2). In this regard Jenkins (1979) offers some useful guidelines on how nurses and doctors can remain responsive to their patient's psychological needs. He suggests they should:

1. provide continuity of personalized care (that is, a small number of persons known to the patient should be responsible for her care);
2. meet or change patients' expectations of the health-care worker;
3. provide all the information necessary to follow care recommendations in a comprehensible manner;
4. emphasize the importance of health-related behaviour to the patient and (with her consent) to those she regularly interacts with;
5. reduce as far as possible the costs of help-seeking and compliance behaviour while actively finding ways in which the patient can be rewarded for health-care behaviour;
6. instil in the patient a sense of personal responsibility for and control over her health.

These suggestions emphasize how service delivery depends upon good communication which itself relies upon our understanding of how other's see their situation. We shall return to this theme in later Chapters.

CORE IDEAS IN CHAPTER 2

- Health maintenance depends upon our responses to perceived symptoms and the advice. Understanding these behaviours involves modelling people's health-related beliefs.

- Non compliance rates are high and undermine the effectiveness of health care services. Compliance may be improved by understanding the psychological bases of patients behaviour.

- Behaviour in any particular setting is the result of many beliefs about oneself, others and the consequences of one's actions. This can create discrepancies between expressed attitudes and actual behaviour.

- The theory of planned behaviour, the health belief model, attribution theory, an understanding of perceived self-efficacy and Mechanic's model of help-seeking behaviour provide a rough map of the type of beliefs and intentions which direct health-related behaviour.

- An investigation of patient beliefs can enable health educators to target their communications on beliefs which are maintain destructive behaviour or block self-care. Such communications may need to be tailored to the beliefs held by particular groups of people with specific health concerns.

- Our beliefs about the world not only determine health-related behaviour but can also affect our health directly through the physiological mechanisms which underlie our psychological responses to our experiences. This is illustrated by type A behaviour.

- Taking account of patients' beliefs and intentions may mean changing the way nurses and doctors communicate and interact.

3

Understanding others and ourselves

1 Seeing and Knowing Other People
Finding out who thinks what about whom

Much of our everyday experience is shared with, and shaped by other people. However, much of the influence others have upon us is mediated by our perceptions of them. We may be very upset if a close friend devalues our work behind our back but the criticism of a long-standing work rival may even be amusing. The impact of such criticism depends upon our expectations of the person and the value we attach to their opinion. In this chapter we shall look at some of the processes or 'programmes' involved in representing others and our relationships with them.

We readily discuss our perceptions of others. We might say that, 'John is very sensitive', that, 'Ann is intelligent', or that 'Julia is spiteful'. We think of people as having sets of characteristics like houses or landscapes. It seems obvious that those we know have particular personalities, intentions, ambitions, and so on. Moreover, our 'knowledge' about what *type* of people they are enables us to make fairly confident predictions about their abilities, their responses and their relationships with others. Indeed a great deal of our time is spent comparing notes on our representations of others. We want to know if friends and colleagues agree with our views of the new charge nurse and we may even be interested to know what they think of our favourite soap opera character. Such everyday gossip is important in maintaining our relationships. It allows us to work out what our friends think about us and others and to discover how these views compare to our own (see Chapter 6, Sections 2 and 4). This enables us to form expectations about what others are likely to do and say which we can use to plan our own behaviour.

Conversations about a new charge nurse or a recently admitted patient can shape future relationships and contribute to the establishment of shared representations of these people within particular social circles. In this way gossip can influence the judgements people make about others and how they relate. This could mean, for example, that assessments of a person's abilities, their promotion prospects, and even the standard of care they receive in hospital could be affected by views swapped informally in coffee rooms or corridors.

Seeing others through our own assumptions

We tend to regard our representations of others as arising naturally from their behaviour, that is as mere descriptions of how they really are. However, much of what we think about others can be traced back to our own assumptions about the world. In other words our perception of any particular person is *constructed* out of a background of representations of people in general. Our culturally shared views on what is appropriate and inappropriate behaviour in certain situations, our particular responsibilities in a situation, our expectations of people of a certain sex, age, race, religion all influence how we regard those we meet or hear about. Thus, to a large extent, 'seeing' others involves fitting them into a network of assumptions which we hold about the social world. This is why people have serious disagreements about what sort of person someone else is. They disagree because their different perceptions of the other person are partly their own creations!

A study which neatly demonstrates our active construction of representations of others was conducted by Dornbusch, et al., (1965).

They asked children to describe one another and recorded the type of descriptions (or categories) they used, that is, whether they mentioned the other child's race, sex, relationships, moods abilities and so on. Using 69 categories they compared the degree to which the same categories were used when:

1. two children described the same target child;
2. one child described two different target children;
3. two children described two different target children.

If our perceptions of others are merely the result of how others actually are then we would expect the greatest category overlap in (1) when the same target child is described by two others. In fact, Dornbusch and colleagues found that the *greatest overlap occurred in (2) when one child described two others,* suggesting that it is *the perceiver and not the person who is perceived who provides the categories* used to represent others. Thus our knowledge of others is to a large extent the result of our imposition of our own categories onto their behavior.

Dornbusch and colleagues found that descriptions produced when two children described the same child showed the next greatest overlap but also noted that there was little difference between this overlap and that found when two children described two different children (where there is no obvious reason for overlap). This suggests that the *situation in which we make judgements* about others can have an important impact on our perceptions regardless of who is judging whom. In this study the children were describing fellow campers. Their attention would therefore be directed towards aspects of other children most evident in a camping situation. The characteristics we think are important about other people change as we move from one situation to another. For example, the characteristics which attract us to someone we meet on a beech holiday are likely to be quite different to those which we value in a colleague on an intensive care unit.

Inferring personality – implicit personality theories and stereotypes

Asch (1946) explored the processes involved in building up impressions of others out of our stock of general characteristics. He showed that when we are presented with categories describing a person we tend to *infer* that they also have other characteristics (not on the list). In other words *we go beyond what we have been told to assume characteristics which have not been mentioned*. When given the list 'intelligent, skillful, industrious, warm, determined, practical and cautious' Asch's participants inferred that the person was persistent rather than unstable, serious rather than frivolous, honest rather than dishonest and so on. Asch also found that *some characteristics have more impact on our inferences than others*. Characteristics which help us anticipate how a person relates to others such as 'warm' and 'cold' seem to be especially important. Finally, Asch showed that the order in which we hear about a person's characteristics affects the type of inferences we make (see also Luchins, 1957). This seems to be because the meaning of later characteristics is affected by the ones we have already attributed to them. Being 'calm', for example, is usually a good quality but notice how different it sounds in 'warm, humorous and calm' and 'cold, humourless and calm'. In the first it makes the person seem more attractive whereas in the second it seems to make them even less so. In general positive descriptions of others lead us to infer that they have further positive characteristics which have not been mentioned while negative descriptions prompt negative inferences (Osgood, 1962). This tendency is often referred to as the 'halo effect'.

Bruner and Tagiuri (1954) used the term *implicit personality theory* (IPT) to describe the unconscious inference processes which enable us to form impressions of others on the basis of very little evidence. They proposed that we each have our own general 'theory' or set of expectations about others. We use this general theory to fill in gaps in our representations of particular people. This IPT is partly derived from our primary socialization. Harré (1983), for example, notes that Eskimo and Maori languages embody very different theories about people to those embodied in the English language. Thus Eskimo and Maori perceptions of others will be very different to our own because they begin from a different set of basic categorizations. As well as this background culture our individual history of making judgements about people and interacting with them provides us with sets of assumptions and inferences which we may not share with others. One person may, for example, feel intimidated, or even hostile, on hearing that a new work colleague is 'very intelligent' whereas another may may feel pleased and interested. Thus we share a basic theory of others through our language but we develop personal variations through our particular social experience. This common-sense theory directs the inferences we make about which characteristics are likely to go together and defines the meaning we attach to those characteristics. In this way it shapes our representations of others.

As well as IPT's defining which personal characteristics go together we have theories about broad groups of people. We can use these theories or *stereotypes* to infer characteristics once we have placed a person in one of our groups (Allport, 1954). Our stereotypes may refer to different kinds of groups defined in many different ways, for example, a person's sex, their age, their race, their religion or their work role (see Chapter 4, Section 1). Taking the example of work role, a person might hold the view that nurses are 'patient caring, feminine, and unambitious'. When such a person is told that someone is a nurse they can apply their stereotype and assume that this particular person is patient caring, feminine, and unambitious. We assume that the individual will display the characteristics typical of the group in which we have placed them. This process provides the basis for many of our everyday social judgements and sustains many social prejudices, divisions and discriminatory practices. Duncan (1976), for example, has shown that when a white audience watched a film of a white man pushing another person they were less likely to judge the man to be aggressive than when they watched a film of a black man behaving in an identical manner. As with IPTs people from similar backgrounds tend to share stereotypes. Shared stereotypes change and develop over time (Karlins, et al., 1969) and as individuals we elaborate on the stereotypes we acquire through primary and secondary socialization to develop our own personal stereotypes. Understanding stereotyping can be useful in making broad predictions about how members of different groups will view one another. This can help us explain certain types of intergroup conflict.

The characteristics we use to represent others allow us to build up expectations because they help us explain the causes of events. If, for example, we believe that Julia is spiteful then we can explain a breakdown in one of her friendships in terms of this 'dispositional attribution' (see Chapter 2, Section 3). Indeed attributional studies suggest that we have a general tendency to explain events in terms of peoples' personal characteristics rather than aspects of the situation they find themselves in. This is known as the *fundamental attribution error*. Even when we know that a person has been specifically instructed to give a speech, or write an essay expressing a particular view we still tend to believe that the attitudes expressed are their own (Jones and Harris, 1967; Yandrell and Insko, 1977). Jones and Nisbett (1972) and Watson (1982) point out that although we are aware of situational determinants when explaining our own behaviour we underestimate their influence when considering others' behaviour.

Initial impression formation is important because these early appraisals may persist and guide later behaviour towards others. Once we have categorized a person as cold and humourless, for example, we may be prepared to discount contradictory evidence to keep our established view of them intact (Kelley, 1972). Indeed we tend to remember information that fits with our established view of the person better than that which contradicts it and to think that we have received information consistent with our view even when we have not (see Cantor and Mischel 1977, 1979). In general then our impressions of others only change slowly, so once we think we know them it is hard for them to alter our opinion. Our perceptions of them affects how we behave towards them so that seeing them as cold and humourless, for example, we are likely to be fairly unfriendly towards them. They in turn may see us as unfriendly and remain cold and aloof so strengthening our negative view of them. In this way our perceptions of others can result in the very responses we expect. In other words they become *self fulfilling prophecies*. Automatic inferences about other people based on our IPTs and stereotypes can mislead us and lock us into destructive relationships. An awareness of these processes and their implications is especially important for nurses since communication with, and assessment of, others is central to their work.

Stereotyping patients – good and bad patients

Nurses share a common secondary socialization through their training courses (Davies, 1975; Simpson, 1973). They also encounter their patients in similar settings and relationships. We might therefore expect them to share patient stereotypes. Many studies have explored the positive and negative inferences nurses make in their perceptions of different types of patient. Larson (1977), for example, asked nurses to look at slides and read descriptions depicting a fictitious patient. The descriptions were varied so that they portrayed the patient as, either middle or lower class and having a more or less serious, and more or less socially acceptable illness. Larson found that manipulation of each of these three independent variables generated differences in responses to questions about how the nurse participants saw the patient, how they expected him to learn about his illness and how they thought she would manage self-care. Patients described as lower class, for example, were seen as more dependent, passive, unintelligent, unmotivated, unsuccessful, lazy, careless and unreliable in comparison to those described as middle class. By inviting nurses to think of a patient as belonging to the group 'lower class' Larson prompted the application of a fairly typical stereotype of 'lower class people'. Similarly those with less socially acceptable illnesses (for example, alcoholism) were thought to be more sensitive, rigid and resistant while those with more serious illnesses were thought to be less motivated to learn and less likely to comply with suggested self-care programmes. Larson's findings confirm other studies showing that nurses make attributions about their patients based on shared stereotypes. Research of this kind has tended to contrast the way in which some patients are positively represented by nurses while other are regarded more negatively and it has therefore become known as the 'good and bad patient' literature. Stockwell (1972) reported that 'unpopular patients' tended to be those who complained, implied they were suffering more than nurses thought they were and had conditions nurses believed would be better cared for elsewhere. More recently, Kelly and May (1982) reviewed studies in this area and concluded that patients who have particular kinds of problems (for example, malnutrition, incontinence or long-term illness), who engage in certain behaviours (for example, over-dependency or non-compliance with clinical advice), who are older or who are unappreciative of nursing care tend to be viewed more negatively.

A worrying implication of these findings is that nurses may behave differently towards 'good' and 'bad' patients and those who are negatively stereotyped may receive a less caring, tolerant and professional service. Few studies demonstrate this perception-interaction link though Morimoto (1955) observed that nurses limited themselves to businesslike, physical care with 'bad' patients but attended to the psychological and social needs of their 'good' patients. Similarly Sudnow (1967) noted that the effort devoted to resuscitation of 'dead on arrival' patients in casualty wards was related to their attractiveness and Hollingshead and Redlich (1958) found that social class was a better predictor of recommended treatment for psychiatric patients than their diagnosis. We also know that teachers expectations of how rapidly students will learn affects teaching techniques and can influence the performance of their students (Brophy and Good, 1970; Rosenthal and Jacobson, 1968). Thus while it has not been clearly demonstrated it is plausible that nurses' perceptions of their patients affect their interaction with them. In this way unintentional communication of expectations about patients could become self-fulfilling prophecies. Expectations generated by stereotypes of lower-class patients, for example, might result in slower acquisition of self care skills.

Kelly and May note that many researchers in this area have recommended further training for nurses aimed at eliminating such patient stereotyping. However, they also point out that such stereotyping may not be due to everyday stereotypes and prejudices contaminating professional judgement but rather an aspect of nurse socialization itself. They argue that 'bad' patients may be perceived in a negative manner precisely because nurses find it more difficult to nurse them. In other words it is the demands of the nursing interaction itself that leads to the differentiation between 'good' and 'bad' patients. This analysis finds support in the results of Worsley's studies of how student nurses describe favourite and disliked patients. Worsley (1980) found that patient stereotypes were based on two major dimensions, 'cooperativeness' and 'state'. In other words attributions in these two areas formed the basis of these student nurses' patient stereotypes. Favourite patients tended to be characterized as cooperative and friendly while 'emotional distress' was especially important in identifying disliked patients. Worsley relates both dimensions to the notion of 'demandingness', that is, how much effort it takes to nurse patients. If a patient is 'friendly, helpful, understanding, cooperative and thankful' then nursing her is likely to be rewarding whereas if she is 'worried, tense, anxious, frightened and nervous' it may be a difficult and draining process (Worsley, 1980). Thus the ease or difficulty with which nurses can fulfil their nursing aspirations in relation to particular patients appears to provide an important foundation for the perception of those patients. Since we know that initial impressions tend to persist and that people spend much of their time passing on their impressions of others we might be well advised to behave in a friendly, cooperative and thankful manner when we first enter the patient role (see Chapter 4, Section 2)!

If a 'bad' or 'unpopular' patient is essentially one who, for whatever reasons, is less rewarding and more demanding, then it seems unrealistic to suggest that nurses should not recognize this. All workers identify rewarding an unrewarding aspects of their work and this kind of distinction may be important to maintaining work motivation. Of course, we must ensure that nurses' person perception processes do not lead to a deterioration of care for unpopular or negatively stereotyped patients. This will not be achieved through prescriptive recommendations about how nurses should think about their patients.

Developing an awareness of how our judgements of others are based upon our own IPTs, stereotypes and work role aspirations is the best guarantee of professional consistency. Enhancing awareness of the personal nature of our assessments of others can enable us to monitor the effects of our perceptions on our professional behaviour. This in turn allows us to take responsibility both for our judgements and for ensuring that they do not unthinkingly affect our relationships with others. If, for example, we regard Jim as ungrateful and bad tempered further negative inferences, reduced interaction and feelings of neglect and resentment on both sides may result in a self-fulfilling prophecy and a self-perpetuating destructive relationship. If, however, we recognize that it is *our need* for appreciation that makes nursing Jim *difficult for us* then we take responsibility for our feelings and can plan our approach to Jim accordingly. We can break the often automatic connection between perception and action thereby driving a wedge between prejudice and discrimination. Nurses, psychologists and all other 'interpersonal professionals' need to be able to monitor their patient perceptions and relationships in this manner. Critical reflection on our judgements about patients is prerequisite to providing a professional service. Moreover, by maintaining a positive and helpful approach, we may engender a more rewarding response from even the most trying patients. This consideration of self-reflection and professional behaviour emphasizes how social psychology can promote personal development. We shall return to the idea that awareness of our own psychological functioning can help us gain control over our thoughts and behaviour (see Chapter 7, Section 4).

Negotiating assessments – sharing records

A controversial topic touched on by the psychology of person perception is the issue of patient access to medical and nursing records. Some doctors and nurses open their files and notes to patients while others only allow other professionals to see them. Frunkel and Wilson (1985) argue that allowing patients access to their files provides a safeguard against well-intended but inaccurate record-keeping, and against unsubstantiated speculation and prejudice. They cite evidence suggesting that medical records can be mistaken in such simple details as date of birth and such major items as whether or not a patient has undergone brain surgery! The more general issue here is to what extent professionals (including nurses, psychologists and lecturers) should share their assessments with their clients. Our discussion of person perception emphasizes that we must be vigilant in our monitoring of how our categorization of patients affects our own and other professionals' behaviour towards them. The argument that professionals would be more likely to monitor their judgemental processes and take their patient's perspective into account if their assessments were open to examination is therefore a strong one in favour of open access.

Over-confidence and rigidity in our assessments of patients can lead to inappropriate and unprofessional service delivery. Yet our particular professional perspective may lead us to draw the wrong conclusions about our patients motivations and concerns. Johnston (1976, 1982), for example, has shown that nurses' perceptions of patients' worries do not match patients' own reports of their worries. Nurses tend to overestimate how many worries their patients have and to focus on the wrong ones. Indeed Johnston demonstrates that fellow patients tend to be more accurate at assessing patients worries than nursing staff. Thus, in assessing anxiety, pain or psychological well-being greater dialogue with patients is likely to overcome stereotyping and promote greater accuracy. This in turn will allow nurses to offer more effective counselling and treat-ment. Since service delivery depends upon our judgement of others and their problems, and since interaction is inherently constituted by different perspectives, it is crucial to question the accuracy of our judgements through negotiation with others. This necessitates client participation in the the construction and maintenance of records and plans relating to their case.

2 Managing Others' Impressions of us.

Representing others representing us

As well as forming representations of ourselves and others we also try to understand others' representations of us. Indeed this ability to represent others' representations of us is crucial to our management of our own behaviour (see Figure 5). In Chapter 1, Section 3 we noted that the infant's entry into our social world depended upon learning to represent herself. However, in order to become a fully functioning person she must be able to monitor her own behaviour and reflect on what others' think of it (Henry and Tuxill, 1987). In order to feel guilty for example, we must know that others would judge our actions to be wrong. It is not the presence of others which counts. We can feel guilty even when unobserved because we have developed a conscience, that is an internal representation of others' judgemental criteria. As soon as we are able to anticipate others' impressions of us we begin to modify our behaviour in order to influence these impressions. This is known as 'impression management' and it shapes much of our everyday interaction (Tedeschi, 1981). Snyder (1979) distinguishes between 'high' and 'low' self monitors, where high self monitors are people who are especially concerned with their impression management and more likely to change their behaviour as they move from one social situation to another. However, even low self monitors must pay attention to the impression they make. They must, as Goffman (1955) put it, work at maintaining positive social value or 'face'. Harré (1979) has emphasized these 'expressive' aspects of everyday life and argued that the avoidance of others' contempt and the gaining of their respect is a fundamental principle guiding much of human behaviour. It is hardly surprising then that we find gossip so seductive. As well as keeping track of who thinks what about whom we need to gather information about how we can most effectively manage our impressions.

Interaction as mutual impression management

To complicate things further interaction consists of mutual impression management; as we try to control what others think about us they are simultaneously shaping their behaviour in order to make particular

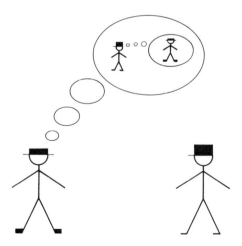

Figure 5   Our behaviour is affected by our representation of others' perception of us.

impressions on us. Furthermore, each side is capable of representing others' impression management tactics. We may, for example, regard another's compliments as ingratiation, aimed only at establishing positive reputation with us and, in order to let them know that we have not been taken in, inform them that flattery will get them nowhere (see Chapter 6, Section 2)! Such everyday interaction depends upon our ability to represent ourselves and others in fairly sophisticated ways. We need to be able to form impressions of others, represent their representations (or impressions) of us and understand the strategies they may be using in attempts to influence our impressions of them. Social psychologists face the difficult task of developing second order models which take this complexity into account. We noted in Chapter 2, Section 2, that simple attitudes-predict-behaviour models had to be modified to take account of what people thought other people expected of them and how much they valued others' approval (that is, we needed to measure subjective norms). It is equally important to bear this complexity in mind in our professional practice and to consider the ways in which we encourage our patients to engage in particular kinds of impression management in order to obtain our attention and services!

The management of reputation has crucial consequences for the individual. If we attract others' disapproval they may withhold both emotional and material support. Thus, people, and indeed institutions, will often willingly suffer inconvenience and cost in order to maintain positive reputation or 'face'. People borrow money they cannot repay in order to buy others presents, go on hunger strike to support groups they belong to, and a hospital with a one million pound shortfall in funds may spend tens of thousands to replace a carpet before a flying royal visit (*The Guardian* 14/9/87). The moment-to-moment, day-to-day maintenance of reputation regularly takes priority over other motivations.

Successful impression management depends upon good social judgement and behavioural control skills. Staring at others, touching them inappropriately or saying the wrong thing can ruin the impression we hoped to make. Similarly we need to be skilled at interpreting the voice intonations, expressions, pauses, sighs, and eye movements of others so that we can assess their impressions of us and modify our behaviour appropriately. The use of such 'social skills' is foundational to health assessments and the promotion of health behaviour (Davies, 1981). Dimatteo, et al., (1979) for example, have demonstrated that patients tend to be more satisfied with doctors who show greater sensitivity through their use of non verbal communication (see Chapter 5, Section 5). The importance of such satisfaction is emphasized by Dimatteo, et al., (1986) and Ley (1982) who have shown that satisfied patients are more likely to keep their appointments and comply with medical advice.

Interviewing - assessing or influencing?

Interviews are widely used as a means of individual assessment in personnel selection and health care planning. In either case the interview is a process of continual and mutual impression formation and management (Schmidt, 1976). Interviewers tend to believe that they can 'see' what sort of person they are interviewing but should be more sceptical because their judgements may be based upon their own IPTs, stereotypes or expectations about interviewees (Carlson, 1971; London and Hakel, 1974; Arvey, 1979). Moreover, the manner in which interviewers phrase their questions, change their tone of voice and use *non-verbal communication* (see Chapter 5, Section 5) can affect the interviewee's behaviour (Greenspoon, 1955; Rosenfeld, 1967; Argyle, 1972). Initial expectations can affect interviewers' questioning style and impression formation which may be communicated to interviewees and influence their behaviour. By smiling, nodding, offering encouraging 'mmm hmm 's' or by telling the interviewee that her responses are interesting or in agreement with the interviewer's own the interviewer can communicate that the interviewee is successfully maintaining a positive reputation. This is likely to bolster the interviewee's self-esteem and may result in more active, enthusiastic and expressive participation (Greenspoon, 1955; Verplanck, 1955). This type of encouragement can, of course, be very useful in gaining insight into the interviewee's perspective but if such techniques are used differentially in job selection interviews then the assessment of candidates may become a self-fulfilling prophecy and unfair discrimination may result (see Arvey, 1979 for a review).

The vulnerability of the interview process to interviewer influence has cast doubt on its reliability and validity as a personnel selection method (see Chapter 1, Section 4). Mayfield (1964) and Ulrich and Trumbo (1965) reviewed a number of studies of the selection interview and found that the person perception processes involved could lead to unacceptably low inter-rater reliabilities. This suggests that the interview is not a valid measure of candidates' ability to do the job. Kelly and Fiske (1951) for example, showed that interviewing for clinical psychology courses did not improve predictions about future success made on the basis of written tests and questionnaires. Mayfield concluded that we should have more confidence in written tests than the judgements of interviewers and more recent research suggests that cognitive tests which do not discriminate against 'minority' group members but are reliable and valid measures of candidates job-relevant abilities can be developed for many jobs (Ghiselli, 1973; Schmidt and Hunter, 1981).

Interviewing is nevertheless important in health assessment. Skilled interviewers who have clear objectives and use explicit judgemental criteria may be able to assess patients' beliefs, expectations, social skills and health status in a more detailed and efficient manner than written assessments would allow. However, as interviewers we must remain aware of the threats that our person perception processes pose to making reliable and valid assessments. Moreover if we wish to use interviews or consultations to promote particular patient behaviours then we must be aware of various ways in which interviewers can influence interviewees. We shall return to the processes involved in communication with patients but it is worth noting that research on medical interviewing suggests that further training in these areas might enhance health care delivery (Raines and Rohrer, 1955, Maguire, 1979; Ley, 1988).

Examining impression management highlights the misleading nature of our bias towards attributing the causes of others' behaviour to stable features within them. We perceive stable personalities but, in reality, social behaviour is primarily directed towards impression management for particular audiences in particular social settings. We therefore underestimate the way in which social situations (for example, being interviewed by a nurse in a clinic) affect people's behaviour and overestimate the degree to which know them and can predict their behaviour in different situations. These person perception and impression management processes have important implications for nurse–patient interaction. Riehl's (1980) *'interaction model of nursing'*, for example is based upon a symbolic interactionist view of everyday behaviour and recommends a nursing role which is sensitive to the subtle interpersonal influences we exert upon one another (see too Wood, 1980; Aggleton and Chalmers, 1986). This social psychological perspective on nursing recommends a need for self-awareness in nurse–patient interaction. In assessment, for example, nurses need to make deliberate efforts to seek out patients perspective and develop a skilled, self-questioning approach to making judgements. They must also remain aware of how their perceptions may be influenced by patients' attempts to manage impressions within what they take to be their appropriate role. Nurses therefore need to monitor the expectations they are communicating to their patients and try to negotiate the adoption of a health-promoting patient role (see Chapter 4, Section 2).

3 Group Membership, Self Categorization and Social Identity

Social and personal identities

If you try answering the question 'Who am I?' by writing down a series of statements which begin 'I am ...' you will probably find that it is fairly easy to distinguish between two types of answers, those that categorize you as belonging to a *social group* and those which describe some *per-*

sonal characteristic. Consider the following, 'a woman, a nursing student, Scottish, a hockey player, a person with a good sense of humour and generous'. We can see that sex, occupation, nationality and playing a particular sport all categorize this person as belonging to various groups while having a sense of humour and being generous refer to personal characteristics. We can speak of women, nursing students, Scots and hockey players but, although many people may be generous and have a good sense of humour, these characteristics do not identify particular social group. Turner (1982), building upon Tajfel's (1978) *'social identity theory'* proposes that our self-concept is made up of both social and personal representations of ourselves and that these can operate quite independently. The ideas of Tajfel and Turner give us some insight both into what we mean by a 'group' and the way in which our self-representations guide our everyday behaviour. We shall see in Chapter 8, Section 1 that groups usually consist of two or more people who interact regularly, and share values, aspirations and social norms. However, Turner points out that the most fundamental aspect of a group is that two or more people categorize themselves as members, in other words, self-categorizing members make a group. Belonging to a group then does not depend primarily upon meeting people regularly or living close to them. We may meet the same people on a bus or train journey but we are unlikely to identify ourselves as 'a bus 34 commuter'. On the other hand we might belong to a political party, an international religious group or a union and identify as a member even if we had not attended a group meeting or met other members.

Switching social identities across situations

These self categorizations, or social identifications, constitute a major part of our self representations. Thus who we are is to a large extent determined by the set of groups to which we feel we belong. Of course we belong to many such groups and different identifications become important or 'salient' to us in different situations (Turner,1982; Reicher,1984). In a conversation about the levels of pay within nursing a nurse may be very aware of her registered nurse status but at an international sporting event her nationality may become the most salient aspect of her identity. Brown and Turner (1981) suggest that certain aspects of the social situations we find ourselves in may 'switch on', or make 'salient' particular social identities. Being the only member of our group present or being in a large crowd of group members both make it more likely that we will identify ourselves as members of that group. When a social identity becomes salient for us we wish others to see us in terms of that particular social category. In other words salient social identities determine the of kind impression management strategies we employ. At different times, then, we may be trying to manage our impressions in order to live up to being a good student, a good nurse, a 'real' man or woman or a patriotic citizen. As we move from one situation to the next we act in accordance with different self categorizations because these different situations switch on different social identities (see Figure 6). This helps explain why our behaviour may be inconsistent across situations and again emphasizes the unreliability of inferences about others' behaviour in unfamiliar situations.

Of course, in some situations it is not our social identity but our personal identity which is most prominent in our self representation. In an intimate conversation with a family member or a lover we may behave in accordance with our view of ourselves as having particular personality traits or on the basis of a particular personal history with that person. Tajfel (1978) therefore, proposes that social interaction takes place along an *interpersonal-intergroup dimension,* where the interpersonal end is characterized by interaction directed primarily by people's personal representations and the intergroup end refers to interaction directed by peoples' social identities. It is important to understand here that *intergroup interaction* refers to the manner which people think about themselves and can occur even when two people interact. Thus when two rival football fans behave aggressively towards one another we do not wonder if this is a personality clash or if one did not like the other's sense of humour. Their behaviour is intergroup in the sense that they are acting as members of competing groups. It is in this sense that Turner (1982) claims that when a particular social identity is salient for us it serves to 'depersonalize' the way in which we regulate our behaviour; we act as a group member rather than a personal being.

Shifting self-categorizations means that the basis for our interaction with other people changes as different aspects of our (and others') personal

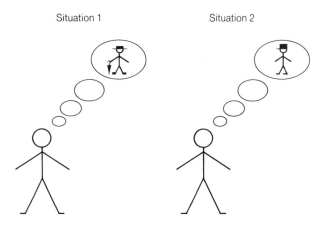

Figure 6   Different social identities become salient in different situations.

and social identity become salient. Thus a family group may relate well with one another at a reunion so long as they engage in conversations about old times and what personality traits best describe various family members. In this way they can become intimate by sharing aspects of their personal identities. However, the social situation can alter when new topics of conversation arise. If, for example, the conversation turns to politics and they discover that they support opposing parties then their political social identities will become salient and the conversation may become competitive or even acrimonious. Even close friends can become opponents or enemies if competing social identities are adopted. At the same time, we may feel an affinity with those we hardly know when we discover a shared social identity. The implications of this for relationship development are considered further in Chapter 6, Section 2.

Many nursing models (for example, Johnson, 1980; Riehl, 1980) promote the idea that nurses should aim to build up a rapport with their patients so that the are able to relate to them on a personal and individual basis. In identity terms then nurses try to interact with their patients on an inter*personal* basis. However, nurses also need to know how a patients identity and self-esteem are based in her various social identities (or group memberships). A mastectomy may threaten a woman's sense of being 'a women' and a keen marathon runner may find feel she has lost an important part of her identity after a knee injury that prevents further running. Nurses own identifications may affect their interactions with patients and nurse–patient interaction may slide towards the intergroup end of Tajfel's dimension. This will undermine rapport and result in fairly stereotyped behaviour. It is therefore important to be aware that others' behaviour towards us may change as a result of changes in identity saliences and that our own behaviour may be directed by social identity needs.

4 Social Identity, Self Esteem and Intergroup Conflict

Maintaining self-esteem through valued social identities

To maintain any particular social identity we must strive to behave appropriately, and if possible excel, as a member of that group. If, for example, we do not live up to expectations as a nurse then our job and perhaps our qualifications may eventually be jeopardized (see Chapter 4, Section 1). We therefore manage our impressions so that others will continue to categorize us as a member of the groups we wish to belong to. We saw (in Chapter 2, Section 4) how important self-esteem is to our everyday functioning and Tajfel (1978) and Turner (1982) suggest that positive self- esteem gained through self-categorization motivates us to work to maintain group memberships. This means that sometimes the audience with whom we wish to maintain a reputation may be fellow group members who are not present, that is we act to preserve reputation with valued but absent members of our group. A student nurse for example, might carry out a procedure in a different manner to that practiced by her colleagues because she is identifying with her college tutors or classmates. By doing so she maintains her self esteem by living up to the standards she regards as important to these other group members. This kind of identification can, however, become difficult if the person has little contact with the group she identifies with. Self esteem may diminish if no recognition is forthcoming from those with whom she regularly interacts.

Deriving positive self esteem from our social identities depends upon our belief that the groups we categorize ourselves as belonging to are themselves valuable. If the group does not confer a valuable identity then we will try to leave (Tajfel, 1978). If for example a hospital becomes known for being badly resourced and providing poor care it will have difficulty keeping and attracting staff who will prefer to find a work identity which offers them greater self esteem. However, it is often difficult or impossible for us to swap our group memberships for more prestigious ones. We therefore try to enhance our self esteem by promoting the value of the groups we belong to. We try to persuade others that our group is worthwhile and deserves respect. Indeed many conflicts including industrial strikes may be primarily concerned with the establishment of a group's dignity and respect (Harré, 1979; Lopez, 1990). Tajfel (1978) and Tajfel and Turner (1979) point out that this commitment to the valuing of our own group has important implications for everyday interaction. It means, for example, that we tend to favour members of our own group over members of other groups. Experiments by Tajfel et al., (1971) and Billig and Tajfel (1973) suggest that we favour members of our own group even when we have been placed in the group for very trivial reasons and when there is no reason to assume that other members of the group are similar to ourselves! Moreover, these studies show that we tend to distribute rewards in a way that maximizes the relative difference between our own group and others even if this means our own group gets less in absolute terms. Brown (1978), for example, demonstrated that shop stewards, making simulated decisions about wage negotiations would choose lower overall levels of pay for members of their union in order that they could continue to earn more than other workers who they thought were less deserving. Thus we not only promote our own group but seek to *positively differentiate* our group from others. In other words we look for positive features of our group which make it different from other groups and try to maintain these differences (Tajfel, 1978; Tajfel and Turner, 1979). We are particularly prone to do this with other groups which are similar to our own. Nurses, for example, will tend to compare themselves with other nurses and health care workers. Maintaining our self- esteem therefore involves a perpetual round of social comparisons; we feel good about ourselves by construing our team, our religion or our work group as better than others' teams, religions or work groups. Prejudice and discrimination can result from this need to maintain a positive view of ourselves through the various groups to which we belong. This again alerts us to the importance of monitoring our judgements of others while offering professional service; it is not in patients' interests if professionals engage in competitive and even hostile relationships in order to promote their own esteem (see Chapter 5, Section 1).

Social identity and intergroup competition in nursing

van Knippenberg and van Oers (1984) illustrated the way in which these self-categorization processes affect nurses judgements of themselves in relation to other groups of nurses. Comparing student nurses studying for degree-level qualifications with registered nurses in the Netherlands they found that the groups' perceptions of one another's skills could be summarized along three dimensions; practical skills, skills in interpersonal relationships and theoretical insight. Their results showed that the degree students rated themselves as having better theoretical insight and practical skills but poorer interpersonal skills whereas the registered nurses rated themselves as better at interpersonal relationships and practical skills but having poorer theoretical insight. When the groups were asked to evaluate these different skills the degree students rated theoretical insight as most important while the registered nurses saw interpersonal relations as being most important. In this way each group identified an area in which they regarded themselves as superior and defined this as central to nursing. However, each group also thought the other had some career advantages. Degree students thought registered nurses had more prestige and better incomes whereas the registered nurses viewed graduate nurses as having better promotion prospects, better incomes and better access to specialized training. van Knippenberg and van Oers explain this by suggesting that we tend to portray our own group as more worthwhile and more deserving. Thus although both groups saw themselves as more skilled in central areas of nursing they saw the other group as better off in some respects. This perspective leaves both groups ready to argue that their skills should receive more recognition and greater rewards!

A somewhat similar set of intergroup relationships with in nursing was revealed by Skevington's (1981, 1984) study of registered and enrolled nurses in the United Kingdom. She found that both groups saw registered nurses as more intelligent, better educated, better organized and more responsible. Both groups saw enrolled nurses as more cheerful, thoughtful and practical. However, although the two groups could therefore seek positive differentiation on the basis of these different characteristics, Skevington found that both groups regarded registered nurses enjoying greater privileges and suffering fewer disadvantages. Even the enrolled nurses accepted the higher value of the registered status. Moreover, when asked how similar they felt themselves to be to their own group the registered nurses identified more strongly with their group than the enrolled nurses. This ambivalence about their occupational identity was further underlined by the fact that 28% of the enrolled nurses intended to re-train as registered nurses, that is, leave their group for a higher status one. This example illustrates the general point that despite our attempts to value our own social identities we must at times accept that other groups have established greater status, income, or influence than our own. Of course such realizations are damaging to our self-esteem and are not usually suffered contentedly. They may lead to resentment, competition and hostility between groups and Skevington reports that enrolled nurses do express resentment about the limitations of their work roles in comparison with those of their registered colleagues.

The evolution of group conflict

As cultures evolve the positions of groups in relation to one another change. Taylor and McKirnan (1984) have developed a five-stage model to help us understand such changes. Their model considers a situation in which one group has great power over another and where there seems to be no possibility of members of the lower status group moving into the higher status group. They suggest that this situation may change when an individualistic or meritocratic ideology emerges, that is, where people's position in life is thought to be the result of their own efforts rather than a consequence of the group (such as a race or caste) which they are born into. This development may gradually lead to a third *social mobility* stage in which some members of the low status group pass into or gain positions within the higher status group. Relating this to Skevington's study we can see that the possibility of enrolled nurses retraining as registered nurses means these groups have reached this stage. However, if only a few select members of the lower status group are allowed to join the higher status group then a forth *consciousness raising* stage emerge. In this stage members of the lower status group begin to realize that they are unfairly disadvantaged as a whole and that the solution to their problem lies in collective action which will benefit the whole group, and not just the few who successfully joined the higher status group. When this happens the search for respect and positive social differentiation becomes a shared group struggle which may involve attempts to create new, more positive, social identities for the lower status group. This will involve revaluing the group's characteristics and encouraging members to stand up for equal rights and recognition. Declarations, such as, 'sisterhood is strength', 'black is beautiful' and 'its good to be gay' represent consciousness raising activities among women and black and gay people. These activities lead to the final stage in which members of the lower status group, who have come to see themselves as oppressed, engage in competition with their oppressors. They try to ensure that their identities and opportunities are not illegitimately damaged by the oppressing group through campaigns to change beliefs, attitudes and laws. Enrolled nurses may be regarded as having reached this stage to the extent that they have campaigned for the Briggs (1972) report recommendation that training should lead to an amalgamation of enrolled and registered nurses. Such a move is unlikely to be popular with registered nurses who will lose positive differentiation in relation to their enrolled colleagues and may feel that their social identity will be devalued by such a merger.

Health through valued social identities

We have noted that illness and injury may threaten valued social identities. Reestablishing self esteem through reclamation of discarded social identities or discovery of new ones is therefore integral to patients' recovery. Riehl's model of nursing suggests that assisting the patient in this enterprise may be a central nursing intervention. Wills (1981) notes that 'downwards comparisons' may be a useful way of bolstering self-esteem in the face of threat and Taylor (1983) observes that patients may maintain self-esteem by seeking positive differentiation between themselves and other patients who they regard as worse off, or coping less well. Adapting to the consequences of illness may therefore depend upon being able to regard ourselves as 'well off' in comparison to others. Perpetually comparing ourselves with others who we regard as more fortunate is likely to result in lowered self esteem and impaired coping. Taylor also points out that overly optimistic, internal attributions of control and expectations regarding present and expected improvements may play an important part in successful adaptation to illness. It seems that optimism, rather than realism, about ourselves and others' perceptions of us is the key to optimum psychological functioning.

The provision of community care for certain clients has created much debate. People with mental handicaps are one group upon which this controversy has focused. Central to the campaign for community care for people with mental handicaps was the principle of *normalization* which proposed that people with mental handicaps had a right to normal lives in the community and that carers could provide them with the support necessary to attain these normal lives (see, for example, Wolfensberger, 1972, 1983; Jay Report, 1979). This idea has been criticized by Szivos and Travers (1988). Using Taylor and Mckirnan's model they view normalization as a 'social mobility' solution which allows certain people classed as mentally handicapped to 'pass' from their lower status group into the higher status 'normal' group. They argue that people with mental handicaps would benefit more from a stage four, 'consciousness raising' approach. They propose that by becoming more aware of their lack of abilities and their rights, as people with mental handicaps, they could develop a redefined and re-evaluated group identity which would create a more positive self-esteem for individuals and the group as a whole. Corbett (1989) also criticizes the struggle independence which is often integral to normalization programmes, arguing that it can be so difficult that it diminishes peoples' day-to-day quality of life and fails to provide them with the valued personal and social identities upon which positive self esteem depends. Others have criticized the idea of community care because of the assumption that, by living in a particular area, people with mental handicaps will become part of a community, gaining shared social identities through their interaction with others. Abraham (1989) argues that geographical proximity does not imply shared social identities and points out that the search for positive differentiation may make deinstitutionalized people a convenient out-group from which local people can differentiate themselves. In other words people already living in a geographical area may deliberately resist the attempts of people with mental handicaps to integrate into their ('normal') social identity. This can result in isolation, discrimination and victimization which will further damage the person's self-esteem.

Thus we are left with the question of how we can most effectively support people in lower status groups, such as those with mental handicaps, to develop valued social identities. Szivos and Travers suggestion is that any valued social identity must recognize real impairments but re-evaluate the people who have those impairments. This will involve highlighting differences without devaluing people. In the case of people with mental handicaps this may involve reframing the group's psychological characteristics (such special needs for social support and more open expression of feeling) in a positive manner. Highlighting the value of acknowledging feelings and focusing on present relationships may provide a useful starting point. This is a more radical approach than the social mobility solution offered by normalization and creates a greater challenge to non-handicapped people who are asked to accept a new status for people with mental handicaps as *valued people with mental handicaps*.

People with mental handicaps are only one client group whose problems are exacerbated by a low status social identity. There have been similar calls for a consciousness raising approach to combating discrimination against physically impaired people (Brechin, et al., 1981). Indeed Robinson (1980) argues that the creation of new, valued social identities is a central function of self-help groups in general (see Chapter 8, Section 5) Certainly understanding the social identity needs of others is important when planning implementing and evaluating approaches to care.

CORE IDEAS IN CHAPTER 3

- Our perceptions of others are crucially shaped by our own assumptions about people and by the situations in which we encounter them.

- Stereotyping, implicit personality theories and halo effects all lead us to go beyond what we are told about people to infer further characteristics.

- The way people relate to others depends upon their expectations of them. Therefore our behaviour can turn our perceptions of others into self fulfilling prophecies.

- Nurses tend to view demanding patients as 'bad' patients. In order to ensure that such perceptions do not lower the standard of care offered to these patients nurses should be able to reflect on and take responsibility for such stereotyping.

- We tend to overestimate what we know about people and under-estimate the effects of different situations on their behaviour. Sharing our assessments with patients may help us maintain a more sceptical and detached view of our own judgements.

- We perpetually manage the impression we give others and are simultaneously aware that others' are trying to shape our impressions of them.

- This means that interviews are strongly affected by interviewers' behaviour.

- Our identity is made up of social and personal self-categorizations. Social identities become salient in particular social situations and direct our impression management activities in those situations.

- We try to maintain the value of our social identities in order to enhance our self-esteem. This involves us in positive differentiation of our own group from others,

- Over time the relationship between groups may change. In particular consciousness raising strategies may help to redefine the relationships between groups and bring about social change.

4

Fitting into the social world

1 Rules, Roles and Scripts

Understanding social rules

In the previous chapter we examined our representations of ourselves and others and the way in which these shape our interaction through social identifications and mutual impression management. In this chapter we shall look more closely at how such processes affect our social behaviour.

Most social situations are fairly predictable. We tend to be regularly involved in certain types of event (for example, a lecture, a ward round or a meal out). This familiarity means that we know roughly what to do. We can play our part and fit in with others. However in new situations such as the first day on a ward we may not know how to behave. We may feel anxious and search for clues from others as what is expected of us. Over time we discover the patterns of interaction become more confident about our own contribution. In this way shared representations (or intersubjective knowledge) of what to do and how to fit in enables people to interact smoothly and to fulfill each others' expectations in everyday social life. This allows people with different training, backgrounds and experiences to turn up for work and cooperate with a minimum of negotiation or quarrelling about who should do what. The way such shared knowledge about social situations allows us to take aspects of our lives for granted also means that social change is inherently threatening. It threatens to obliterate our understanding of what is appropriate behaviour and indeed who we are in social settings.

Games also have shared rules which guide players actions and we can think of our knowledge of social situations as consisting in part of social rules. Some of these rules may be explicit and officially recorded, for example, rules forbidding smoking or stipulating the wearing of special clothing at work. However, most are implicit and are only referred to when there is a dispute or someone is suspected of having broken them. We know we should thank people for their gifts so we regard anyone who does not as 'ungrateful' or 'rude'. This perception of rudeness is based in our knowledge of what is appropriate behaviour. The offender is seen to have broken an unwritten social rule so we think badly of them. This example highlights the connection between shared social rules and the maintenance of social reputation. When we break social rules people tend to make unflattering inferences about us and our reputation is endangered.

Goffman is perhaps the most revealing investigator of the unspoken everyday rules which govern our everyday interactions. In *Relations in Public*, for example, he discusses rules personal space and gaze. Personal space concerns the distance at which we feel comfortable relating to others and the amount and type of touching we regard as appropriate. If, for example, we step too close to someone while talking they are likely to step back and if we lean back during a seated conversation our conversational partner may lean forward to maintain the appropriate distance. In this way we unthinkingly maintain a comfortable distance for the kind of interaction at hand. Of course, this is not always possible. When travelling in trains, buses or lifts, for example, we may be forced into closer contact with others than we would normally choose. Goffman points out that in these circumstances controlling where we look is crucial. In order to manage the forced 'violation' of personal space we must avoid eye contact. If we look into the eyes of the person we are crushed against on a train we emphasize our inappropriate intimacy and are likely to cause offence! In a similar manner we must strive to maintain the rules of conversational privacy even when we are in fact overhearing others' conversation. In a cafe, for example, we may overhear people nearby but we must not look from one to the other smiling and nodding as if we were enjoying their conversation! Of course rules regarding personal space, touching and gaze differ across cultures and types of relationship. Jourard (1966), for example, reports that people observed in cafes in Paris touched 110 times an hour whereas those observed in London did not touch at all! It is clearly important to to know what social rules apply when arriving in a new city.

Breaking and changing social rules

The complexity and subtly of these social rules mean that even when we are very careful we inevitably break some of them. We bump into people, stare at them without thinking, interrupt them when they are talking, keep them waiting and forget their birthdays. In this case we want to minimize the damage to our reputation, we want to convince others that we do not usually break rules, that we can be trusted and that we are worthy of respect as polite, considerate and competent member of our culture. Goffman points out that there are remedial procedures for doing just that. We can *offer an account* of our rule breaking, *apologize* for it or ask that that it be looked at differently or *reconstrued*. When offering accounts we show that we are not to blame by making excuses which show we could not help it ('I tripped over your bag') or claiming our action was justified by special circumstances ('I had to let the policemen through') (see Scott and Lyman, 1968). Apologies, on the other hand, accept at least part of the blame and distance us from our old blameworthy selves ('I'm sorry that was stupid, I don't know what's wrong with me today'). An apology then is an implicit promise that we are now a new person who can be trusted not to go around breaking rules. Finally, we can try to persuade others to regard our behaviour as something other than rule breaking ('I was only a joking', 'I just wanted to get your attention'). Of course, some rule breaking is so serious that social sanctions will follow and reputation will be tarnished even after attempted remedial action. A neighbour may convince you that they are sorry they chopped your tree down while you are on holiday but you may nevertheless remain outraged. However, even in these cases some vestiges of reputation may be retained by properly executed remedial action. An admission of guilt and an apology may not be enough to earn a pardon but at least we will appreciate that the person had the good grace to be sorry!

Such remedial action reveals that social rules are somewhat different to those of games. Players may claim not to have broken the rules but it is usually very difficult to persuade others that although you have cheated everything is alright and the game can continue without further problems! Social rules and social violations are more flexible. They are open to discussion and debate in a way that the rules of chess, for example, are not. Social rules can be changed and violations can be reinterpreted as something else. Hospital administrators might decide that nurses should wear mufti rather than uniform, a family might decide not to celebrate birthdays and people in a therapeutic group might decide to sit touching each other while talking. Similarly if we respond to someone who has just bumped into us with 'Can we do that again' we suggest that instead of unintended rule breaking we were involved in deliberately becoming more intimate. If the other person agrees to this suggestion then something quite different from 'bumping into someone' is happening! However, other people limit our power to rewrite the rules. The person who bumped into us might reply 'Sorry I tripped' and walk on thereby redefining the event as a 'bumping into'. Moreover, our role may limit the control we have over local social rules, note that it was *hospital administrators*, not nurses on the ward, who we suggested might decide to abandon nurse uniform.

The rules we have discussed above are general social rules but we know that social rules are specific to particular types of relationships. If a stranger touches our cheek we will expect some fairly convincing remedial action but he same gesture by a lover may be welcomed and need no explanation. Argyle and colleagues have begun to explore how certain types of rules apply differently across different types of relationships. Argyle, et al., (1985) studied people's views of the importance of 33 rules in 22 different types of relationship. These relationships included intimate ones such husband, wife or parent as well as professional ones such as doctor and patient. The rules which applied to most of these relationships concerned privacy, keeping confidences, sexual relations, making eye contact and how one should behave in public towards the other person. Unsurprisingly they found that respecting the other's privacy and keeping confidences were thought to be important in intimate and nonintimate relationships. However showing affection in public, intentionally touching and asking for material help were approved of in intimate relationships but not nonintimate ones. Some behaviours are expected in certain relationships but prohibited in others. Sexual behaviour, for example, is strongly prohibited between relatives and constitutes an incest taboo. Argyle and colleagues conclude that there are three broad categories of

- relationship rules;
- coordination of behaviour;
- regulation of intimacy;
- avoidance of relationship-specific sources of conflict.

These rules help maintain relationships by providing a stable framework within which people can predict one another's conduct and cooperate to achieve joint goals relevant to their particular relationship.

Understanding social roles

Our understanding that different rules apply to different social relationships is encompassed by the idea of a 'social role'. The dramaturgical analogy highlights the way in which our behaviour changes as we move between relationships in a similar manner to an actress who switches from one stage role to another (see Chapter 1, Section 2). As soon as we become aware of the social world we learn that different behaviour is expected within different relationships. Indeed, Shatz and Gelmen (1973) suggest that the beginnings of such understanding can be observed in four year olds.

In Chapter 3 (Section 3) we discussed the concept 'social identity'. The terms social identity and social role are derived from different theoretical traditions within social psychology and to some extent overlap. We shall regard a social role as forming part of and belonging to a particular social identity. For example, maintaining the social identity of 'nurse' requires that the individual be accepted as to able relate to others within the nurse role. However, there are many particular roles within nursing, involving different types of relationship. 'Social role' then refers to the kind of interaction which is identified as sustaining a particular social identity or selfcategorization. It encompasses the rules and expectations which define a set of relationships and so goes beyond the idea of categorization of self in relation to others. Indeed during the secondary socialization process (see Chapter 1, Section 3) by which we acquire roleappropriate behaviours we usually take on the social identity (for example, 'student *nurse*') before we are officially admitted into the social role (that is, become qualified).

Social roles then consist of shared rules or expectations which shape our behaviour towards particular others. We learn how to fit into these roles by attending to others' expectations (Goffman, 1961). Most roles are defined by a particular role partnership, that is two roles which complement one another. For example nurse–patient or lecturer–student. It is difficult to continue in the nurse role if there are no patients requiring nursing care or to be a lecturer without students. The expectations governing such complementary roles must be coordinated. The nurse is expected to provide good nursing care for the patient and the patient is expected to cooperate with the nurse in the delivery of that care. Secord and Backman (1974) offer a useful analysis of social roles and use the terms *rights and obligations* to refer to this coordination of expectations. The patient has the right to expect good nursing care and it is the nurse's obligation to provide it. On the other hand the nurse therefore has the right to ask the patient to cooperate with this care and the patient is obliged to do so. One partner's role-related rights are the other partner's role-related obligations.

These role-related rights often include the right to break certain general social rules. In delivering nursing care, for example, nurses must touch and look at their patients in a manner which would be quite unacceptable outside this relationship. Emerson (1970) shows how, when conducting gynaecological examinations, nurses and doctors employ particular forms of interaction such as maintaining a nonchalant demeanour and ignoring inappropriate responses such as embarrassment. This professional approach sustains the patient's view of the examination as a routine, matter-of-fact procedure having no sexual or emotional connotations. This invites the patient to fulfill a complementary and cooperative role and prevents the interaction being sees as a violation of privacy. Our knowledge of particular role relations defines what situational rules apply. One function of uniform, for example, is to announce the particular role relationships between individuals. We will allow those dressed as nurses and doctors to question and examine us because we assume they have particular care-orientated intentions derived from their role-related obligations. Of course this willingness to assume intentions on the basis of uniform can be exploited by impostors as when newspaper reporters pose as medical staff in order to obtain information they would be denied as reporters.

Role strain, role change and role conflict

To maintain ourselves as competent and accepted members of our culture we must understand general social rules and the detailed structure of the various social roles we hold. Our reputation as a 'nurse', for example, depends upon convincing others that we are able to carry out our role-related obligations in a competent and pleasing manner. However, it is not just our immediate role partners we must convince. There are many different role-occupants who will have expectations about how a nurse should behave. These include senior nurses (for example a ward sister or charge nurse), doctors, auxiliaries, clinical psychologists and for student nurses their nurse tutors. Merton (1957) referred to people whose expectations define a role as the *role set*. The expectations role set members communicate have a crucial impact on our role performance. Stockwell (1972) for example, found that some nurses avoided talking to patients for fear that their colleagues would think they were slacking! Unfortunately role set members do not always agree about how we should perform our role and this can lead to confusion and stress for the person trying to retain reputation amongst all role-set members. For example, a patient, a ward sister and doctor may all have somewhat different views about how a nurse should relate to the patient and how she should relate to the doctor! We shall refer to these contradictions within a particular role as *role strain*.

We can attempt to resolve role strain by acting on the old adage that you cannot please all of the people all of the time. The role occupant, the nurse in this case, can evaluate which of the role-set members is the most legitimate judge of her role performance in any one area. She can also estimate which role set member has most power to punish or sanction her, she might, for example, consider the extent to which loss of reputation (with any particular roleset member) would affect her future career. Taking legitimacy and power into account she can then decide who it is most important to please. Of course this will not always, or even usually, be her primary role partner. The patient's perspective may not be regarded as the most legitimate definition of the nurse role and may not be supported by powerful sanctions. Moreover, for some aspects of the nurse role it may be unclear whether medical or senior nursing staff have the most legitimate claim to define what is appropriate nursing conduct (Mauksch, 1966).

Consideration of the potential differences between role set members' expectations reveals the way in which role definitions, like social rules, must be negotiated on a day-to-day basis within particular relationships. This means that roles can evolve and change through a process of negotiation. A duty that used to be considered part of our role may be claimed by another role-occupant and we may take on new duties. Within nursing various nursing models identify different sets of core goals and duties and the way these models are adapted for practice results in quite different role expectations in different wards and institutions. This means that we are not only engaged in trying to perform our roles competently, we are also a part of the process by which they are developed. Returning to the dramaturgical model for a moment, we are not just actors but playwrights and directors as well.

The complexity of such role performances reveals the potential for misunderstanding, conflict and confusion at work. This in turn helps us understand why we and others can feel stressed and oppressed by work demands (see Chapter 9, Sections 3 and 4). When individuals make internal attributions for failing to comply with perceived expectations lowered self efficacy and reduced coping may follow. In the extreme people may abandon chosen careers to escape such stress. We can alleviate role strain by reducing the seriousness of our role performances through what Goffman (1961) calls *role distancing*. This is the process by which we indicate to others that there is more to our lives than this particular role or that we are not really trying to perform to the best of our ability. This is especially useful when we are learning a new role and do not wish others to judge by the same standards as those who are more experienced. It can also serve to reduce anxiety about role performance for oneself and others. We can also introduce a lighter note into our lives by stepping out of our real social roles and playing according to another set of rules. This is the fun of game playing. Goffman points out that by adopting a new set of rules which exclude much of what is important in our everyday reality we can engage in new activities (some of which which might require remedial action if undertaken in our everyday roles!). If we take the rules of the game seriously we can enjoy ourselves by escaping for our usual obligations into a temporary social reality created by the rules of the game. Of course the fun can be spoilt by a player who reminds us that the game is only an escape ('This is silly, I've got to get back to work...') because by doing so she invokes everyday rules and roles which flood in to destroy the game's temporary reality.

As we move from one situation to another we may occupy the roles of nurse, club secretary, team member, mother, daughter, and political campaigner. In each case we have to take account of the expectations of role set members who we regard as having the right to define part of our role and who have differing sanctions in relation to our position within that role. In each case we are concerned to maintain our reputation as competent and to defend whatever acceptance and recognition we have gained. The demands of these roles compete for our time and energy, leading to *role conflict*. A typical source of such role conflict is between obligations to family members and to those at work. When we find it difficult to simultaneously correspond to the expectations of important role set-members across two or more roles we may become anxious about potential loss of reputation. This can lead to stress, loss of self-esteem and reduced coping.

Roles and rules – knowing the script

Overall then we strive to fit in and play our part within a framework of agreement about what is appropriate behaviour within particular situations in relation to particular others. The shared understanding of social rules and roles which we gain through interaction with others constitutes our particular culture and as we gain such understanding we become socialized as culture members. Much of this understanding can be taken for granted and Schank and Abelson (1977) have used the term *scripts* to refer to well known pieces of interaction which involve rules and role relations. If, for example you read the sentence 'Jim asked the waiter for the sweet menu' you are easily able to infer that Jim is in a restaurant, that he has probably finished his main course and that the waiter will ask him if he wants coffee to follow his sweet. You know this 'restaurant script' and many others. Thus we do not have to think too much about breakfast, our route to work in the morning or why a man in peaked cap is pushing envelopes thought slots in doors. We can rely on our scripted knowledge to guide us (on autopilot) thought whole sequences of perception and behaviour (Langer, et al., 1978). This is just as well when we consider how much potential stress role strain and role conflict may generate!

2 Negotiating Nurse and Patient Roles

Nurse socialization – learning the role

In order to be accepted as a nurse one has to undertake an official (secondary) socialization process, that is, nurse training. Davies (1975) divides student nurses' socialization into stages. In the first stage of 'initial innocence' the student nurse must rely a on lay knowledge of nursing which Davies found to be dominated by Christian or humanitarian values concerning altruism. In other words, the student wants to learn skills which would allow her to do things for others who are less able. However, students may find that instead of being taught discrete helping skills their tutors emphasize general nursing principles such as the nature of the nurse–patient relationship and the overall scope of nursing. This may produce frustration with the training and a feeling that they are not being taught 'proper' nursing. Such feelings mark Davies' second stage in which student nurses recognize discrepancies between their initial expectations and those of their tutors. Students them embark on a process of observation aimed at defining exactly what it is their tutors want them to do. Davies calls this third stage the 'psyching out' stage. Discovering what type of behaviour is valued and rewarded by tutors leads to a period in which students simulate this behaviour but feel that they are only pretending or doing it to please tutors. We might expect to see a lot of role distancing during this stage which Davies refers to as 'role simulation'. As this proceeds the student nurse is learning the role-related rights, obligations and values of nursing as well as specific sets of relevant situational rules. This will include the development of what Travelbee (1966) called a 'nursing conscience'. The student will regularly categorize herself as a nurse and have to respond to demands resulting from role-set members' expectations. She will also begin to develop standards of good and bad practice and judge her fellow nurses in these terms. This is the process of 'internalization' through which the necessary cognitive representations of the nurse's role are developed (see Chapter 1, Section 3). Once these are in place the student is able to function within the nurse role and the socialization process is complete. Only official recognition (through passing examinations) is then required to become a nurse.

Student nurses have to integrate their initial expectations with those of role-set members into an understanding of the nurse role. This may be difficult, especially if role-set members disagree. Ogier (1984) discusses a body of research which suggests that nurse students experience role strain and confusion. Quoting the Briggs Report (Briggs, 1972) she points out that discrepancies between college and ward based definitions of nursing practice may mean that students must learn two versions of techniques and remember who expects which version. She also points to evidence that students are unhappy with supervision and teaching on the wards, that they are uncertain as to whose expectations they should comply with and that they are unsure whether they are primarily learners or workers. Both Orton (1981; 1984) and Ogier (1984) point to the importance of the ward sister as a key role set member. The manner in which she teaches learners, her awareness of learner's needs and her commitment to ward teaching all have an important effect on learners' experience. Orton also emphasizes the importance of an accepting ward climate. This corresponds to Parkes (1982) finding that social support leads to lower stress levels (see Chapter 6, section 3). Parkes shows that the type of placement affects student stress. She found, for example, that medical wards generated greater stress than surgical wards. Medical wards were perceived as making greater emotional demands and students felt they had less control over their work (that is lower self-efficacy) than in surgical wards where they felt they had greater opportunity to learn and apply technical skills.

The role ambiguities encountered by student nurses in the United Kingdom may be alleviated by the implementation of 'project 2000' proposals. These will make student nurses supernumerary and thereby clarify their 'learner' role. However, role strain is unlikely to be eliminated because of the very nature of education. As Ruano (1971) points out colleges of nursing aim to train nurses who will become innovators within nursing and help change and develop nurse roles. Such change inevitably conflicts with well-established practice and students and newly qualified staff find themselves unable to live up to the expectations of both their tutors and their more experienced colleagues. Colleagues are powerful role set members and often conformity with accepted practice is the easiest resolution of such role strain. As Ruano points out educating individuals cannot in itself bring about institutional change.

The medical model – patients as bodies

Nurse role ambiguities are, of course, not confined to student nurses. Anderson's (1973) study of nurses' patients' and doctors' views revealed ample scope for different interpretation. Reviewing the application of role theory to nursing she notes the potential conflicts between perceptions of nurses as 'mother surrogates' and 'healers', between the role of carer and technical expert and between between nurses' patient-orientated and managerial concerns. The importance of these various elements may be differentially valued by patients, doctors, colleagues, and those responsible for promotion. Anderson also reported that while nurses' and patients' valued nurses' provision of psychological care (such as emotional support) this was less important to doctors. This is a classic source of nurse role strain. As Anderson's puts it 'where the patient's demand for support conflicts with the doctor's demand for efficiency the nurse is faced with a dilemma'.

The influence of medical staff and a medical model of health care on both nurse and patient roles has been widely considered. The medical model is characterized by its emphasis on the efficient delivery of treatments to diseased body systems. This approach has been challenged as a basis on which to offer help to those with mental illnesses or mental handicaps. Indeed the the very concept of mental illness has been questioned. Szasz (1961) has argued that these problems stem from either physical malfunctioning of the brain or 'problems of living' which are not founded in physical disorders. In terms of the computer analogy he has argued that so called 'mental illness' must be viewed as either hardware (neurological) or software (psychological) problems and that in either case 'mental illness' seems to be something of a misnomer. The critical psychiatry movement has challenged basic assumptions within psychiatry (Laing, 1959; Ingleby, 1981). However, in general traditional medical perspectives have persisted within psychiatry and their impact on psychiatric/mental handicap nursing appears to mirror that of general nursing (see Barker, et al., 1989).

Even where there is no debate about the physiological bases of health problems the medical focus on biological systems has come under attack. It has been seen as diverting attention away from the psychological needs of patients and thereby downgrading the importance of interpersonal skills in nursing practice (Faulkner, 1985a). In his book *Psychological Care in Physical Illness* Nichols (1984) argues that this focus prevents health care workers from recognizing the need for psychological care and results in unnecessary and unnoticed distress amongst those who are treated as 'patients'. He describes this medical perspective as follows;

> To a large extent the 'person in the body' is an inconvenience and an irrelevance since the requirements for optimum technical medicine often clash with the requirements of the person. To this end, people and their needs are banished by turning them into something less distracting called patients. (Nichols, 1984, p. 26)

The passivity of the patient inherent in the medical model is reflected in Parson's (1951) characterization of how we tend to treat those categorized as ill. He outlined a 'sick role' which described some of the assumptions and expectations involved. He proposed that those people defined as sick (usually by a doctor) have two special rights, exemption from other social-role responsibilities and exemption from responsibility for the illness itself. These are combined with two obligations, to want to recover and to seek technically competent help. This generalized view of our social response to illness incorporates the idea of transferring responsibility to those qualified to restore health and thereby corresponds to the medical definition of the patient. If medical and nurse training incorporate this view of illness then trained staff are likely to communicate expectations regarding passivity and the assumption of control over recovery to their patients. Certainly patients feel that they are expected to minimize their needs and potential criticisms and behave in a passive and cooperative manner (Tagliacozzo and Mauksch, 1972).

The negotiation of such a 'patient role' has, however, some fairly negative consequences. It may lead nurses to define patients as 'good' or 'bad' patients based on their own technical definition of treatment rather than an analysis of patient needs (see Chapter 3, section 1). This may also mean that some patients are not regarded as legitimate recipients of care because they are not seen as wholly exempt from responsibility for the illness itself, for example, those suffering as a result of addictive behaviour ('Nursing': Survey Report on Nursing Ethics, 1974). An emphasis on treatment tasks may render nurse–patient communication irrelevant so that nurses regard it as a waste of time and avoid having to address patient inquiries Chapter 5, Section 4). Limited communication may alienate nurses from their patients' perspectives. They may become less aware of patient's worries and psychological distress may go unnoticed (Johnston, 1976, 1982; Nichols, 1984). The feeling that their perspective and expectations are not being met may lead to low compliance amongst patients and so undermine the effectiveness of health-care delivery (Ley, 1988).

Nichols refers to the reciprocal role relationships which may develop when a strict medical regime is imposed by those in authority as 'ESO medicine'. He explains the term as follows;

> This particular label is used to signify a social system wherein experts (doctors) administer to objects (patients) through the agency of servants (nurses and other para-medical professionals). The experts do their own thing and keep their own counsel. Quite often even the servants do not know what they are planning and thinking and certainly the objects do not. There is inevitably resentment and tension from the servants (nurses) to the experts (doctors), and the objects (people) are often wounded by not being given sufficient information (Nichols, 1984, p. 113)

The demands of such a social system may have many damaging effects on patients. Taylor (1979) has argued that patients who lose control of their lives in hospital environments may first resist this by exhibiting what Brehm (1966) referred to as psychological reactance. However, if such resistance fails because they cannot change the established role relationships in operation they may succumb, suffering from a loss of self efficacy and learned helplessness (see Chapter 2, Section 3) which leads to impaired psychological functioning and reduced coping. The opposite of improved health. Taylor's proposals have received support from a study showing that reduced cognitive functioning and inreased depressive symptoms are associated with longer periods of hospitalization (Raps, et al., 1982). Similarly, Miller's (1985) study of geriatric nursing showed that task allocation nursing promoted dependency, that is, patient dependency was *iatrogenic*. Since dependency is related to higher mortality Miller concluded that these nurses may be 'nursing their patients to death'. Miller also found that individualized care based on the nursing process was associated with lower dependency, shorter periods of hospitalization and better survival chances in hospital. These findings suggest that nursing practice which promotes patient passivity may be detrimental to health.

Beyond the medical model patients as clients

Those wishing to reject a passive definition of the patient role may abandon the term 'patient' altogether and refer to those they care for as 'clients'. Client connotes a consumer role and therefore implies much greater responsibility and control. Some health-care workers regard a consumerist role as inappropriate because it suggests market-place ethics and loss of a traditional sense of trust. McWhinney (1989) compares this to a mutuality role relationship between patient and health-care worker in which power is equalized so that the client's experience of her problem is recognized as a source of equally important expertise to be drawn upon in planning, decision making and treatment management. Butterworth and Skidmore (1981) consider the role of clients in the community noting that they must be involved in planning and decision making so that they are actively participating in their own care from the beginning. Clients are allowed to impose their own rules on meetings with professionals, they expect to be fully informed and instead of becoming depressed by threatening encounters they will become angry and dispense with the professional services. Such a client role can will of course require new health-care worker roles.

Oakley (1984) argues that nurses may be able to reformulate the patient role by defining their own roles in relation to patient needs and distancing themselves from the needs of the medical profession. Certainly, many nursing models propose mutual role relationship between nurses and their 'patients'. Orem's (1985) self-care model, for example, involves negotiations with the patient about control of a care plan which is aimed at maximizing the client's own care efficacy and responsibility. Reihl's (1980) interaction model begins with a consideration of role taking and focuses upon the nurse's ability to help clients to make sense of the demands of their social world. Wood (1980) argues that one application of this model is the adoption of a nurse advocacy role directed towards assisting the client in understanding and gaining control over the social demands of hospitalization. This might imply assisting the patient in resisting the imposition of a medical focus on her problem and thereby avoiding any onset of learned helplessness. These models describe nurse and client roles which entirely reject the passivity and loss of control which pervade the traditional medical view of the patient role. It is worth noting that they do not simply emphasize psychological care but propose *negotiation with the client about her needs and preferences*. This is important because in some settings clients may value technical skills more than nurses. Mayer (1987) and Larson (1984), for example, showed that cancer patients valued nurses' instrumental and technical skills most whereas the nurses themselves regarded their interactive and expressive behaviour as most important.

Nursing models will, however, only determine everyday nursing practice if hospitals and nursing institutions fully endorse new role definitions. We have noted that role change is difficult to instigate and innovation easily dissipated. When widespread re- definition of roles is required within a social system many *change agents* must be working simultaneously in order to overcome resistance in interlocking parts of the organization. Nichols sees the organizational procedures within hospitals as inherently promoting medical styles of relating and, comparing nursing and medical roles in hospitals and hospices, concludes that hospices free staff to relate to their clients in a more open and psychologically sensitive manner. The challenge then is to mount a concerted effort to remove the institutional structures which limit the participation of patients/clients in their own health care.

3 Obedience and Authority in Role Relations

Doctors as authority figures

Relationships between nurses and doctors are important because doctors' role-related rights include giving orders to nurses. They have authority over part of the nurse's work and therefore expect nurses to obey them (Coser, 1962). This inequality in doctor–nurse relations was exemplified by Stein's (1968) observation of the 'doctor–nurse game'. The rules of this interaction prohibit nurses from giving doctors direct advice on treatment but allow them to offer indirect indications of their views. Such communication ensures that doctors' authority and expertise remains unchallenged while they can still take account of nursing advice. Nurses' experiences of this relationship were illustrated by the findings of a survey undertaken by the American journal *Nursing* ('Nursing': Survey Report on Nursing Ethics, 1974). Nineteen per cent of their sample (of 11,000) nurses indicated that they seldom or never 'felt used as a servant by a doctor', 18% indicated they did so occasionally, 45% indicated they often did with some doctors but not with others, 13% indicated that they frequently felt used in this way and 2% indicated that they almost always felt used as a servant. Interestingly, this data indicated that nurses with higher academic qualifications were more likely to feel treated like a servant. Younger nurses were also more likely to feel used as servants than those over 40. It may be that more recently trained nurses with higher academic qualifications are more sensitive to being ordered about because their training has led them to expect greater autonomy and equality in their dealings with doctors. It would be interesting repeat this study in the 1990s.

Studying obedience – shocking results

Our response to authority was the subject of one of the most notorious investigations in the history of social psychology. Milgram carried out a series of experiments on people's response to orders given by those in authority (Milgram, 1974). He recruited participants by means of a newspaper advertisement offering people payment for taking part in a study of memory and learning. When they arrived they were introduced to another participant by the experimenter and told that the study would assess whether punishment enhanced learning. They were told that one person would play the role of a learner, learning to associate pairs of words while another would act as teacher testing the leaner and punishing any mistakes. In fact the experimenter (a 31 year-old man) and the other participant (a 47 year-old man) were always actors who had learnt to play out predetermined parts. Real participants were led to believe that they were allocated to the teacher role by chance, that is that they might have been given the learner role. In fact the procedure was arranged so that they always became the teacher.

The experimenter then explained that the punishment was to take the form of electric shocks and participants watched while the learner was strapped into a chair and had electrodes attached. They were told that these were connected to a shock generator in the adjoining room and taken next door to see what was really a mock shock generator. It had 30 levers each labelled in 15 volt intervals (15 volts, 30 volts, 45 volts and so on) up to 450 volts. These levers were also labelled with increasingly serious warnings from 'Slight Shock' to 'Danger: Severe Shock'. To persuade participants of the reality of this apparatus they were given a real shock of 45 volts delivered by pressing the appropriate (third) lever.

The real point of Milgram's experiment was to see to what extent participants would continue to punish the learner with electric shocks when instructed to do so by the the experimenter. They were instructed to deliver a shock each time the learner made an error and to increase the voltage with each mistake (so the third mistake would be responded to with the 45 volt lever and so on). They were also asked to announce which voltage was being applied before pressing the lever. Of course, in reality, the learner received no shocks. However, his voice had been recorded so that he appeared to be responding to the shocks in a manner which is clearly audible by the teacher in the next room. After the 75 volt lever is pressed (following the fifth wrong answer) he is heard grunting, after 120 volts he shouts that the shocks are painful, after 150 volts he shouts to the experimenter that he wants out and that he refuses to continue with the experiment. As he gives further 'wrong' answers and the 'teacher' continues to press levers he is heard crying out and after 180 volts he shouts that he cannot stand the pain, by 270 volts he is screaming in apparent agony and at 300 volts he says he will not answer further questions. The experimenter instructs the teacher to regard his failures to respond as wrong answers and deliver higher voltages. The learner screams again after 315 volts and is then completely silent, neither answering nor responding as the voltage is increased up to the maximum of 450 volts. When the (teacher) participants asked questions about the procedure the experimenter used prompts or orders of increasing insistence. He would begin with 'Please continue' and if the participant was still reluctant after two even more insistent prompts, he would say, 'You have no other choice you *must* go on'.

The surprising and controversial outcome of the experiment was that almost two-thirds (62.5%) of Milgram's 40 male participants were prepared to obey the experimenter and continue pressing levers until they has delivered 450 volts. Female participants were found to be equally obedient with 65% continuing to 450 volts. Even when the 'learner' mentions that he has a heart condition and shouts that his heart is bothering him at 330 volts two-thirds (65%) of participants continued until they had delivered 450 volts. Obedience was reduced when teachers were brought closer to their 'learner' victim. When the victim was in the same room and could be seen and heard responding to the shocks 40% of participants continued to 450 volts. This was reduced further to 30% when teachers had to physically press the learner's hand onto what they were told was a live plate! It appears then that the further away we are from another person's suffering the easier it is for us to inflict pain on them.

The crucial point of the experiment is the power the experimenter exerted over the teacher participants. When the experimenter left the room and gave his prompts by telephone obedience dropped dramatically to 20.5%. Participants also misled the experimenter over the telephone, telling him they were delivering higher voltages than they really were but if the experimenter returned to the room he could again command their obedience. Milgram showed that it is the perceived authority of the experimenter and not the orders themselves which elicit obedience. When the experimenter volunteered to be the learner (on the pretext that it is difficult to get participants to play this part) and the orders to continue delivering shocks are given by an 'ordinary man' (who the teachers thinks is another participant in the same position as themselves) *none* of the teacher participants continued beyond the point at which the experimenter asks them to stop. The efforts of the 'ordinary man' to get them to continue are useless once the authority figure decides he has had enough.

The power of legitimate authority

Milgram argues that the authority of experimenter role derives from three attributes. First he is seen as a *legitimate* authority. In volunteering to participate in an experiment one expects to find someone who is organizing and directing the procedure and no one cast any doubt on the identity of the experimenter. Secondly, he is acting *within his jurisdiction* or appropriate domain. In other words he only gives orders which are relevant to those things he is seen to be in charge of. He instructs participants only about what they must do in the experiment. He does not, for example, order them to sell their cars of change jobs! Thirdly, he has the advantage of being able to draw on a *widely accepted justification* of his orders. He is after all engaged in a scientific endeavour which will reveal aspects of learning which may be of benefit to humankind in general. He does not, for example, claim to be carrying out the study merely to enhance his own fame and career. Perceiving him as legitimate, operating within his proper domain and supported by the accepted ideology of 'science as progress' the participants are confronted with a true authority figure of the kind their socialization has taught them to obey.

Yet obeying an authority figure who asks you to do things you do not approve of is not easy. Milgram's transcripts show that many of the obedient participants questioned the experimenter, protested against the learners suffering and found the experience very stressful. Nevertheless, they could not bring themselves to disobey. Milgram explains that once the authority of another is acknowledged we change the way in which we attribute responsibility for our actions. We no longer feel that our actions flow from our own intentions, we become an instrument of the intentions of the authority figure and regard our task as performing her will competently and efficiently. In other words, we strive to be perceived as behaving appropriately in our subordinate role. We accept the authority figure's definition of the situation, relinquish responsibility and strive to perform in a loyal and dutiful manner. In this state which Milgram calls the *agentic state* we evaluate our actions in terms of how well they correspond to what we have been asked to do rather than in relation to our personal values and morals.

Disobedience only becomes possible once we leave the agentic state and again assume personal responsibility. Only then can we come to the conclusion that we should not be doing the things we have been asked to do. Milgram shows how difficult it is for his participants to extricate themselves from the agentic state. He outlines a series of stages by which the subordinate may gradually challenge authority. First, she must acknowledge to herself that the stress she feels in an indication that her actions are problematic. Secondly, she must express this doubt to the authority ('Are you sure this is okay?'). Then as the authority persists, she must express disagreement or dissent ('I do not think this is right'). Next, as the authority ignores her dissent she must threaten to withdraw cooperation ('I am not going to do this'). However, even at this stage she may remain obedient feeling unable to finally withdraw from her role obligations. The final act of ceasing to carry out orders is very difficult because it rejects what seem to be legitimate role-related obligations and may result in severe sanctions when the authority responds. It is only if the person can manage this that they will be able to disobey.

Milgram applies this idea of an agentic state in which we are 'locked into' obedience to the immoral and destructive actions of soldiers during wartime. Using examples from Nazi Germany and Vietnam he argues that soldiers of ordinary moral calibre are capable of carrying out senseless and ruthless executions when ordered to by a legitimate authority, in an appropriate situation (in wartime), justified by an accepted ideology (for example, the notion that communism is evil and oppressive). Interestingly, Kilham and Mann (1974) show that those who pass orders in hierarchies such as those found in military and nursing organizations are even more obedient in transmitting orders that those who are asked to carry them out. This suggests that it is relatively easy to set up an *obedient organization* in which people playing *transmitter roles* become legitimate authority figures for those who are asked to act on orders from above.

Psychiatrists asked to predict the behaviour of Milgram's participants agreed that participants would disobey the experimenter when the learner asks to be let out (at 150 volts). Indeed most of us also tend to think that we would disobey such orders. These predictions are based on the assumption that our sense of fairness and beliefs concerning the rights of others will prevent us from delivering shocks to an unwilling victim. However, Milgram shows that it is not the individual's beliefs but her understanding of how she should carry out her role as a subordinate which determines her behaviour. Therefore it is the plausibility of the authority and the authority's commands, and not the individual's beliefs and values which explain and determine behaviour in the subordinate role. The psychiatrists' predictions and our own confidence about our behaviour are examples of the fundamental attribution error (see Chapter 3, Section 3). They are based on attributing the causes of the behaviour to something internal to the participant (or ourselves) and underestimating the importance of external social factors.

Of course, there may be limits to the manner in which we can generalize from Milgram's results. There may, for example, be important variations in how authority is responded to within particular cultures and in how we respond to commands to hurt different types of victim (Kilham and Mann, 1974). Mixon (1972) has argued that in psychological experiments the experimenter has an implicit role obligation to ensure the safety of participants. He argues that this enables participants to trust the experimenter and that this is an important factor in Milgram's demonstration of obedience. If Mixon is right and we assume that soldiers in wartime cannot count on their commanding officers to prioritize the welfare of 'enemy civilians' then we may need to consider other processes involved in the destructive obedience of soldiers during wartime. In particular we may need to consider how 'the enemy' is socially constructed as a dehumanized outgroup (see Chapter 3, Section 4). For example, within days of war being declared between the United Kingdom and Argentina a popular newspaper carried the headline 'Kill an Argie and Win a Metro'. Here enemy pilots are viewed as mere targets in a competition to win a car. Such social derogation of 'the enemy' may be an important additional factor in destructive wartime obedience.

Milgram's study concerned orders to inflict pain directly upon another. However, as Meeus and Raaijmakers (1986) point out destructive obedience may often concern more subtle and indirect forms of violence, that is, 'psychological violence'. We may, for example, be asked to withhold information from people or give them false information which may in turn create anxiety and interfere with their plans and intentions. Meeus and Raaijmakers (1986) found that a higher proportion of participants were prepared to obey such orders than had obeyed Milgram's 'experimenter'. In this study participants were asked to create a stressful social situation for an unemployed person who they knew might do badly on a test and thereby fail to get a job as a result. Thus destructive obedience may be even more pronounced in situations where we are asked to act against another's interest but are not involved in physical harm.

Milgram's demonstration of the power of the experimenter to overrule participants' consciences is a disturbing reminder that in fitting into what we see as our appropriate roles we are capable of surrendering our independent judgement and simply following orders. The study also underlines a central theme in social psychology, namely that the role relationships we find ourselves in may be more important in shaping our behaviour than our personal beliefs. As Milgram concludes: 'it is not so much the kind of person a man is as the kind of situation in which he finds himself that determines how he will act'. This same point was highlighted by Zimbardo's famous prison roleplay study (see Haney, et al., 1973). Young male students without criminal records volunteered to play the role of either guards or prisoners in a twoweek simulation. All were offered a small daily payment and 'guard' or 'prisoner' roles were allocated randomly. During the simulation the guards' used their authority harshly and antagonism between the 'guards' and 'prisoners' escalated quickly. After six days many of the 'prisoners' were suffering from serious anxiety and depression and the study was terminated for ethical reasons. The behaviour and responses of the individuals in the simulation can be understood by examining arbitrary authority relations existing between them but it is not appropriately explained by personal dispositions or beliefs.

Obedient nurses?

Milgram's work may be especially relevant to nurses because of the type of role strain described by Anderson (1973). Nurses may be subject to conflicting obligations as patient advocates on the one hand and as subordinates to medical staff on the other. One of Milgram's women participants who obeyed until the end of the experiment was a nurse. Milgram quotes Nurse Dontz comparison of her obedience in the experiment to her obedience of medical instructions which she does not agree with:

> If I question the dose of a drug, I can ask the doctor three times, 'Is this the order you want?....And if he keeps on saying 'Go ahead' and I know this is above the average dosage I may call his attention to the fact that its too much. . . Then you still have the right to bring the question up with the supervisor'(Milgram, 1974, p.78)

Nurse Dontz feels she can question the doctor's prescription but is unable to disobey or even threaten to disobey within her nurse role. It is interesting to ask how Wood's (1980) idea of nurse advocacy (see Section 2 above), can be applied to this type of role strain. Competing and complex ethical considerations are involved. Clients' rights to information and control, the minimization of client anxiety, and the nurse's obligations to medical staff are all relevant to the nurse's decision-making.

A number of studies have examined nurses responses to such role strain. Raven, et al., (1982) report that nurses may find themselves in such dilemmas in relation to infection control. In such circumstances nurses may feel they cannot correct doctors' infringements of the rules or fail to act on a doctor's request when it contravenes infection control procedures. Hofling, et al. (1966) tested nurses obedience to doctors' prescriptions on the ward. Nurses received telephone calls from a doctor they did not know asking them to prescribe a drug they were unfamiliar with. Hospital rules stated that prescriptions should not be made over the telephone and that prescribed drugs had to be on a ward stock list. The doctor asked the nurses to find the drug and then administer twice the maximum daily dose as clearly stated on the pill box. Twenty-one out of 22 nurses agreed to give the drug and had already prepared the excessive dose when the study was revealed to them. In the Milgram study the authority of the experimenter was reduced when he communicated by telephone. However, in this case where use of the telephone violated hospital rules nurses obeyed doctors' orders to administer an excessive drug dosage.

Hofling and colleagues terminated their study if the nurses involved attempted to check the order with their fellow nurses or superiors. They do not report what proportion of nurses actually tried to check in this way. Rank and Jacobson (1977) regarded this as an important element in nurses responses to medical orders and repeated the experiment allowing such checking. They also changed the prescription to 30 milligrams of Valium, a drug which the nurses would be familiar with. They found that out of 18 nurses only two were prepared to administer the drug without checking, a further ten prepared the drug but then attempted to recontact the doctor, the pharmacy or their supervisor and six tried to check the order before preparing the drug. Rank and Jacobson found that nurses discussed the dosage with other nurses and whether or not they should check it. Thus when nurses are familiar with a drug and are able to discuss a prescription with colleagues it seems that they are much more likely to check an excessive dose before administering it. This suggests that providing nurses with a good knowledge of treatment procedures and encouraging them to ask questions and seek social support when unsure may reduce the level of destructive obedience in nursing. This in turn suggests that educational programmes used to socialize nurses should emphasize questioning, consultation and the assumption of personal responsibility for one's actions.

4 Helping in Emergencies

Failure to help – apathy or indecision?

People do not always receive help when they most need it. There have been many reports of people sustaining injuries or dying when others were available to help but did not. The case of Kitty Genovese has become famous in social psychology because it prompted Latané and Darley's (1970) investigations into why bystanders do not help in emergencies. Kitty Genovese was beaten, sexually assaulted and finally stabbed to death over an extended period in front of a New York apartment block. Although 38 people witnessed the assault, no one called the police or tried to intervene. The image of people watching such a brutal attack without feeling impelled to help led media commentators to conclude that city dwellers had become apathetic, callous and uncaring. Latané and Darley's work rejected this generalized internal attribution (see Chapter 2, Section 3) and focused upon the social and situational features which can prevent helping in emergencies.

They point out that emergencies by their very nature are unscripted occurrences in which people must take responsibility for unusual and perhaps frightening events in brief decision-making spans. The absence of appropriate rules, roles or scripts disables potential helpers in a similar manner to an uninformed visitor on a ward (see Chapter 1, Section 3). When we do not how to behave appropriately and are unsure about how others may judge us we are vulnerable to social influence which often inhibits helping.

Latané and Darley propose a fivestage decisionmaking model which describes representations of the emergency and ourselves which need to be in place before we can offer help. We must

- *notice* that something has happened,
- correctly *interpret* it as an emergency requiring action,
- *take personal responsibility* for helping,
- *plan* our response,
- and finally *intervene*.

This process may break down at any stage and result in a failure to help. Progression through these stages seems to be strongly influenced by other people and by our perceptions of the costs and benefits involved. Latané and Darley found that people approached on the street were generally helpful in the case of simple straightforward problems such as someone in need of directions. However as the potential costs of helping increased, for example when people were asked for small amounts of money, fewer people offered help. This finding corresponds to Schwartz and Howard's (1981) more general model of altruistic behaviour which proposes that before we help others we evaluate the potential costs of doing so. When the psychological and material costs are high then we may enter a *defence stage* in which we rethink our inclination to help and decide not to intervene.

Noticing an emergency may seem easy enough. However, Milgram (1970) points out that living in cities leads to a constant information overload which people may cope with by limiting their attention to those things which they feel concern them. In doing so they learn to block out many events occurring around them. This may explain why people who come from smaller towns have been found to be more likely to intervene in emergencies than those from cities (Latané and Darley, 1970). Of course noticing that something is going on does not guarantee that we will interpret the information correctly. Goffman (1974) provides some striking examples of the mistakes which can occur. He reports an incident in which a teetotaler suffering from a seizure was thought to be drunk and died in a police cell instead of being taken to hospital. Her slurred voice, vomiting and use of a mouth wash had led bystanders to misinterpret her need for help. In another example a priest who heard screaming during a rectory robbery ignored it because he knew that one of his fellow priests was always singing in a loud voice! Emergencies take us by surprise and the information available may often be ambiguous. There is, therefore, a tendency to assimilate our experiences into what we are familiar with, that is to assume that we are witnessing some ordinary occurrence rather than a rare and dramatic event. Thus we may act as if nothing special is happening even in the middle of an emergency we have noticed but misinterpreted.

If we understand the need for help then we are faced with the question of whether we should take responsibility or leave it to others. We may conclude that others are better placed to intervene, more competent or already taking charge of the situation and so feel no obligation to get involved. Even if we decide that it is our responsibility we may find that helping is too difficult or complex when we begin to plan our intervention. We may not be able to decide whether we should act directly or call upon others. In either case we may be unsure whether we have the skills and resources to help effectively. As we begin to worry about the costs and consequences of our actions time slips away and we may enter the defence stage and conclude that our help is not needed after all.

Social inhibition of helping behaviour

Latane and Darley demonstrated that the social influence of other people at emergencies makes decision-making breakdown more likely. Many studies have shown that we are more likely to help when we are alone than when we are with others (Latané and Nida, 1981). One reason for this is that others' uncertainty may make the situation more ambiguous. We may see that others are not responding and assume that nothing is really wrong. Moreover, if someone else declares that everything is alright we may welcome this as a resolution of our puzzlement about the situation. This tendency for groups of bystanders to collectively influence each other to deny emergencies is known as *pluralistic ignorance*. In this case the presence of others leads to a breakdown at the interpretation stage of the decision-making process. The presence of others may also discourage us from taking personal responsibility, we may assume that others are already involved in helping and conclude that our efforts are unnecessary. If all bystanders make this assumption this leads to *diffusion of responsibility* and a lack of helping.

A third source of social influence results from our concern with impression management and reputation maintenance (see Chapter 3, Section 3). Audiences make us apprehensive about how others' will judge our performance and if the task is a difficult this tends to impair our performance. Other bystanders will therefore inhibit helping because they trigger this *evaluation apprehension*. Only where we are well practiced and sure of our response will this effect promote helping behaviour (Zajonc, 1965; Carver and Scheier, 1981). In this case we may believe that intervening will lead to an enhanced reputation as others recognize our competence and decisiveness. However, because emergencies are unusual and unanticipated we are rarely practised and well prepared.

The impact of these three processes was demonstrated by Latané and Rodin (1969). In this study participants saw a woman go behind a curtain into an adjoining room. They then heard her fall off a chair, shout out about having hurt her foot and moan in pain. The independent variable in this experiment (see Chapter 1, Section 4) was whether the unwitting participants were alone or with other people. When alone 70% of participants intervened. However, when pairs of participants heard the accident together only 40% of these pairs generated any intervention and when participants were with a person who had been instructed to remain passive only 7% of the real participants intervened. A similar study highlighted diffusion of responsibility amongst a group of potential helpers. Darley and Latané (1969) invited student participants to discuss the difficulties of student life. They were told that they would communicate with other students using an intercom system in order to preserve confidentiality. Different participants were led to believe they were involved in a discussion with one other person, two others or five others. In each case the other voices were taped and participants heard one of them discuss his epilepsy and then begin to have a seizure. The need for help was fairly unambiguous and 85% of those who thought they were the only person who could hear the appeal responded while the victim was still speaking. However when they thought someone else could hear only 62% responded and this dropped to 31% when they thought four others could also help. Moreover, even those who did help when they thought others could hear responded more slowly, with participants in the 'six-person group' taking three times as long to intervene.

Our mood and feeling of empathy may also affect our willingness to offer help in an emergency (Shaffer and Graziano, 1983). This can be changed by our attributions concerning the cause of the victim's distress. Just as attributions concerning our own symptoms affect help-seeking and preventive behaviour so our understanding of others' plight may affect helping behaviour. Piliavin, et al., (1969) found that a man who collapsed on an underground train carrying a cane was more likely to receive help that a man carrying a bottle of alcohol. Attributing a person's need to an internal and controllable cause such as drinking may lead us to conclude that they are more responsible and less deserving and may elicit disapproval and negative feelings. By contrast attributing their need to an uncontrollable cause, for example a disability may lead us to regard them as less responsible and more deserving which may generate feelings of sympathy (Weiner, 1980). Such attributional processes may also affect health-care workers' responses to their patients' requests for help. Brewin (1984) for example, reports that medical students were more willing to prescribe psychotropic drugs for patients who had experienced uncontrollable life events such as bereavement than those suffering because of more controllable events such as getting into debt.

Since we have a general tendency to to attribute events to others' internal dispositions (that is make fundamental attribution errors, see Chapter 3, Section 1) we may also overestimate the degree to which people deserve what they get. Lerner (1980) has referred to this tendency as our 'belief in a just world'. Regarding others' as in some way responsible for their fate will reduce our obligation to offer help. Moreover, we can justify failing to help by the belief that everyone has the right to to pursue their own interests. Thus our perception of others' need for help and the degree to which we feel obligated to help are affected by attributional processes and intersubjective beliefs about justice, morality and self-interest.

Some of the costs of helping in emergencies cannot be removed. Piliavin and Piliavin (1972) for example, found that victims who bled from the mouth were less likely to receive help that those who did not. Potential contact with blood may be seen as an important cost for many people. The time involved in helping is also an important cost for people who feel rushed. Baston, et al., (1978) showed that participants who were in a hurry were less likely to help especially if they felt their presence elsewhere was important. Nevertheless the research in this area suggests that preparing people to intervene increases the likelihood of helping. Shotland and Heinold (1985) found that people who had taken a 'Red Cross' training course in first aid and emergency intervention were much more likely to help someone who seemed to be bleeding from a cut artery than those who had not taken the course. Moreover, the trained individuals were less likely to be inhibited by the presence of others. Similarly, Huston, et al., (1981) found that training was an important factor differentiating those who had and had not intervened in incidents of violent crime and Clark and Word (1972) demonstrated that those with relevant training were more likely to help and take proper precautions in an emergency which seemed to involve electric shock. Thus courses which train large numbers of the people in simple first aid and emergency intervention may be very effective ways of ensuring that we receive prompt help in emergencies.

Becoming aware of the situational barriers involved in helping may help us modify our decision-making process in emergencies and pause before concluding that everything is alright. Practice in the helper role will also make it more likely that we translate our good intentions into helpful action. Finally, it is worth noting that victims can also increase their chances of receiving help if they are able to address others and clarify their needs. In such cases it seems important to focus on one's need for help rather than the other person's obligation. Langer and Abelson (1972) showed that victim-orientated requests (for example, 'I'm hurt') were more likely to elicit help than target-orientated requests (such as 'Would you help me. .?').

5 Sex, Gender and Nursing

Gender – femininity and masculinity

An important social identity is derived from our awareness of ourselves as men and women and of culturally based expectations concerning sex appropriate behaviour. We can therefore consider *sex roles* in much the same way as we have discussed occupational roles. Learning about these roles leads to the development of sex role stereotypes used to understand others and to the construction of a personal *gender identity* used to regulate our own behaviour (see Chapter 3, Section 3).

A common-sense view of men and women might suggest that the biological differences between them are responsible for any differences in their patterns of behaviour. However, a more detailed consideration reveals this to be a simplification. Biological sex itself is made up of several components which tend to vary along dimensions rather than falling simply into male and female categories. Money and Ehrhardt (1972) point out that the inheritance of sex chromosomes from parents, the development of either testes or ovaries, the secretion of male or female hormones and the development of male or female genitalia are all involved in the complex developmental process which leads to the designation of sex at birth. Moreover, variation can occur at each of these stages. In rare cases for example, individuals with the usual (X plus Y) male chromosomes may be insensitive to the action of the male hormone testosterone. This results in the development of a female physique and genitalia (with a non-functional male reproductive system). People with this condition will be regarded as female and although they will be infertile can live very successfully as women despite their male chromosomal constitution. Money and Ehrhardt (1972) and Money (1974) also report on a case of genetically and genitally male twins in which an accident during circumcision led to a reassignment of sex of one twin. Cosmetic surgery and hormone treatment allowed this biological male to be successfully socialized as a girl and resulted in the development of behaviour patterns which distinguished her from her boy twin. Adults may also engage in crosssex behaviour and request cosmetic surgery and hormonal treatment which will allow them to engage in sexual activity as members of the opposite sex. These unusual cases illustrate that the adoption of a sex role is dependent upon social perceptions of a person as a girl, boy, woman or man, the person's own categorization of themselves and their perceptions of what type of behaviour is appropriate to that sex categorization. Our social status as women and men is based primarily upon our presentation in terms of behaviour, clothes, gestures, and communication and this is not determined by simple biological differences.

It is therefore useful to distinguish between the terms *sex* and *gender*. Sex is made up of the biological dimensions mentioned above. These can used to designate people into two biological groups, *females* and *males*. Gender, on the other hand, refers to representations of how males and females should behave. These include shared representations within cultures (that is sex roles) as well as individual representations of self in relation to sex roles. Gender then refers to a set of beliefs which map out *feminine* and *masculine* behaviours which are thought of as being appropriate for females and males respectively. Thus although they are importantly related sex and gender must be considered separately. Different cultures define femininity (behaviours appropriate for women) and masculinity differently and a person's biological sex does not determine their gender identification.

Oakley's (1972) *Sex, Gender and Society* provides an interesting introduction to this area and illustrates the way in which different cultures have developed varying and contradictory definitions of masculinity and femininity. Despite crosscultural similarities, questions concerning differences in the behaviour of men and women should be addressed in relation to particular cultures. There has been much research into such sex differences in industrialized, Western societies. In an important review of this work Maccoby and Jacklin (1974) concluded that only four of the proposed differences between boys and girls could be reliably substantiated. They concluded that girls have better verbal or language abilities while boys have a greater facility for acquiring mathematical skills, have better spatial representations of their environment and are more aggressive. They found no evidence that girls were less analytic, less motivated to achieve, have lower self-esteem or are more likely to conform.

The importance of the sex differences identified by Maccoby and Jacklin and the implication that they are due to biological rather than socialization processes have since been questioned (see Deaux, 1985). It is extremely difficult to isolate biological predispositions from the effects of socialization differences because the designation of sex may prompt different parenting approaches. Moss (1970) found that three-week old boys were held for longer by their mothers than girls of the same age and Condry and Condry (1976), showed that adults' perceptions of a nine month-old's behaviour differed according to their perception of the child's sex. Responses identified as fear when the child was thought to be female was more likely to be seen as anger when the child was categorized as male. Our sex stereotypes may therefore become self-fulfilling prophecies as we modify our behaviour towards infants on the basis of their designated sex. This means that boys and girls may be socialized into different social worlds from a very early age.

Psychologists have tried to describe these stereotypes with a view to understanding the different expectations we have of men and women and how these affect our construction of gender identities. It seems that we can readily distinguish between characteristics which we associate with women (feminine attributes) and those we associate with men (masculine attributes). Masculine characteristics tend to imply dominance, activity and independence (as indicated by adjectives such as, self-confident, blunt, loud, competitive, assertive and self-reliant) while feminine characteristics imply interpersonal sensitivity, 'connectedness' and gentleness (as indicated by adjectives such as, understanding, warm, tactful, cooperative and tender) (see, for example, Bem, 1974; Spence and Helmreich, 1978; Deaux, 1985). There is evidence that we agree upon these stereotypes and that they are similar across cultures (Williams and Best, 1982). However masculinity and femininity are not opposite ends of the same dimension. Instead it seems that they are quite separate dimensions and that we can identify different degrees of both masculinity and femininity in ourselves and others.

Towards psychological androgyny

Bem (1974) argued that we can measure the degree to which people identify themselves as masculine and feminine and thereby divide the population into four broad categories; those who are primarily masculine (*masculine sex typed*), those who are primarily feminine (*feminine sex typed*), those who have few of either characteristics (*undifferentiated*) and those who have a lot of masculine and feminine characteristics (*psychologically androgynous*). Spence and Helmreich (1978) have estimated that about 30% of the population may be psychologically androgynous and Bem (1975) has argued that such people are more adaptable to changing social contexts because they can contentedly display both masculine and feminine responses as the situations demand them. Williams (1979) argues that this adaptability allows psychologically androgynous individuals to deal more effectively with a wider range of social situations and therefore makes them less vulnerable to stress and psychological problems. Later studies have suggested that our model of gender identity needs to go beyond Bem's fairly straightforward categorization system (Deaux, 1985). However, there is little doubt that the structure of our gender identities affects the way in which we perceive and interact with others.

   Gilligan's (1982) has adopted a more developmental perspective on gender identity. Criticizing psychologists for ignoring the psychological development of women she argues that widespread gender expectations encourage boys and girls to develop different views of interpersonal relationships and moral issues. Women are encouraged to develop an identity which is based on an 'ethic of care' in which looking after others and maintaining close intimate relationships are central to decision-making. Men, on the other hand, tend to develop a social sense of justice which is based on a respect for other's rights, an obligation of non-interference and a sense of separateness. Gilligan argues that these feminine and masculine paths through social development give rise to different social difficulties for men and women. For women the importance of close caring relationships may mean that they have difficulties in dealing with competitive and hierarchical relationships in which differences in power and prestige separate and divide people. This provides an explanation for Horner's (1972) observation that women showed a fear of success when this was measured in terms of competing with and beating others. Such success may be unattractive for women because it threatens their feminine self-representations. Men, however, may not be troubled by competition but threatened instead by relationships which infringe on their independence and separateness. This is illustrated by the results of a study carried out by Pollak and Gilligan (1982). They asked men to write stories about a picture of a tranquil scene in which a couple seemed to be enjoying time together and found that 21% of these stories included unexpected violence. Gilligan regards this violent imagery as an expression of the threat which intimate relationships pose to masculine gender identity. In her developmental model men and women who gradually come to terms with these problems achieve emotional maturity through an amalgamation of masculine and feminine approaches to interaction. Women become better at dealing with competition and separateness while men learn to deal with closeness and intimacy. This view of maturity corresponds closely to Bem's portrayal of the adaptable psychologically androgynous individual.

Devalued femininity and sexism

Different expectations and parenting practices may provide different social and physical environments for boys and girls (Rheingold and Cook, 1975). However, this does not mean that masculine and feminine characteristics are equally valued. Rosenkrantz, et al., (1968), for example, found that masculine characteristics were more highly valued by students while Fabrikant (1974) reported that male and female therapists rated the majority of feminine characteristics negatively. In a similar study Broverman, et al., (1970) asked practicing clinicians (psychologists, psychiatrists and social workers) to describe the characteristics of three categories of people; a healthy woman, a healthy man and a healthy *person* (of unspecified sex). Healthy persons and healthy men were characterized in masculine terms (for example dominant, active and independent) and were thought to be fairly similar. However, the feminine characterization of the healthy woman was different to the description of the healthy person. This suggests that therapists may regard masculine characteristics as the standard against which healthy behaviour is judged. Femininity may therefore be regarded as tending towards deviancy or sickness and be less valued as a result. There have, however, been debates about the measurement of our evaluation of feminine and masculine characteristics and suggestions that feminine characteristics are more valued now than in the past (see for example, Eagly, 1989).

Such differential evaluation can be observed in the way in which boys and girls are socialized into sex roles. Parents tend to be more concerned about boys who display feminine characteristics than girls who adopt masculine behaviour. 'Tomboy', for example, is a more positive stereotype than 'sissy'. Archer (1989) notes that masculine girls may be seen as gaining 'promotion' into more positively evaluated activities, but boys must avoid femininity in order to maintain a positive reputation. If society encourages women to develop a primarily feminine approach to interpersonal relationships and decision-making but values masculine behaviours more highly this may create difficulties for women's develop-ment of self-esteem. It may also limit their opportunities because others view them in terms of a stereotype which devalues them in relation to men. Such sexist stereotyping may lead to discrimination against women when they are in competition with men. Goldberg (1969) for example, found that women students were more likely to think an article was high quality when they thought it was written by a man than a woman. Early feminine socialization and experiences of such discrimination may have adverse affects on the way women represent themselves and their behaviour. For example, there is evidence that men and women make different types of causal attributions. Men tend to attribute their failures to external factors whereas women tend to make internal stable attributions (Simon and Feather, 1973; Dweck and Licht 1980). Recalling Bandura's work on self-efficacy we can see that such attributions will damage women's sense of self efficacy and may even become a self-fulfilling prophecy (see Chapter 2, Section 3).

The acknowledgement that our gender stereotypes and the socialization practices which they support may make it difficult for women to achieve valued reputations in our society is one of the foundational ideas of *feminism*. This feminist perspective portrays women as disadvantaged or oppressed by gender stereotypes. Spender and Sarah's (1980) *Learn-ing to Lose* for example, argues that the school system socializes girls into interpersonal and work roles which are less highly valued. Scott (1980) demonstrates how educational policy has developed curricula that emphasize caring and self-sacrificing roles for girls and Sarah, et al., (1980) argue that because sex-role differentiation is especially evident in mixed sex schools, single sex schools may provide better academic opportunities for girls. Feminism seeks to promote more positive images of women both by emphasizing the positive features of femininity (for example, the importance of interpersonal intimacy and a caring morality) *and* by asserting women's capacity to adopt typically masculine behaviour. From an intergroup perspective we can regard feminist activities as representing both consciousness raising and intergroup competition in relation to men's privileged position (see Taylor and Mckirnan, Chapter 3, Section 4)

Gender in nursing – from femininity to androgyny

The social psychology of gender is relevant to nursing because patients' gender identity may affect their communication about health problems and willingness to engage in preventive and curative behaviours. Sextyped men, for example, may find acknowledging distress or dependency more difficult than most women but may suffer just as much. The perceived costs of treatment or prevention may also be assessed differently by men and women if the behaviours in question are seen as more appropriate for either sex. Thus an understanding of gender identity may enhance the nurse's sensitivity to patients' gender-linked beliefs, behaviours and anxieties.

Nursing has traditionally emphasized the relationship between feminine socialization and nursing skills. The delivery of care has been viewed as a vocation for which women are especially suited to because of their femininity. Nightingale herself defined nursing as the expression of women's 'natural' talents of mothering and caring. The work of nursing was therefore portrayed as part of womens' feminine role obligations and nurses were expected be altruistic and obedient so as to conform to shared expectations of feminine behaviour (see Gamarnikov, 1978; Webb, 1982; Oakley, 1984). Nursing was defined in relation to the authority of the almost exclusively male medical profession which highlighted the femininity of nursing. Girl's magazines and nurse recruitment literature alike have presented nursing as a 'natural' job for girls; a job for which feminine socialization provided vital preparation. This has also led to a rejection of feminism within nursing because of the potential opposition between feminist goals and the feminine role upon which nursing was founded (Reverby, 1987a).

More recently, however, debates concerning the nature of the nurse role and the need to expand the traditional pool of potential recruits has led to a re-analysis of the relationship between femininity and nursing. Nurses have developed role definitions which stress independent, decision-making in relation to nursing tasks. The technical and scientific basis of nurse education and practice has expanded. The proportion of male recruits has increased and feminist analyses of nursing and nursing research have been undertaken (see, for example Webb, 1984), Reverby (1987b) describes this as progress from an 'obligation to care' to 'altruism with autonomy'. The shift mirrors Gilligan's portrayal of the emergence of increased self-worth and independence within feminine gender development and constitutes a reassessment of the appropriate balance of feminine and masculine skills required for nursing competence.

This reassessment has led to some interesting gender-linked debates within nursing. It has been argued that increased masculinity may damage nursing by undermining core caring values and, alternatively, that it may enhance nursing by introducing new competencies, for example greater independence and leadership (Dingwall, 1977; Brown and Stones, 1973). Since these debates focus on gender they they are not primarily about the recruitment of male nurses but rather the skills required of both male and female nurses. Even where there is evidence of differences between men and women in relation to relationship management (see Chapters 6, Section 2; Chapter 8, Section 2) these differences may not be evident amongst nursing applicants because men who wish to enter nursing may not be typically sextyped (Brown and Stones, 1973; Choon and Skevington, 1984). The degree to which female nurses characterize themselves in terms of traditionally feminine and masculine characteristics will also vary and Joseph (1985) suggests that those who describe themselves in masculine terms are more willing to make independent decisions about nursing matters. Moreover, appropriate nurse education programmes may diminish gender differences relevant to nursing practice. Thus, while an awareness of gender may have implications for selection of nurse students (for example a degree of psychological androgyny may be considered desirable for both male and female entrants) it has greater implications are for the process of nurse training (Webb, 1982).

There are, however, some questions which specifically concern the entry of men into nursing. The recruitment of men necessitates campaigns which do not associate nursing exclusively with womanhood and femininity. However, Cottingham (1987) points out that an overly technical portrayal or one which emphasizes physical strength could discourage suitable women applicants and attract sextyped men who may not be ideally suited to nursing. Male nurses also raise the question of sex interchangeability amongst nurses. It can be argued that male and female nurses are equally capable of performing any nursing task. However, patient's preferences and the views of nurse managers are likely to be influenced by sex and nurse stereotypes. This may mean that certain nursing tasks are regarded as appropriate only for nurses of the same sex of the patient. This may be particularly true for female patients and may impose a limitations on what male nurse's are allowed to do (Thompson, 1989).

Perhaps the most controversial aspect men's entry into nursing is their better promotion prospects. Gaze (1987) demonstrates that although less than 10% of nurses in the United Kingdom in 1987 were men this small group held more than half of promoted posts. This was true of nurse unit manager posts, chief nursing posts and director of nurse education posts. Many explanations have been offered for women's poorer promotion prospects. Choon and Skevington (1984) suggest that differences in attributions for success and failure may indeed become self-fulfilling prophecies so that while men continue to maintain high self-esteem and apply for promoted posts women become discouraged and settle for less prestigious posts. This corresponds to Hackett and Betz's (1981) use of Bandura's work on self efficacy. They suggest that attributional patterns encouraged by feminine socialization, a limited array of successful women role models and the lower expectations of those advising women on career choice (including teachers and counsellors) results in diminished self-efficacy and career ambition. However, wider social factors are also likely to assist men's promotion prospects in nursing. As a minority group men are more noticeable in nursing and stereotypes may lead managers (whether men or women) to favour men because they are viewed as being more motivated by salary increases and less committed to family roles which might distract them from nursing obligations. A comprehensive analysis of discrimination against women would require an analysis of gender roles in relation to child rearing and housework as well as work roles (Oakley, 1974).

CORE IDEAS IN CHAPTER 4

- Everyday social behaviour is guided by a shared knowledge of rules which define appropriate behaviour. Breaking social rules results in loss of approval and reputation. This can be minimized by offering accounts, apologies or reconstructions.

- Rules only operate in relation to particular role relationships. Such roles give us certain rights and obligations in relation to role partners. We try to perform these in accordance with the expectations of role set members to enhance role-related reputation.

- Social rules and roles can be re-negotiated through interaction but they are largely taken for granted.

- The nurse role incorporates ambiguities which may result in role strain. This may be especially true during training.

- A traditional definition of the patient role promotes dependency which may be detrimental to patients' capacity for self-directed coping. Many nursing models suggest a re-definition of this role implying that nurses should negotiate with patients and promote joint decision-making. Such changes may, however, threaten established health care practices and may be resisted.

- Role obligations to authority figures may override our individual judgements allowing us to engage in destructive obedience. This is especially likely if the authority figure is seen as legitimate, acting within her appropriate jurisdiction, and can offer a culturally valued justification. Authority hierarchies within nursing may create conflicts between taking personal responsibility for patient care and following orders.

- Nurses are more likely to question orders they are unsure about if they are familiar with the treatment in question and can discuss the problem with other nurses.

- Emergencies are ambiguous social situations for which we have no available rules, roles or scripts. This makes it difficult for us to know what to do.

- We are also susceptible to social influence which often inhibits helping. Others' failure to respond may lead us to assume that nothing is wrong (pluralistic ignorance) or that someone else is dealing with the matter (diffusion of responsibility). Others can also make us anxious about how we will be judged as a helper (evaluation apprehension). Training in intervention strategies appears to increase helping behaviour.

- We learn culturally specific expectations concerning appropriate behaviour for men and women. Many sex differences are therefore due to socialization processes. Gender refers to this social construction of biological sex.

- Expectations of boys and girls may create separate developmental paths, with different challenges, for boys and girls. However, emotional maturity and social adaptability may be maximized in psychologically androgynous individuals who categorize themselves as both masculine and feminine and can exhibit both types of behaviour according to situational demands.

- The historical links between femininity and nursing raises interesting questions concerning the amalgamation of positive masculine behaviours and traditionally feminine obligations within a modern nurse role. These have implications for recruitment and especially for training.

5

Communication and health care

1   Introduction

Communication in interaction

All interaction involves communication. Even ignoring another person may communicate unfriendliness, busyness or a lack of concern. Communication is also foundational to person perception (see Chapter 3), interaction co-ordination (see Chapter 4), relationship management (see Chapter 6) and facilitating change in others (see Chapter 7).

We noted in Chapter 3 (Section 2) how we use communication to manage our impressions and safeguard our reputations. When we feel someone accepts and approves of us we are more inclined to disclose our thoughts and feelings. In such a relationship we can express our concerns without fear of rejection. This in turn means that the relationship is likely to flourish encouraging further communication. (see Chapter 6, Section 2). If, on the other hand, we think someone is indifferent or disapproves of us we are unlikely to expose ourselves to potential rebuffs by revealing our thoughts and feelings. In such relationships we may learn to deny or distort our needs in order to avoid disapproval. If this happens regularly, failing to express our feelings may become a habitual way of coping with others and have damaging consequences for our representation of ourselves and our sense of self-efficacy (see Chapter 2, Section 3). Communication with others determines how we understand our social world, what we think we are capable of doing and what opportunities actually arise. It is the basis of our social existence.

Communication takes place within social contexts defined by particular sets of rules and roles (see Chapter 4, Section 1). Most of these rules are unspoken and specific to our own cultural groupings. Different groups use different rules to regulate communication and this can lead to serious misunderstandings (Labov, 1973). We tend to take these rules for granted until they are broken, for example, when we are spoken to very loudly by a person standing only a few feet away. When such rules are broken we seek to explain the 'deviation". We may achieve this by attributing certain characteristics to the rule-breaking person, for example regarding them as deaf, drunk or attention seeking. If they belong to our cultural group and become aware that they are breaking the rules they are likely to engage in remedial action to maintain reputation. However, if different rules apply to communication in their own social groups they may not be aware that we perceive them to be behaving unusually. In such cases our attributions may be misleading and generate further misunderstanding.

Communication between nurses and patients

Nursing has been traditionally regarded as a 'doing' discipline and has been managed through task allocation. Task allocation on wards involves each nurse carrying out one procedure with all patients. This type of organization minimizes nurses' contact with individual patients and focuses communication upon the procedure being performed. This results in superficial communication and a failure to identify the individual needs and and concerns of patients (see Chapter 4, Section 2). However, nursing models are increasingly rejecting this traditional framework and proposing new nurse–patient role definitions which prioritize understanding patients' concerns. The patients' interpretations and feelings are regarded as factors which may be responsible for the problems being presented and therefore vital to their resolution. Nursing models such as Roy's (1984) adaptation model, Orem's (1985) self-care model and Neuman's (1982) system model place the establishment of open communication between nurses and patients at the centre of effective nursing intervention.

The nursing process further highlights the importance of nurse–patient communication. Assessment and evaluation rely upon communication concerning patients' experiences and needs. Joint planning depends upon detailed communication to achieve shared understandings and commitments between nurse and patient and many nursing interventions also depend upon the quality of nurse–patient communication. Although some procedures involve acting directly upon the patient most will require a degree of participation or at least cooperation from the patient. This means that the effectiveness of health care depends upon the patient's own behaviour. This behaviour is in turn guided by the patient's beliefs and understandings (see Chapter 2, Section 1). *Thus effective health care ultimately relies upon health-care workers understanding of, and influence upon, their patients' beliefs.* This is why health education is so important to health promotion. Communication aimed at exploring patient's beliefs and at educating or persuading patients is therefore foundational to nursing.

We noted in Chapter 2 that about 45% of patients do not carry out treatment procedures as recommended. This dramatically reduces the efficiency of the health-care system and results in much avoidable illness and expenditure. In his book *Communicating with Patients; Improving Communication, Satisfaction and Compliance*, Ley (1988) discusses studies which suggest that (in addition to patients' adoption of appropriate health beliefs) patients' satisfaction with communication concerning their problems and their perception that their expectations have been met by health-care workers are important factors in promoting compliance. Thus the failure of many patients to carry out treatment may be partially due to poor communication with health-care workers. The problematic nature of such communication is further highlighted by research evidence suggesting that about a third of all patients are dissatisfied with communication concerning their health problems.

Communication amongst health-care workers

Communication between health-care workers is also vital to effective health-care delivery. Increases in the number and specialization of health-care workers makes coordination vital and highlights the importance of open communication between nurses, doctors, psychologists, physio-therapists etc. Patients in hospital and primary health-care settings are faced with an array of different professional groups with a variety of grades and role-related responsibilities. Integrated communication is therefore essential to the coordinated delivery of care. In hospital, for example, a nursing goal might be to educate a patient in stoma care but if a doctor is unaware of this goal the patient may be discharged before this goal is achieved. Failure to coordinate may disrupt the sequence of activities carried out by different disciplines causing unnecessary stress and confusion to patients through the imposition of different professional demands at the same time. Services may also be omitted or duplicated causing disruption to the continuity of care. This is particularly common where responsibility for care is transferred from one setting to another, for example from hospital to home.

Communication between health-care workers about their separate com-munications with patients is therefore vital. It is important, for example, that all staff are aware of the patient's current thinking and needs. For example, if a doctor discusses a terminal illness or a permanent handicap with a patient it is important that nurses are made aware of this so they can offer appropriate support and counselling. Communication and coordina-tion problems escalate dramatically when multidisciplinary teams become competitive. Multidisciplinary working involves the maintenance of sepa-rate professional identities and any breakdown in mutual respect may result in staff belonging to different professions engaging in intergroup conflict (see Chapter 3, Section 4). Such conflict may result in intentional failures to communicate motivated by a desire to preserve privilege and power (Graham, 1981; Fielding and Llewelyn, 1987). Once this occurs poor communication may be deliberately perpetuated between agencies. This will lead to a disintegration of services and generate dissatisfaction, disillusionment and low compliance amongst patients. Thus the time and energy required to maintain good professional relationships within multidisciplinary teams may be a good investment when measured against the damage done to health-care delivery by poor communication.

2   Communication and Persuasion

The S-M-C-R model

We can begin to understand the communication process by dividing it into parts and stages. Berlo (1960) proposed the 'S-M-C-R' model which analyses the communication into the *source* (or sender), the *message*, the *channel* and the *receiver*. This type of analysis allows us to ask questions about particular aspects of the process, for example what features of the sender affects the receiver, what type of message will be most persuasive, what channels are available, what difficulties does the receiver face and so on. It also emphasizes the fragility of the communication process. The sender must translate her ideas into some kind of message which the receiver must understand in the same way as the sender in order to achieve successful communication. These processes are often referred to as encoding (by the sender) and decoding (by the receiver).

The idea of different channels refers to our ability to use different senses simultaneously in decoding messages. We can listen to what someone is saying, see their smiling face and feel their reassuring touch at the same time. They have encoded their message in three channels and we understand what they mean by decoding in all three. The use of channels is often broadly divided into *verbal* communication involving spoken or written language and *non-verbal* communication which includes facial expression, touch, gaze, tone of voice and body posture. These different channels can be used to send different messages. For example, we might tell someone how useful a meeting had been using spoken verbal communication while at the same time indicating that we wish to end the meeting by glancing at our watch and beginning to lean forward in our chair as if to stand up. Indeed, most everyday communication involves simultaneous verbal and non-verbal encoding and decoding. Verbal and non-verbal channels are therefore interdependent aspects of an integrated communication system.

A five stage model of persuasion

Involving patients in decision-making and encouraging independence are key elements of many nursing models. However, involvement in health promotion means that nurses are likely to want to *persuade* patients to consider and perhaps adopt certain beliefs. We might wish to persuade a patient to acknowledge and accept responsibility for the health consequences of, for example, smoking. We might also seek to persuade a patient to change her behaviour for the sake of her health. Nurses are therefore likely to engage in persuasive communication aimed at educating patients and promoting health-enhancing behaviours. Patients who are persuaded through open communication do not lose their independence but gain the freedom to appraise their views and lifestyle in new ways. Indeed communication which acknowledges the patient's responsibility and control is likely to be *more* persuasive because it does not provoke deliberate resistance. We noted in Chapter 4 (Section 2) that patients may engage in such resistance (or 'psychological reactance') in response to loss of control. Thus health promotion may be best served by persuasive communication aimed at ensuring that the patient's choices are based on beliefs which have been formed in the course of open discussion about their health.

McGuire (1969) proposed a five-stage model of persuasion. First, the receiver has to *attend* to the message, otherwise it will not even be decoded. Secondly, she has to *comprehend* it through successful decoding, thirdly, she has to *yield* to its sense by changing her beliefs, and fourthly, she has to *remember* it if it is to prompt *behaviour change*. The third stage involving belief change may depend crucially upon the receiver's perception of the credibility of the source. Credibility is greatest when the sender is seen as both trustworthy and expert (Hovland, et al., 1953). Competent and knowledgeable nursing combined with a demonstration that the patient's needs are the nurse's priority should therefore establish nurses as credible sources for their patients. Interestingly, a fast and dynamic presentation of the message also appears to enhance credibility, probably because it gives the impression that the sender is knowledgeable (Miller, et al., 1976). Of course speed of delivery must also be matched to the receiver's decoding speed if comprehension is to be achieved.

Factors affecting persuasion

Our perception of the sender may affect yielding and in particular the manner in which we respond to the relationship between our beliefs and those they are expressing. Heider's (1958) balance theory proposes that if we like the sender we will want to match our beliefs to hers. If, for example, we like Nurse Smith and she approves of one technique and rejects another then we will feel most comfortable if we do the same. However, if we dislike Nurse Brown or regard her a member of an outgroup we may be unconcerned to find that we disagree with her. Indeed disagreement may be expected and merely reaffirm our commitment to our original contrary belief. Thus attempted persuasion by a disliked sender can have a counter-productive or boomerang effect. If we later find that Nurse Smith supports a political party we disapprove of then we will be in a state of cognitive imbalance; we like the sender but our views do not match. We can remove this imbalance by deciding that we do not after all like Nurse Smith or by rethinking our view of her political party. This of course means that there is a tendency for us to like people who have beliefs similar to our own (see Chapter 6, Section 2) and that by challenging others' beliefs we may reduce our popularity which may in turn jeopardize our credibility. Establishing rapport with patients and presenting oneself as trustworthy and expert is therefore a prerequisite to the difficult process of exploring and challenging patients' health beliefs.

The cognitive imbalance mentioned above is an example of the more general principle of cognitive consistency which seems to affect persuasion and belief change. Festinger (1957) proposed that when we are confronted with the inconsistencies in our belief systems we experience *cognitive disonnance* and are motivated to change beliefs. For example, if someone feels she cannot enjoy life without regular drinking sessions she may experience cognitive dissonance when it is pointed out that the amount she drinks is damaging her health. Much health education is aimed at creating such cognitive dissonance. However, dissonance does not ensure persuasion. Changing our beliefs in the direction suggested by the message is only one way to resolve dissonance. We can also search for other beliefs which support the challenged belief or try to minimize the importance of the inconsistency. In the case above the person may remind herself of others who have drunk as much as she does for many years and are still healthy, or she may decide that a longer healthier life is not as valuable as an enjoyable one. Unfortunately these alternatives are all too readily available to receivers of health education messages which induce dissonance. Moreover, the inconsistencies creating dissonance may not persist across social situations. Conversations with health-care workers may create genuine dilemmas and lead to intentions to change our behaviour but when we return to our friends and peers our old beliefs may be strongly supported and our new health-related resolutions may seem dissonant and misplaced. This reminds us that we need to understand the patient's social identities and subjective norms if we wish to have any lasting effect on health behaviour (see Chapter 3, Section 3; Chapter 2, Section 2). One way of combating the influence of others who may undermine our message is to expose the receiver to potential counter-arguments and provide ready-made refutations. It appears that such exposure and refutation can *inoculate* the receiver against later counter-arguments (McGuire, 1969).

The extent to which messages induce fear may also affect yielding. Discussion of important health beliefs such as perceived susceptibility and severity may induce fear. However, we can design messages which maximize or minimize such fear. Overall the evidence suggests that use of fear-inducing messages does promote belief and behaviour change. However, we must consider the effects of fear on particular receivers. If the receiver becomes very frightened then coping with this fear may be as important as responding to the health threat (see Chapter 9, Section 3). This may result in attempts to ignore or deny the threat. Receivers with low self-esteem and receivers who do not know what to do about the threat may react badly and resort to denial rather than yielding. Thus we should assess our receiver's coping capacity before we employ high fear-arousing messages. We should also advise patients on how to deal with fear-arousing threats and where possible try to enhance their self-efficacy. Leventhal (1970) showed that compliance is likely to be greatest when fear-arousing messages are combined with specific instructions on how to respond to the threat. We also need to consider the degree to which patients are repeatedly exposed to such messages as research suggests that belief change is reduced with multiple exposures to fear-inducing messages (Ley, 1988).

Even if we are successful in promoting belief change McGuire's model reminds us that this will have no effect on behaviour unless the receiver remembers the message. Ley (1988) discusses how we can improve patient's memory of health-related messages. *Stressing the importance* of different aspects of our message, for example information concerning treatment may enhance recall. We can also *repeat* messages and tell people what we are about to tell them before we tell them, that is use *explicit categorization*. Ley offers the following example of a doctor using explicit categorization;

> Now I'm going to tell you:
> What is wrong with you;
> What tests and investigations will be necessary;
> What the treatment will be;
> What you must do to help yourself get better;
> and what the outcome will be,
>
> First what is wrong – I think you've got bronchitis.
> Secondly, what tests and investigations are
> necessary – you will have to have an X-ray and a
> blood test to make sure.
> Thirdly what the treatment will be. . .(Ley, 1988 p. 80)

Memory is also likely to be improved if we use *simple language* and *specific rather than general* instructions, for example 'do not drink more than two pints of beer a day and do not drink any spirits' is more likely to be recalled than general advice on 'limiting units of alcohol consumption'. Also, *the things which we say first* may be remembered better due to what is known as the primacy effect. Finally, but importantly, memory may be greatly improved if we can provide readable and easily understood materials which patients may refer to later when they are alone.

To summarize then there are a number of factors which nurses must take into account if they are to communicate effectively with patients and influence their health behaviour. First, they must establish a good working relationship so that they are perceived as liked and trustworthy communicators. Secondly, they must explore the patient's health beliefs and shape their communications to build upon or perhaps challenge these beliefs. Thirdly, they must remain aware of the multiple channels which the patient may be using in decoding their messages and where possible use both verbal and non- verbal channels in an integrated fashion. Fourthly, they must assess the patient's ability to decode different kinds of messages and encode their message in a manner which it will be easy for the patient to understand. This may include choosing a time when the patient is in an optimum state to receive and understand communication. Finally, our tendency to forget what we have been told means that our messages should be encoded in a manner that makes them easy to remember.

3 Psychological Care and Communication

Informational care

Studies of patients' anxiety have demonstrated that psychological interventions may be an essential part of patient care even when the main
problem is identified as physical. Patients' psychological reactions to
physical illness can themselves constitute a serious threat to health
requiring nursing attention. Nichols (1984) reviews evidence suggesting
that illness-induced anxiety and depression may be widespread amongst
patients receiving physical treatment. Yet, because doctors and nurses
focus upon the physical illness and its treatment they may fail to acknowledge and respond to this psychological distress (see Chapter 4, Section 2).
Nichols points out that such distress may reduce compliance, increase
the probability of future illness, increase health service usage and at worst
lower patients' survival chances. Thus neglecting these psychological
reactions not only leads to patient suffering but also undermines the
efficiency of health-care services.

Monitoring and responding to such psychological reactions requires
specialized nurse–patient communication. Communication in which the
nurse takes time to ask about, and listen to the patient's, fears, worries,
health beliefs and feelings about herself. This involves offering the patient
emotional support and information which is directed primarily towards
maintaining their *psychological* well being. Nichols emphasizes that such
communication is central to the provision of care and refers to it as
informational care. He argues that it should be regarded as an important
role-related obligation for health-care workers and given greater priority
in the planning and provision of patient care. Communication aimed at
helping the patient to *cope effectively* with their condition may be necessary *before* nurses can communicate about compliance or preventive
behaviour.

Health-care workers often attempt to minimize patients' anxiety by not
telling them the whole truth about their prognosis or possible side-effects
of treatment. Such secrecy may be well intended but its effectiveness
as informational care is not supported by available evidence. Nichols
(1984) and Ley (1988) review a number of studies examining patients'
wishes concerning the communication of bad news. These studies not
only demonstrate that patients want to be told but that when they are
given bad news they do not generally react in a destructive and distressed
manner. Indeed the evidence suggests that distress is caused by a lack
of information. Patients who are not told the truth are unlikely to remain
in blissful ignorance of their condition. Rather their fears may be even
worse than reality and without reliable information they are likely to
feel uncertain and unable to take appropriate action. This is likely to
lower self-efficacy, promote helplessness, maintain high anxiety levels

and inhibit interaction which might generate social support (see Chapter 6, Section 3). Even in the case of a terminal prognosis the knowledge that time is limited can enable patients to arrange their affairs, see important people and seek support in preparing for death. These active coping responses which may include expressing sorrow and upset are likely to enhance the patient's sense of self-worth and minimize distress. Thus we must conclude that withholding information from patients is not in their interests. Informational care requires open communication and support in dealing with bad news.

Communication-based nursing interventions

Many studies have demonstrated that appropriate communication can reduce patients' anxieties. Hayward (1975) for example, found that providing extra information could reduce patients' reported pain and use of analgesics as well as helping them to sleep. Many other studies have shown that communication-based interventions can reduce anxiety, reported pain, analgesic use and duration of hospital stay for surgical patients (Egbert, et al., 1964; Boore, 1978; Wilson-Barnett, 1984). Weinman and Johnston (1988) point out that it is important to identify the nature of patients' anxiety and provide corresponding information at the appropriate time. They distinguish between *procedural* anxiety which includes worries about what will happen and what will be felt during a procedure (for example an operation) and *outcome* anxiety which refers to worries about the findings or results of a procedure. In reviewing 22 studies of communication-based interventions with surgical patients Mathews and Ridgeway (1984) divided the interventions into provision of:

1. *procedural* information which helps patients to understand what will actually happen during a procedure;
2. *sensation* information which helps them to anticipate how they will actually feel during or after a procedure;
3. *instructional* information which helps them control their actions or behaviours appropriately;
4. *relaxation training* which helps them to deliberately relax and reduce muscle tension and;
5. *cognitive coping training* which helps them anticipate and deal with their psychological responses.

It is worth noting that last three of these categories include interventions which go beyond providing information and aim to act directly upon the patients' thinking and behaviour (see Chapter 7, Section 4). Mathews and Ridgeway concluded that the provision of information, including sensation information as well as cognitive coping and relaxation training can be effective in reducing patient anxiety and promoting recovery.

Despite the evidence suggesting that communication-based interventions are effective their impact on nurse clinical practice appears to be minimal (Wilson-Barnett, 1984). This may be because nurses and indeed doctors have difficulties of their own in establishing open communication with their patients.

4 Problems in Communicating with Patients

Effects of health problems on communication

Patient's health problems may of course interfere with their capacity to encode and decode messages and patients with mental illness or mental handicap may have special difficulties. Lebet and Levinson (1973) report that those diagnosed as depressed have lower levels of verbal activity and communication initiation as well as slower response speeds. Argyle (1988) showed that those diagnosed as having schizophrenia are poorer than average at using non-verbal channels and Bryant, et al., (1976) found that almost one-third of their sample of people diagnosed as neurotic lacked basic conversation-maintenance skills.

People with reduced intellectual functioning due to dementia or mental handicap have difficulties in learning and may have limited communication skills. Stansfield (1986) reported that nearly 76% of adults attending mental handicap training centres had some difficulty with communication. Communication skills also deteriorate when people live in institutions which provide little opportunity for discussion and self-expression. Communication skills training may therefore be an essential component of rehabilitation programmes preparing patients for community care. People with mental handicaps, especially if these are compounded by sensory impairment or neurological problems, may, however, show slow progress in developing communication skills. Their development may need to be monitored through detailed assessment procedures. Nursing patients with special communication difficulties will usually involve careful assessment of understanding and flexible exploration of the effectiveness of different types of message using various communication channels.

Patients' physical health problems can also affect their capacity to communicate. Motor dysfunctions can prevent the transmission and reception of messages, for example the sending of verbal messages may be inhibited by temporary localized conditions such as laryngitis or by long-term general conditions causing dysphasia such as cerebral vascular accidents. Non-verbal communication may be affected by difficulty in initiating or controlling movements caused by motor-neuron disease and injuries to the nervous system as in cerebral palsy. Sensory impairments affecting patients' abilities to see, hear and feel also affects their ability to send and receive messages. Temporary impairment may result from treatments such as the application of dressings to eyes or ears, the removal of spectacles or hearing aids and the side-effects of drugs while irreversible impairments may be the result of disease, trauma or aging. Sensory aids and the development of new skills to compensate for the loss of function in a specific channel (e.g. loss of hearing) may restore the patient's capacity to communicate and thereby greatly enhance their quality of life. Assessment of such communication difficulties and interventions designed to facilitate communication may be an essential first step in patient care.

Patients' psychological responses to their condition (for example, pain) and the care environment (for example, a busy hospital ward) may affect their memory and lead to defensiveness or avoidance in their communication with nurses (Nichols, 1984). Anxiety is one of the most common reactions to illness and anticipated treatment or tests. Johnston (1980, 1987) has shown that surgical patients may be unusually anxious for many days before and after an operation and may worry not only about the outcome of the operation but about what will happen afterwards and the effect on their families. If such worries are not addressed they may disrupt nurse–patient communication. Weinman and Johnston (1988) reviewed studies suggesting that anxious patients may attend more closely to bodily sensations and signs of threat than non-anxious patients. Anxious attention of this kind can perpetuate high levels of anxiety and cause misinterpretation of health status. This can in turn affect the way in which patients report their experiences, feelings and symptoms and may distort assessment procedures which rely upon patient reports. Unnoticed anxiety may also lead to decoding and memory failures which mean that patient's do not understand or remember instructions, advise or explanations. Thus failure to accurately perceive and monitor patients' anxieties can also seriously disrupt nurse–patient communication.

Jargon and comprehension

In addition to tackling role-related, communication barriers nurses may need to reflect upon the language they use in communicating with patients. Professional socialization provides health-care workers with useful technical vocabularies which facilitate efficient communication amongst themselves. However, use of such vocabulary with patients may create barriers if patients have not learnt to decode this technical language and are therefore unable to understand health-care workers' messages. From the patient's perspective such language may be incomprehensible jargon serving only to highlight her ignorance and lack of control. Ley (1988) reviewed a number of studies which have shown that patients' understanding of medical terminology used by doctors and nurses is limited. In a well-known study Boyle (1970) showed that although doctors were able to agree amongst themselves about the meaning of common medical terms and the location of organs within the body many adult patients did not share these understandings. For example, only 52% of the patients in the study chose the same definition of 'palpitation' as the doctors and only 20% chose the anatomical location of the stomach. Only 46% chose the doctor's position for the kidneys and surprisingly 3.5% located the kidneys in the testicles! Clearly then doctors and nurses must be very careful to assess patients' understanding of their bodies and illness processes before discussing these issues. This problem may be even more acute with children. Eiser and Patterson (1983) suggest that children below the age of 10 may have very vague ideas about the construction and functioning of their bodies. Nursery school children's understandings may be even further from medical orthodoxy. Wilkinson (1987) reports that they tend to think of 'germs' as round, blue, between 1 and 9 inches in diameter and able to move between people by crawling up their legs without being noticed! If these differences in understanding between health-care worker and client are not acknowledged then mis-understanding, incomprehension and low compliance may result.

Inappropriate use of technical language also has important implications for patients' feelings about themselves, their perceptions of nurses and the kind of relationship they wish to develop with them. Technical language can be thought of as particular kind of 'language code'. Argyle, et al., (1981) described language as having a high and a low code which were more or less appropriate in different social situations. High code is characterized by complex and jargon-filled language is most appropriate in formal settings involving specialized expertise, for example in educational settings or official reports. Low code, by contrast, is informal, casual, direct and simple. It is most appropriate for interactions in day-to-day encounters. The use of such language codes carries messages about role relations and the nature of the social situation in addition to the meaning of the words used. Use of high code may convey high social status, expertise, power and social distance. This may alienate patients not accustomed to high code. For example, a patient may attempt to use medical terminology to describe her illness or treatment in order to establish a reputation of being interested, informed and motivated. However, if she fails in this attempt she may have to resort to low code again and may suffer embarrassment and a sense of powerlessness (Hauser, 1981). Equally, patients who are conversant with high code may feel insulted when health-care workers use low code, for example referring to genitals by gesturing downward, and asking 'How are things down below?' Ideally the health-care worker listens to the terms used by the patient and encodes her messages in these terms, introducing new terms with full explanations only when clarity demands it. A sensitive matching of professional language to patient understanding is crucial to successful relationship building and patient satisfaction.

Doctor–patient communication

Studies of doctor–patient communication are informative because they demonstrate general points about communication with patients and highlight patient difficulties arising as a result of doctor–patient communication (Hauser, 1981). Doctors' professional socialization may encourage them to view communication with patients as a means of checking the validity of a diagnosis and providing treatment instruction. Helfer (1970), for example, reported that first-year medical students were better able to elicit interpersonal information about a child's illness from mothers than more senior students. He suggested that medical education focused doctors' attention on factual information and thereby reduced their capacity to explore other important aspects of patients' experience. Byrne and Long (1976) studied a large sample of general practice consultations and found that individual doctors displayed a consistent communication style across different patients thereby failing to adapt to patient needs. Such inflexibility may be the result of limited opportunities to study and develop communication skills after qualifying. Byrne and Long observed seven communication styles which they arranged along a dimension from patient-centred to doctor-centred. At the patient-centred end doctors tried to discover and make use of the patient's concerns, health beliefs and expectations regarding treatment. In these consultations patients became informed decision-makers drawing upon the doctor's expertise. However, such styles were rare with more than three-quarters of the doctors using doctor-centred styles. These consisted of doctors making decisions, giving patients information and instructions and then terminating the consultation. Most patients were therefore reduced to passive recipients of doctors' judgements and directions.

Doctor-centred approaches to communicating with patients may be widely adopted as a means of maintaining control over consultations and minimizing the time they take. This justification is clearly expressed by one of Byrne and Long's doctors who was also responsible for training other general practitioners:

> The doctor's primary task is to manage his time. If he allows patients to rabbit on about their conditions then the doctor will lose control of time and will spend all his time sitting in a surgery listening to irrelevant rubbish. . . (Byrne and Long, 1976, p. 93).

The mistake in this logic is that the patient's views are not irrelevant. They affect interaction within consultations and more importantly compliance with treatment advice beyond the consultation. Short consultations which leave concerns unresolved and key beliefs unexplored may actually undermine the efficiency of health care by reducing compliance. Byrne and Long emphasize the importance of greeting patients and establishing rapport. This is an important way of influencing patients' first impressions of the doctor which may in turn determine the patient's willingness to discuss their problems. The following greeting, for example, is unlikely to facilitate relationship building and communication;

Doctor: Good morning. The weather is nice outside isn't it? Sit down, I'm just finishing these notes.
Patient: It's raining.
Doctor: That's nice.
(Byrne and Long, 1976, p. 34)

Encouraging patients to feel at ease and express their views is vital because they find it difficult to raise concerns and are reluctant to ask for information (Korsch, et al., 1968; Ley 1988). Overcoming this reluctance and discovering the patient's real reasons for attendance is, however, essential to successful consultations. Byrne and Long show that consultations are more likely to go wrong if the doctor fails in this task. Time may be wasted because the patient only raises her main concern at what seems to be the end of the consultation forcing the doctor to begin the problem-solving process all over again. Worst still the patient's main concern may not be addressed at all creating dissatisfaction. As Korsch and colleagues put it;

a few minutes spent getting acquainted with the patient's ideas and expectations would save the physician time later on and make for a more satisfactory doctor–patient relationship (Korsch, et al., 1968, p. 868).

Supporting this view Hughes (1983) compared two practices which arranged consultations of different average lengths. He found that the practice employing longer consultations required fewer patients to make follow-up appointments and had fewer patients who made new appointments within four weeks.

Combining data from a number of studies of doctor–patient communication Rotter (1989) concluded that time spent on partnership-building and information-giving increase patient recall, satisfaction and compliance whereas question-asking appears to reduce recall and compliance. Establishing rapport and addressing patients' concerns appear to be more important to consultation effectiveness than fact finding.

Nurse–patient communication

Inadequacies

Nurses may try to compensate for limitations in doctor–patient communication (Hockey 1976). However, there is substantial evidence that nurse–patient communication is also also problematic. Studies by Menzies (1970), Stockwell (1972) Hayward (1975), Faulkner (1979; 1985), Macleod

Clark (1981; 1984) Speedling (1982) and Ashworth (1982) have consistently underlined inadequacies in nurse–patient communication. Collectively these studies suggest that nurse–patient communication remains enmeshed within the role-relations of ESO medicine and fails to provide informational care (see Chapter 4, Section 2).

Menzies (1970) reported that a task-focused, rather than a patient-focused, interaction style undermined relationship continuity and personalized care. This was combined with a denial of feeling and emotion which served to objectify patients. Stockwell (1972), Faulkner (1979) and Macleod Clark (1981) found that nurse–patient conversations tended to be short and to concern the performance of nursing tasks rather than exploring patients' beliefs or anxieties. MacLeod Clark (1981), for example, found that nurses spoke more than twice as much as patients and that less than 2% of their conversations concerned psychological or social aspects of the patient's condition. These studies also reveal strategies used by nurses to actively avoid acknowledging patients' concerns and answering their questions concerning prognosis and treatment. MacLeod Clark (1981) found that nurses often asked closed questions requiring only a 'yes' or 'no' answer or leading questions which suggested a particular response. Such communication tactics severely limit patients' opportunities to widen the conversation or introduce their own concerns. This is especially unfortunate since studies of nurse–patient communication mirror those of doctor–patient communication in showing that patients are reluctant to ask questions or trouble nurses with their anxieties. Even when patients' do introduce their problems they may be ignored. Nurses may resort to platitudes, pleasantries or irrelevant distractions in order to avoid confronting patients' concerns. MacLeod Clark (1981) refers to such stereotyped responses as 'nurse-ese' and offers the following example of a nurse failing to respond to a serious concern by abruptly terminating the conversation with a distraction:

Nurse: There you are dear OK? (gives tablet)
Patient: Thank you. Do you know I can't feel anything with my fingers nowadays at all.
Nurse: Can't you? (minimal encouragement)
Patient: No I go to pick up a knife and take my hand away and it's not there any more.
Nurse: Oh broke my pen! (moves away)
(Macleod Clark, 1981, p. 16)

Clearly nurse-ese is not directed towards the provision of informational care and undermines the aim of holistic care promoted by many nursing models. Indeed it may increase patient anxiety and distress (Nichols, 1984; Wilson-Barnett, 1986). It is, nevertheless, widespread. Even in psychiatric nursing where communication might be regarded as a primary therapeutic resource nurse–patient communication is surprisingly infrequent.

Studies by Altschul (1968), Cormack (1975) and Oppenheim (1955) showed that no more than 13% of psychiatric nurses' time was spent talking to patients. Similarly in the care of people with mental handicaps Oswin (1978) and the National Development Group (1978) reported that mentally handicapped people in residential care spent many hours each day without any contact with staff. These latter findings are particularly disturbing as good communication is prerequisite to facilitating the psychological and behavioural development which can maximize independence and coping amongst people with psychiatric problems or learning difficulties (see Chapter 7, Sections 2 and 4).

Explanations

One explanation for these findings is that nurses' good intentions regarding nurse–patient communication are undermined by a lack of time and staffing resources (Hockey, 1978). Undoubtedly nurses are often hard pressed to deal with their workloads and would benefit from better resourcing. However, this does not provide an adequate explanation of their poor communication with patients. In many studies *nurses who had time* to interact with patients used this time to avoid doing so. Macleod Clark (1981) and Wells (1980), for example, found no correlation between the quality of communication and the time available. It would seem that this pattern of nurse–patient communication is not imposed upon nurses but created by them. An alternative explanation of this seemingly destructive communication pattern is required.

Just as doctor-centred communication with patients may be an attempt by doctors to retain control of their consultations so nurse-ese can be seen as an attempt to control nurse–patient relationships and the nature and timing of nursing work. We noted in Chapter 3, section 1) that nurses' stereotypes of patients tended to be structured around perceptions of cooperativeness and that unpopular patients were often those perceived to be demanding. If nurses define their role primarily in terms of obligations to deliver physical treatments within fairly fixed timetables then aspects of nurse–patient interaction which interfere with this work will be viewed as disruptive and unwelcome. Thus within the framework of ESO medicine (Chapter 4, Section 2) nurse-ese is an effective way of discouraging interaction which might divert the nurse from her primary role responsibilities. Nurses, like Byrne and Long's general practitioners, control and limit patient communication in order to protect themselves and their time from potentially distracting but apparently peripheral aspects of nurse–patient interaction.

There are many aspects to this control and protection. At a simple level the time taken to explore patient concerns may disrupt routine time-keeping (Waitzkin and Stoekle, 1972). Patient controlled communication may also generate unpredictable emotional responses. Menzies (1970) suggests that a task focus and the depersonalization of nurse–patient relationships serves to protect nurses from acknowledging the emotional reality of their patients' experiences, thereby minimizing nursing stress. Limited nurse–patient communication may also contribute to impression management by protecting nurses from discussion of the limits of their expertise and knowledge. Bond (1983), for example, noted nurses' anxieties about their abilities to deal competently with patient inquiries. Such anxieties may be especially prevalent amongst inexperienced nurses who may have most face-to-face contact with patients (Melia 1981; Macleod Clark, 1981). Nichols (1984) argues that nurses' concerns regarding their competence and the possibility of making mistakes leads them to protect themselves from responsibility by limiting communication. Patients inquiries may be redirected to doctors who are portrayed as both expert and responsible. This protection from responsibility is one of the main benefits of adopting an obedient or servant role in relation to an authority figure. By following orders we, like Nurse Dontz, (see Chapter 4, Section 3) can absolve ourselves of responsibility for decision-making. This is one of the attractions of the nurse's position in Stein's (1968) doctor–patient game (see Chapter 4, section 2).

The function of nurse-ese in controlling patient communication and thereby protecting nurses from threatening aspects of their work underlines the need to consider nurse–patient communication in the context of wider issues of nurse and patient role definition. The approach to communication advocated by recent nursing models and encapsulated in Nichols' conception of informational care has wide ranging implications for the role of the nurse in relation to both doctors and patients. Adopting such patient-centred approaches to communication involves redefining the core elements of care and the role-related responsibilities of the nurse. This has implications for nurse training and the organization of nursing work and could have an important effect on patient satisfaction and compliance.

Improvements

An awareness of problems relating to nurse–patient communication is foundational to understanding nurse–patient relationships. One approach to improving communication would be to extend the amount of time devoted to these issues in nurse training programmes. Traditionally the development of communication skills has been given low priority in both general and psychiatric nurse training (Faulkner, et al., 1985a; Shanley and Murray, 1986). However, there are signs that this is beginning to change. For example, a recent three-module post-basic course for staff nurses in Scotland includes a compulsory module on interpersonal and communication skills. A focus on the relationships between nurse role-definition, nurse–patient communication, patients' beliefs and health behaviour during basic training would enable nurses to clarify the functions of communication before registration. Such study could be enhanced by greater attention to the teaching and practicing of patient-centred communication skills.

An important element in communication skills teaching is the development of self-insight. Awareness of our own feelings offers insight into others' perceptions and emotional experiences and a heightened awareness of how we regularly communicate with others provides the opportunity for conscious efforts towards change. The use of verbal and video feedback provide powerful techniques for prompting such development (Trower, et al., 1978). Such training may be especially important if nurses hope to facilitate psychological and behavioural change in patients (see Chapter 7, section 2).

5 Communication Through Non-Verbal Channels

Using non-verbal channels

We have focused primarily upon verbal channels because we have been concerned with descriptive or representational communication about the patient's health. However, nurses might also benefit from training in the use of non-verbal channels because we are often unaware of the messages others receive from us through these channels. In other words our non-verbal messages tend to be 'given off' rather than deliberately sent. The lack of control over these channels is sometimes referred to as 'non-verbal leakage'. We can, however, gain a degree of control over our non-verbal presentation and thereby influence others' impression of us. Reflecting upon our use of non-verbal channels, using video feedback to observe ourselves and practising non-verbal presentation can all increase our control. In this section we shall briefly explore some of the available non-verbal channels and their relevance to nurse–patient communication.

Ironically discussion of non-verbal communication can involve communication problems because of the different categorizations used to describe non-verbal channels (see for example Fraser, 1984). It is useful to begin by reminding ourselves that 'non-verbal' communication includes all communication which does not use language. Thus many aspects of communication using the voice, that is *vocal communication* can be categorized as non-verbal. Our use tone, or *intonation*, for example, is one aspect of non-verbal communication. Other elements of speech such as 'ums', 'ahs', coughs, hesitations, rate of speech, accent, and so on, have been classified as *para-language*. Facial expression and body movements have been grouped together as *kinesics*. This category includes a number of important non-verbal channels such as gaze, facial expressions, hand movements, touch and body postures. In addition we communicate through our clothes, hairstyles, furniture and other belongings. These decorations and accompaniments can be classed as *regalia*.

There has been some debate about the relative importance of verbal and non-verbal communication. However, as Fraser (1984) points out this question can only be answered in relation to particular communication functions. In other words verbal communication may be more important for some messages and non-verbal channels for others. Attempting to explain a diagnosis to a patient through non-verbal channels would be very inefficient. This kind of explanation is an example of *representational communication*, that is a message which serves to describe some aspect of our shared world, for example, the physiological processes which give rise to certain symptoms. Verbal communication is especially useful for this kind of communication in which we seek to convey our representations of reality to someone else.

However, we often use non-verbal channels when we wish to send messages about ourselves or our relationships with others. Fraser refers to this type of communication as *interpersonal communication*. Argyle (1972) and his colleagues have demonstrated that non-verbal channels are very important in conveying messages of this type. Argyle, et al., (1970) showed that non-verbal communications concerning power relationships (for example, superiority or equality) were more effective than verbal messages designed to covey the same content. Similarly, Argyle, et al., (1971) highlighted the importance on non-verbal channels in conveying friendliness or hostility towards others. Such interpersonal information is of course vital to our perception of others. Thus gaining control of non-verbal channels is crucial to impression management and therefore to our social acceptance and the influence we have over others. We manage our regalia by dressing appropriately for different occasions and we can manage our facial expressions, gaze, touch and body postures to ensure that we convey desired impressions and avoid unwanted stereotypes (see Chapter 3). At the same time we must be conscious of our own perceptions based on others non-verbal presentations. In the United kingdom for example English accents may prompt different stereotypes to Scottish ones. Scottish people have been shown to regard a person with an English accent as more intelligent, self-confident, ambitious, wealthy and prestigious while regarding those with Scottish accents as more likeable, friendly and generous (Cheyne, 1970; Giles and Powesland, 1975). This reminds us that nurse stereotypes of patients may be triggered unthinkingly by aspects of non-verbal communication which patients may not have control over. It also explains why some people seek to change their accents!

A third function of communication is the *regulation of communication* itself. If we frown when listening to someone they will usually pause and perhaps repeat or rephrase what they have just said. This because they are watching our facial expression for information on our decoding of their messages. This type of information on how others understand us is often referred to as 'feedback'. Thus our frown provides feedback indicating that something has gone wrong with our decoding. Much of the glancing at one other which goes on during conversations serves to regulate turn taking and check understanding without having to use verbal communication. This use of non-verbal channels is convenient as it allows verbal communication to proceed uninterrupted. Skilled use of non-verbal channels can, for example, allow a chairperson to control a meeting largely through use of gaze, facial expressions and gestures, thereby minimizing disruption to the discussion. We also use intonation and para-language to convey that we want to speak or that we are about to finish speaking (for example, clearing the throat can signal the beginning of a speaking turn).

Context and meaning

It is important to note that non-verbal communication, like verbal com-munication takes place within a context of culture-specific rules which affect the way in which messages are decoded. Thus the same non-verbal messages may mean different things to receivers from different cultures. We have already noted Jourard's observation of the difference in everyday touching across cultures (see Chapter 4, Section 1). In high-contact cultures body contact may be viewed as an expression of friendliness whereas the same contact in the United Kingdom may imply a very intimate relationship. Similarly a British businessman attempting a Black American handshake (that is 'giving skin') or continuing to hold hands while talking (in the fashion of some Arab men) may be thought to be bizarre and disapproved of. Patterns of eye contact also vary across cultures. Direct focus on the eyes is expected amongst Arabs, Latin Americans and Southern Europeans while Asian peoples and Northern Europeans adopt peripheral gaze or no gaze at all (Mayo and LeFrance 1973). Encountering someone from another culture who uses non-verbal channels differently may lead to mistaken inferences about their attitudes or intentions. For example, deviation from direct gaze may lead Latin Americans to suspect someone's motives while deviations from peripheral gaze may make Asians uncomfortable (Watson 1970). Thus working in a multicultural society may pose communication problems unless we attend closely to the different rules which people use to regulate their non-verbal communication. We must be particularly suspect of negative first impressions of those from different cultures.

We have noted that social rules change across situations. Even within the same culture the same non-verbal gesture or sound may mean different things in different situations (even to the same receiver). An example is provided by the case of a young man who was arrested, charged and fined for making the sound 'miaow' to a policeman and his dog. The policeman claimed that in the circumstances the 'miaowing' constituted 'threatening and abusive behaviour' and his interpretation was upheld in court. In other situations, for example, when stroking one's neighbour's cat 'miaowing' might be seen as expressing light heartedness or warmth. However, the meaning of the policeman's uniform and dog (his regalia) in terms of role-related rights and authority is fairly unambiguous and the young man's para-language was decoded as a challenge to the power and authority of the role. In this context then the 'miaow' became a mark of disrespect for the police role and thereby a challenge to law and order. Clearly we must judge the social situation carefully before 'miaowing'! This example illustrates that although we can attach general meanings to particular gestures, postures and sounds they are decoded by others in relation to the particular social situation we find ourselves in. The meaning of our messages depends upon the social context and of course, to make matters complex, the social situation may change as a result of our communications.

Types of non-verbal communication

Unconscious non-verbal communication may impair nurse–patient communication and conscious control of non-verbal channels may improve it (French, 1983). Gaze, body posture and facial expressions are all used to convey messages about our interest in another's communication and our willingness to communicate with them. People communicating with us continually monitor our responses and need constant feedback concerning our understanding and reactions. If, for example, we lean away from someone who is talking to us and look elsewhere they will assume we are not interested and be reluctant to continue. We may appear more friendly, interested and accessible if we adopt *an open body posture* (where our body is not covered by folded arms and legs) and if we orientate our body towards the person we are speaking to. Indeed when we feel comfortable with another person we may find ourselves copying or *mirroring their posture*. Such postural mirroring can communicate interest and friendliness. We also use our facial expressions to communicate that we understand others. If, for example someone tells us about a surprising incident we may raise our eyebrows and then nod to indicate our understanding of how surprised they felt. Using non-verbal channels to communicate *interest and attentiveness* may facilitate nurses' exploration of their patients' beliefs and concerns. On the other hand communication may be prohibited by a lack of such non-verbal encouragement. If we walk in a hurried fashion leaning forward and avoiding eye contact people are unlikely to begin conversations with us. This walk has been called *busy gait* and may be used unconsciously by nurses concerned about work schedules. It sends a clear message to patients that the nurses are too busy to deal with their concerns and thereby reduces nurse–patient interaction.

Patients' health problems may interfere with their non-verbal communication and nurses must again be careful to monitor their person-perception processes in order to avoid misleading inferences. For example, where vision is inhibited the patient may not look at those she is communicating with in the usual manner. This may cause confusion about whose turn it is to speak leading to interruptions and dysfluencies (Wiener et al., 1972). Sustained gazing by patients with impaired vision or inadequate skills in social interaction may seem to convey intimacy or an attempt to dominate or intimidate but may merely reflect an effort to attend and understand. Similarly a failure to make eye contact by a patient who is highly anxious or depressed may not convey dislike or an unwillingness to interact. Loss of control of facial muscles as in Parkinson's disease can also disrupt non-verbal communication and use of other channels may be necessary to fully appreciate the patient's intended meaning. These examples illustrate how patients' non-verbal communication must be sensitively considered in light of their particular difficulties.

Nurses' role-related rights include rights concerning touching. They are 'licensed touchers'. Touch is regularly used in nursing to move patients and their bodies, to support them, to carry out observations, to reassure, to restrain and to communicate. These uses of touching may be divided into functional or *instrumental touch* directed towards another purpose and communicative or *expressive touch* used to convey feelings or intentions. Hollinger (1980) notes that expressive touch may be used to communicate trust, empathy and openness to further communication. It can also clarify and encourage verbal communication and thereby facilitate relationship building and understanding between nurses and patients. McCorkle (1974),for example, showed that touch accompanying verbal communication made it more meaningful to patients and resulted in nurses being seen as more caring. Aguielera (1967) observed that touching psychiatric patients led to increased verbal communication and encouraged patients to approach others more frequently. Expressive touch may also have therapeutic effects. Lorensen (1983) showed that mothers who received stroking and affectionate hugs in a maternity setting had shorter labours and perceived nurses as more helpful in relieving discomfort during labour.

However, nurses do not touch all patients equally. Barnett (1972) found that age affects touching. Nurses between 18 and 25 were found to touch patients most and patients between 26 and 30 were most frequently touched. Interestingly, adult patients who were touched least were mainly over the age of 65 years. Another group of patients who may not be frequently touched are those with with physical impairment (Watson, 1975). This failure to use expressive touch with older and more disabled patients seems unfortunate as they may be particularly likely to benefit if they have difficulties in using other communication channels.

Although expressive touch is a powerful communication channel it must, like all other touching, be managed within a framework of open communication if it is not to be misunderstood. If used insensitively touching may evoke embarrassment or hostility and increase rather than alleviate patients' anxieties and discomfort. Not all patients welcome touching. Patients who have strong feelings of persecution, who are confused or have difficulty in maintaining contact with reality in psychosis may respond negatively to insensitive touch, leading to antitherapeutic reactions. Gender differences mean that men are generally less willing to accept touch and may be especially uncomfortable with with intimate touch by male nurses (DeWever, 1977) Whitcher and Fisher (1979) suggest that being touched implies a degree of dependence which may conflict with mens' attempts to preserve their sense of masculinity during illness. Thus sensitive assessments of patients' moods and needs must proceed effective use of touch.

Regalia in the form of uniforms and the organization of space within care settings may also have important effects on nurse–patient communication. Uniforms may create communication barriers and a number of studies in psychiatric settings suggest that replacing uniforms with mufti has beneficial effects on patients. Walsh and Ashcroft (1974) and Newnes (1981), for example, demonstrated that patients' attitudes towards and interaction with nurses improved when they wore mufti. Furniture and use of space may also create physical and symbolic barriers to communication. Sitting behind a desk or standing at a distance establishes social separation and conveys messages about friendliness and role relationships (Argyle, 1972). Indeed even the orientation adopted when sitting around a table can have dramatic effects on communication. Pietroni (1976) found that when general practitioners sat on the corner of a table at 90 degrees to the patient six times more interaction was observed than when they faced each other squarely across the table. Square-on, face-to-face meeting across a table seems to imply confrontation and inhibit communication. Relationships with others are also represented by use of distance and height. Those with greater authority or rights, for example, are usually entitled to greater space and height (Henley, 1977). For example, a patient lying in bed or sitting in a wheelchair is in a low status position relative to a nurse who is standing up. Literally looking down on patients in this way is likely to discourage dialogue. It may therefore be necessary to adopt a more equal positioning before beginning discussion.

The organization of rooms and buildings may also affect nurse–patient interaction. Communicating with patients in their homes involves different rules to hospital-based communication. The home setting may equalize role-related rights because the nurse who is now a guest in the patient's home. Even within hospitals different areas may be seen as belonging primarily to nurses or to patients. Canter (1984) points out that parts of a ward or clinic may be seen as more or less appropriate settings for particular types of interaction. Patients may, for example, be more willing to approach a nurse near their bed bay and less inclined to do so near a nursing station or office. Thus communication may be inhibited by the separation of nurse and patient areas. Such spatial organization may also inhibit communication between health care workers who have no common territory.

CORE IDEAS IN CHAPTER 5

- Health care workers attempt to enhance their patients' health by influencing their behaviour. Such influence frequently depends upon persuasive communication aimed at altering patients' health understanding.

- Communication can be analysed into stages. The sender encodes her message in various channels which the receiver decodes in order to achieve a shared understanding. Breakdown can occur at each stage.

- Persuasive communication depends upon the receiver attending, comprehending, yielding, remembering and changing their behaviour.

- Establishing sender credibility through perceived trustworthiness and expertise is prerequisite to persuasive effectiveness.

- Confronting inconsistencies in our belief systems creates cognitive dissonance which may prompt belief changes.

- Fear arousing messages may promote change but should be accompanied by information on how to cope with the threat.

- Stressing the importance of messages, repeating them, using specific instructions and providing explicit categorization makes messages more memorable.

- Monitoring patients' psychological responses to illness and providing appropriate informational care may reduce patient distress, enhance nurse–patient communication and promote treatment compliance.

- Health problems and disabilities affecting motor and psychological functioning make communication more difficult.

- Jargon may undermine patient comprehension and thereby reduce compliance.

- Studies suggest that nurse–patient communication is typically brief and task-orientated and that nurses avoid exploration of patients' concerns by ignoring them and using closed questions and distractions.

- This pattern of communication may be the result of nurses' attempts to control the timing and content of their work. Avoidance of patient concerns protects nurses from timetable disruption, emotional upset, challenges to their knowledge and responsibility for decision-making.

- Adoption of patient-centred communication will require re-defining the nurse role so as to prioritize informational care.

- Conscious control of non-verbal communication may enhance nurse–patient communication. Verbal channels are especially useful for representational communication while non-verbal channels can be effectively used for interpersonal communication and interaction regulation.

- The meaning of non-verbal signals can be altered by shifts in the relevant situational rules and roles.

6

Relationships and social support

1 Relationships in Nursing

Nursing as relating

Whether dealing with a person who is experiencing psychological problems, a physical illness or learning difficulties, the nurse's relationship is likely to have a major effect on the person's well-being. Nursing is essentially a reciprocal and dynamically changing relationship between patient and nurse. Most of the major models of nursing, reviewed by Fawcett (1984), view the patient's understanding of their social environment as crucial to their state of health and identify the nurse–patient relationship as a major determinant of the effectiveness of nursing interventions.

The Changing Role of the Nurse

Until the 1970s the caring role of general nurses prescribed in nursing textbooks was largely restricted to physical aspects of patient care in hospital settings. Armstrong (1983) traces the changing role of the general nurse and shows that, psychological aspects of the nurse–patient relationship had been generally overlooked. Quoting from Gordon Pugh's (1969) *Practical Nursing* he notes the limiting roles assigned to the nurse and her patient;

> the passivity of both actors in the relationship is confirmed by the role assigned to the patient: he will abide by instructions and will cooperate in the carrying out of the treatment (Armstrong, 1983, p. 457).

Armstrong also emphasizes the lack of attention given to to nurse–patient communication. With the nurse's role of facilitating change being limited to setting patients' a good example:

> by being graceful, nicely turned out and looking fit and well she (the nurse) could convey a sense of good health, well-being and happiness to the patient (Armstrong, 1983, p. 457)

Many nursing textbooks cited by Armstrong portray a similarly mechanistic view of the nurse–patient relationship. However, since the publication of these late 60s and early 70s textbooks, greater emphasis has been given to the use of interpersonal skills in nursing interventions.

Two factors are primarily responsible in this trend. First, changes have occurred in the philosophy of health care provision towards greater self-reliance and reduced dependence on health service agencies. In this new philosophy the role of the general nurse increasingly involves encouraging change in patients' behaviour in order to increase compliance promoting health through lifestyle changes. Facilitating change in dietary habits, work routines, leisure activities and helping patients develop new ways of coping with stress may all be included in general nursing interventions (see Chapter 2, Section 1, Chapter 7, Sections 1-4 and Chapter 9, Section 3). Thus interpersonal and therapeutic skills which had previously been regarded as part of psychiatric and mental handicap nursing are now recognized as pertinent to all areas of nursing.

The second factor concerns the social needs of the population. Social change has generated increasing diversity and instability in social relationships within our society (Toffler, 1971). This may result in more psychological and physical problems which require interpersonal interventions. According to the Central Statistical Office (1985) figures for the United Kingdom there are one million single parents, one million people aged under 65 years living alone and three million over 65 years living alone. These people may be 'at risk' of inadequate social support and we shall see that those lacking social support in the form of close confiding relationships are more prone to physical and psychological disorders. Instability of social relationships also increases the complexity of people's relationship networks. For example, one in three marriages ends in divorce in the United Kingdom and most of those who get divorced remarry. Men tend to marry younger women and children may be relating to a series of parent figures. Such complexity in relationship networks may have implications for the priorities and motivations of patients and for the effective delivery of care.

The changing position of women has also affected relationship networks and the availability of social support (see Chapter 4, Section 5). In 1951 approximately one quarter of married women were at work or seeking work. Today this figure is two-thirds. Their work is mainly part-time and low-paid and most women have a 'double shift' in that they work in employment and at home. In many cases they may be the sole bread-winner and still maintain this double shift. Role conflict is a major source of stress and increased stress and reduced social support results in a greater susceptibility to illness. Understanding the social context in which patients' health problems arise may improve care planning particularly in the assessment and promotion of patients' social support.

The general acceptance by the nursing profession of a holistic approach to helping patients cope with social and health problems has developed in the context of these social trends. It involves a focus upon health promotion through identifying lifestyle factors threatening patients' health. The main medium through which the nurse promotes health-inducing behaviour change is a helping or enabling relationship which is equally important to those with physical or psychological problems. In the United Kingdom the importance of interpersonal skills and relationship development within nursing has been clearly acknowledged in the recently introduced 'Project 2000' Diploma courses.

2 The Social Psychology of Relationships

The relating self

Our relationships with others are inextricably linked to our self concept. The development and maintenance of our self representations is based on our relationships with others which are in turn shaped by how we see ourselves (see Chapter 3, Section 4). William James (1890) was one of the first writers to consider our self-concept and included in it our representations of body and mind, clothes and home, spouse, children, ancestors, friends, perceived social reputation and personal possessions. Experiences involving any of these may affect our sense of well-being and self-worth. James recognized that our awareness of self developed through interaction and Cooley (1956) extended this idea coining the term 'looking-glass self' to describe the way in which our self-representations incorporate others' evaluations of us (see Chapter 3, Section 3). Mead (1934) continued this work, proposing that we see ourselves in terms of our perceptions of how others see us, that is through 'reflected appraisals' (see Chapter 1, Section 3). Of course not all these appraisals are of equal value to us. Early in our lives our parents or other caretakers have the most important effect on our sense of self, in later childhood our peers' opinions of us have an increasingly greater impact, and in later life our sexual partners' perceptions will greatly influence our self-concept. The self-concept then consists of a range of social identities which develop and become salient in relation to particular others throughout our lives (see Chapter 3, Section 3).

When a person is subjected to constant criticism by others whose opinion matters to her, the result is likely to be a lowering of that person's opinion of herself. Lowered self-esteem, in turn, affects our confidence and motivation in interaction with others. Similarly, when a person experiences constant approval, the result is likely to affect her relationships with others. She is likely to assume others feel positively about her and to feel good about herself. Perceived self-efficacy (see Chapter 2, Section 3) is also important to our self-representation (Gekas and Schwalbe, 1983). For example, a nurse who discovers that she runs a ward or community service effectively is likely to commit this knowledge to her self-concept, thereby raising her self- esteem and enhancing her ability to relate to others.

The patient's self-concept may be adversely affected by illness, injury or treatment. Patients' self-concepts incorporate many social identities and roles, some of which are more valued than others (see Chapter 4, Section 1). For a patient whose sense of self is founded on being athletic an injury that disables her may result in considerable identity problems. She can no longer value herself for her strength and agility and will have to identify new aspects of herself which are worthwhile and perceived as valuable by others. Nursing assessment and intervention should therefore explore the effect of illness and treatment on patients' self-concepts and identify ways in which patients can successfully consolidate or recreate a valued sense of self. Stereotyping may threaten such assessment because our stereotypes may include mistaken assumptions about what patients' value. For example, dismissing the loss of sexual responsiveness as unimportant for an elderly person may result in a failure to recognize his considerable adjustment problems.

Impression management and relationship building

We noted in Chapter 3 (Section 2) that we manage our social reputation by deliberately presenting a particular view of ourselves to others. The impression management strategies we employ will depend upon how we think others regard us and on how we see our role-related rights and obligations. These strategies have particular implications for our power, self esteem and relationships with others. Many strategies which result in short-term influence over others or a temporarily elevated sense of self esteem may undermine attempts to develop a trusting and enabling relationship. Jones and Pittman (1982), for example, identified five major self presentational strategies, namely, ingratiation, intimidation, self-promotion, exemplification and supplication that may be counter productive.

Ingratiation is employed to appear likeable, for example by complimenting the other person and agreeing with her opinion. Use of this strategy involves many positive self-presentation features such as friendliness, listening to others and seeking agreement. However, self esteem gained from such interaction depends upon censoring oneself to please others and giving up rights to influence the course of the interaction. Ingratiation is therefore unlikely to engender any real exchange of views and will not facilitate change or development in others. Moreover a nurse, using this strategy to build a non-threatening relationship may be seen by her patient as sycophantic and perhaps dishonest.

Intimidation involves the use of role-related rights or physical presence to arouse fear in others. It is an attempt to control interaction without regard for the others' views and feelings. The stereotype of the ward sister as a 'dragon' conveys this image of persuading patients to comply with the hospital regimes and treatment programmes with little concern for their needs or wishes. While authority figures may use this strategy effectively within their recognized jurisdiction (for example, on the ward) it is unlikely to promote behaviour change beyond this setting (see Chapter 4, Section 3). For example it is unlikely to be effective when the nurse encounters the patient in her own home, where the nurse must adopt a guest role.

Self-promotion involves presenting oneself as competent and important at the expense of others' interests and achievements. Self-promotion may be accomplished by taking the lead in conversations, describing one's assets and achievements and failing to show interest in others' conversations. Although this may temporarily raise one's self-esteem it makes interaction unrewarding for others and so inhibits the development of trusting or understanding relationships. *Exemplification* also involves elicit attempting self-respect through highlighting one's own importance. In this case through claiming moral superiority for one's opinions and actions. Again this strategy is costly for others who are portrayed as inferior and is unlikely to foster relationship development.

Supplication involves attempts to gain sympathy from others. An example of this approach is the patient refraining from doing things for herself in the hope that the nurse will do them for her. This strategy may generate temporary control over others but it also fosters dependence and may erode self-efficacy. An opposing strategy is to reject help in an attempt to gain respect and approval for self-reliance. Although such independence has many positive aspects depriving others' of legitimate helper roles may lead to resentment and failure to share problem management with others who are trying to maintain caring relationships. For example, patients' failure to allow nurses to assist them deprives nurses' of their legitimate role performance and may thereby undermine the nurse–patient relationship (Kelly and May, 1982).

Clearly none of these self-presentational strategies are likely to promote honest communication or the development of an enabling or helping relationship. Their use by health-care workers is likely to undermine their professional effectiveness by diminishing their ability to understand and influence their clients in the longer term. Their use by patients may, however, express a need to bolster self-esteem in the face of threatening situations which undermine their sense of self-worth. Nurses may be able to meet such needs without rewarding self-centred, distancing or coercive interaction. For example, by clarifying that a patient's views and abilities are important and worthy of respect, without necessarily assuring them that they are correct or extraordinary a nurse may short-circuit self-promotional or exemplification strategies. In this way she may be able support continued relationship development while also modelling communication strategies which facilitate the development of a constructive nurse–patient relationship.

The Development of Relationships

Social psychologists have considered a number of factors affecting relationship development. However, no single factor seems to determine whether people will grow to like one another. Rather, different factors seem to influence particular types of relationships at different points in their development. One way of understanding the influence of these factors is to view relationship development as a series of decision points at which we pursue meeting, talking and sharing with another person or decide to withdraw our time, attention and intimacy. Duck (1977) has proposed that we typically manage our relationships through various types of withdrawal. At different stages of a relationship factors such as living or working closely together, physical attractiveness, common interests, and sharing beliefs and values may influence whether or not we withdraw from a relationship. Other interests and demands also limit the degree to which we engage with people we meet. People are therefore 'filtered out' of our network of relationships at different stages of relationship development (Kerckhoff and Davis, 1962).

Accessibility is prerequisite to relationship development and a number of studies have highlighted its importance. Caplaw and Forman (1950) showed that the greater the physical and functional distance between apartments, the less likely friendships were to develop between occupants, where functional distance refers to factors that bring people into face-to-face contact such as a common footpaths stairway or lifts. Similarly, Nahemow and Lawton (1975) showed that, in a city housing project for the elderly, most friendships developed between individuals living on the same floor. Ebbesen, et al., (1976) found that best friends living on a university campus lived closer together than other friends and Byrne (1961) showed that those who sat together in classes were more likely to develop friendships. The first filter in relationship development then is how easy or difficult it is to interact with another person. Although interaction with people we dislike may generate more intense dislike we generally tend to like people better as we meet them more often and get to know them better (Jorgensen and Cervone, 1978).

Even when we have an opportunity to interact with someone we may choose not to or deliberately limit the time we spend with them because of what we infer about them from their appearance (second filter). Our stereotypes allow us to make assumptions about others on the basis of their age, sex, race and general physical appearance (see Chapter 3, Section 1). For example, people whose appearance corresponds to culturally established ideas about what is 'good looking' may be better liked because others stereotype them as more intelligent, sensitive, kind, outgoing, warm, and so on (Dion, et al., 1972; Berscheid, 1981). An attractive physical appearance colours our first impression to the extent that a physically attractive person is more likely to have his or her written work evaluated favourably, to be successful at job interviews, to be judged effective in counselling others and to be regarded as psychologically well adjusted. Consequently people who are considered unattractive have to work harder to avoid being 'filtered out' of potential relationships at an early stage.

Reiss et al., (1982) suggest that stereotypes concerning appearance may affect the relationships and lives of men and women differently. They found that attractive men and women benefited from such positive expectations and had more enjoyable social contacts. However, while attractive men were found to be more assertive and have a lower fear of rejection (than less attractive men), attractive women were less assertive and less trusting of men (than less attractive women). Attractive men also had more social contacts than less attractive men but this difference was not evident amongst women. Perhaps surprisingly, these results suggest that 'good looking' men benefit to a greater extent form our attractiveness stereotype than good looking women!

The 'what is beautiful is good' inference following from such stereotypes may also shape nurses' initial perceptions of their patients. Damrosch (1982) showed that student nurses' rated attractive adults more positively and Bordieri et al., (1984) found that qualified nurses saw attractive pediatric patients more favourably (than less attractive children). The face is a major source of inference about people's behaviour and personality. For example adults whose facial features resemble those of a child, that is, relatively large eyes situated low on the face are assumed to *be* childlike, being seen as less dominant, less astute, more honest, warm and kind (Berry and McArthur, 1985a, b). Clearly, attractiveness stereotypes have an important impact on our first impressions of others. We are more likely to unconsciously withdraw our time and attention from those we regard as less attractive because we expect to find them less rewarding. Since less attractive clients deserve an equally attentive service from health-care workers, it is important that we monitor and question our feelings of attraction and disinterest in relation to particular clients.

Other stereotypes may also determine who we are motivated to develop relationships with. Morgan (1985) for example reported that student nurses had more negative perceptions of black patients than white patients. Student nurses also tend to have less positive attitudes towards the elderly than younger people which is reflected in difficulties experienced in recruiting nurses to work with elderly people (Goebel 1984; Kayser and Minnigerode, 1975). Sex stereotyping is also important (see Chapter 4, Section 5). Healthy men may be stereotyped by health-care workers as independent, active and competitive, while healthy women may be expected to be more submissive, concerned about their appearance and excitable (Broverman, et al., 1970). These stereotypes have particular implications for the rehabilitation of people who have experienced psychological problems. For example, women who display independent, active and competitive behaviour may be regarded as less well adjusted than those who conform to feminine stereotypes.

The development of relationships may also be affected by gender socialization which orientate men and women towards different relationship-management styles. Wheeler, et al., (1983) found that, for both men and women, avoiding loneliness was dependent upon having meaningful interactions and spending time interacting with women. The value of interactions with men depended upon how meaningful the interaction had been to the person concerned but interacting with women tended to be generally positive regardless of the intrinsic worth of the meeting! Moreover, men who had more meaningful interactions with other men tended to be those who had spent more time with women. This suggests that femininity is associated with the ability to create intimacy and closeness in interpersonal interaction and that men who spent more time with women may improve these social skills.

Once we get beyond initial perceptions and begin to develop a relationship a third major filter is the perceived similarity of others' attitudes, beliefs and values to our own. Byrne (1961b) argued that the perception of attitudinal similarity affects interpersonal behaviour in many walks of life. Bank managers tend to authorize bigger loans to people with similar attitudes, jurors tend to be more lenient to defendants who hold similar attitudes and racially prejudiced white people may express liking for black people with similar attitudes. Byrne (1961b, 1971) proposed that we value interaction with those who agree with us because it supports or validates our perceptions of reality. Similarly, Duck (1975) noted that we may prefer those who hold similar attitudes because we assume that they will value us for such support. This corresponds to our discussion of persuasion in Chapter 6 (Section 2). Heider's (1958) balance theory suggests that believing another person shares our views makes it easier for us to like that person because such a relationship produces no cognitive dissonance (Festinger, 1954).

Learning about others' beliefs and attitudes is therefore an important aspect of relationship development. We may choose to spend more time with those who agree with us and as a result may begin to adopt more of their views on other subjects. In this way attitudinal similarity may become more important than geographical proximity once a relationship begins to develop. Newcomb (1961), for example, found that although proximity initially shaped student relationships, attitudinal similarity became more important in determining relationship maintenance over time. In explaining marriage choices Murstein (1977) suggested that although couples may be initially attracted by appearance, attitudinal similarity becomes more important in maintaining or terminating the relationship once it develops. He proposes that if the relationship continues a degree of attitudinal similarity may be taken for granted and the way the couple are able to integrate their various role-related behavioural routines may become more important to continued closeness and intimacy (fourth filter) (see Chapter 4, Section 1). For example, the expectations they have regarding the role-related obligations of a boyfriend and girlfriend may allow them to impress and please one another or alternatively shock and upset each other! Where role performances seem to be incompatible the relationship may break down despite established attitudinal similarity. Murstein refers to these three latter stages of relationship development as the 'stimulus' (or appearance) stage, the 'value' (or attitudinal similarity) stage and the 'role' (or role performance match) stages. The model is therefore referred to as 'S-V-R theory' (Murstein, 1977; Murstein, et al., 1977).

Filter theories apply to situations where people have a relatively free choice about who they interact with. Clearly, they do not adequately account for the development of nurse–patient relationships in which it would be inappropriate for a nurse to disengage from patients because she found that they did not share her values. In order to fulfill her role-related obligations the nurse must continue to foster relationships with patients who fail Murstein's proposed 'relationship tests'. She must continue to relate to those she is not initially attracted to, those she disagrees with and those who challenge her expectations of how patients should behave towards nurses.

However, understanding how and why people pursue and withdraw from relationships may help nurses to understand and reflect upon their feelings towards particular patients. Off duty, the nurse may withdraw from interaction because of attitudinal clashes or role performance incompatibility but in her professional capacity the nurse must continue to look for ways of establishing a constructive nurse–patient relationship. She must seek to understand the patient's perspective and identify what the patient may be gaining from a particular self-presentational strategy. An understanding of judgemental processes involved in relationship development may help her monitor and control her responses to patients and her own self-presentation strategies. This understanding may enable her to cope with issues likely to militate against the growth of a helping relationship and facilitate the development of particular relationships with individual patients.

3 Social Support and Health

Social networks and social support

The amount of support we receive from others depends largely on our social networks, that is, the set of relationships we maintain with family members, friends and neighbours. These networks can be categorized in terms of size and density. Some people have small social networks, interacting only with a few people, while others have large networks involving many relationships. Some networks are dense in that there is a high level of interaction with others while others are loose with less interaction.

The kind of social networks we maintain and therefore the amount of social support we receive has been found to depend upon a number of factors, including the size of our local community, marital status, age and ability to mobilize support (Broadhead, et al., 1983). People living in a community with a population of less than 2500 are likely to enjoy greater informal support than city dwellers. Those who are married generally receive more informal support than those who have never married who, in turn, receive more then those who have been widowed. Those who have been divorced tend to receive least social support. As we get older our social networks shrink in size and the amount of informal support received decreases. Retirement marks a particularly important change in working people's social networks. Our individual ability to mobilize social support also determines how much we receive. We begin to learn support-seeking skills in infancy and people who lack appropriate communication skills or who have learnt to be self-reliant or resigned to helplessness receive less social support than those who actively seek information, advice and emotional support.

Social support is increasingly seen as psychologically complex. Wortman and Dunkell-Schetter (1987) identified several types of support. They include expression of positive feelings, including indications that one is cared for or held in high esteem and, as discussed above, the expression of agreement with or acknowledgement of the appropriateness of one's beliefs and feelings. Invitations to disclose and discuss beliefs and feelings, offers of advice and information or access to new information sources are also forms of social support. These types of support may be vital to the establishment of a helpful relationship, whether this is a friendship or a professional counselling relationship (see Chapter 7, Section 2). In addition to such psychological support the provision of material aid, for example money, or skilled assistance with tasks, such as helping with housework or childcare, are important forms of everyday social support. Finally, reassurance that one is involved in a relationship or a network of relationships which could potentially provide help may in itself be a powerful form of support. Thus we seek to gain different forms of support within the rules and constraints of the different types of relationships which make up our social networks (see Chapter 4, Section 1)

Assessment of social support

By understanding the structure of patients' social networks nurses may be able to maximize health-inducing social support and minimize the detrimental effects of patients' relationships. Such understanding must be based upon an assessment of the patients' social network, the social support she typically receives and the level of demand and stress experienced in her everyday life. Nurses may regularly conduct informal assessments of this kind by observing the patient's interaction with family and friends over a period of time. Such observation may, however, be unsystematic and biased by the nurse's own inferences about patients' relationships. An alternative approach is to ask the patient a series of questions about people who are important to her. Table 1 shows a series of such questions adapted from Dean (1986).

This exploration of the patient's social network may heighten her awareness of those she could approach for help which may in itself have beneficial effects. Cohen and Syme (1985) suggest that such awareness of sources of help is a very important factor in how well people cope with stressful events (see Chapter 9, Section 3). Assessing the nature of the person's social network will also help the nurse identify patients whose health may be 'at risk' due to a lack of social support and may indicate whether the patient is likely to comply with advice or treatment. For example, an obese person with hypertension may be less likely to change her lifestyle if network members regard the discomfort of exercise and the trouble of changing eating habits as too high a price to pay for greater health (see Chapter 2, Section 2). In such cases the nurse may identify members of the patients' network as important health promotion targets.

Table 1   Assessing Social Networks

Question	Dimension assessed
Who are the people who are important to you in some way or with whom you are in touch regularly? Please list them.	Size
What does each of these people do that makes them important to you?	Function
What are their relationships with you?	Composition
How long have you known each person?	Duration of relationship

If you really need help, which of these people would offer it to you?
    financial help
    help at home
    help with family matters
	Perceived social support

In which of these people do you confide?	Intimacy

To which of these people would you offer help?
    financial help
    help at home
    help with family matters
	Reciprocity

Which of these people make you feel good about yourself?	Esteem
Which of these people know one another?	Density
Which of these people agree with your views?	Affirmation

Adapted from Dean (1986)

She may wish to involve the whole family in the health education aspect of treatment and/or refer the patient to a self-help group (see Chapter 8, Section 5).

The impact of social support on physical and mental health

One of the first studies of the impact of social networks on health was Durkheim's (1951) investigation of suicide. He concluded that very low or very high density networks, that is social isolation or too many relationships, could both increase the likelihood of suicide. In another classic study, Faris and Dunham (1939) found a close association between living in run-down areas in Chicago and being admitted to psychiatric hospital. They explained this in terms of social isolation, proposing that a lack of everyday social constraints encouraged inappropriate social behaviour and left people more susceptible to hallucinations and delusions. Such studies suggest that relationships with others are vital to sustained mental health.

It is worth noting, however, that studies, such as Faris and Dunhams', which simply show a relationship between two variables are unable to clarify how these variables influence one another. Although Faris and Dunham proposed that isolation leads to unusual social behaviour or mental illness, the opposite could also be the case. Namely unusual behaviour might result in social isolation. Being able to establish the direction of causal relationship between such variables is one of the strengths of experimental studies (see Chapter 1, Section 4). However, many social issues may not be practically or ethically amenable to experimental investigation. Thus in order to clarify the causal relationships a body of related studies of different aspects of the same issue must be examined.

In the investigation of social support researchers have looked at the protective effects of social support for people experiencing major life changes such as unemployment, retirement or bereavement (see Chapter 2, Section 4). Gore (1978), for example, looked at men who had been made redundant. The men's social support was assessed in terms of their relationships and social activities with partners (if present), relatives and friends. On this basis they were divided into two groups, the relatively supported and the relatively unsupported. The groups showed no difference in length of unemployment or economic deprivation. However, the unsupported group had higher average scores on a measure of depression, reported more physical complaints and showed greater physiological changes such as high serum cholesterol levels. These results suggested that the men who were receiving adequate social support were better able to cope with the stress of redundancy and so suffered fewer ill effects (see Chapter 9, Section 3). Similar findings have been reported in relation to social support for people who have suffered a bereavement (Clegg, 1988 – see Chapter 7, Section 2).

In a large-scale longitudinal study, Berkman and Syme (1979) monitored a random sample of almost 5000 adults aged between 30 and 69 for nine years. They found that the most isolated group of men (measured in terms of marriage, contact with close friends and relatives, church membership and informal and group associations), had a mortality rate which was *two to three times higher* than the men with the most contacts. The difference between socially isolated women and women with most contacts was *marginally higher*. Again these findings suggest that social isolation threatens our well-being.

One of the best-known studies in this area is Brown and Harris' (1979) investigation of the relationship between life events, social support and susceptibility to depression amongst women in London. The researchers conducted in-depth interviews, exploring the women's understandings of various life events and the social support they experienced. They found that life events with long-term threatening implications such as discovering a spouse's unfaithfulness, redundancy at work or a close friend's life-threatening illness were associated with depression. Women who had experienced such a threatening life event were four times more likely to develop depression if they did not have a close, confiding relationship with someone they saw more than once a week. The lack of such a confiding relationship did not in itself predict depression, suggesting that threatening life events may lead to depression but are much less likely to do so if we are supported within a close relationship. In other words unsupported women were able to cope so long as they were not exposed to serious life stress. Similarly, Morgan, et al., (1986) concluded that;

> a strong confiding relationship may be of particular importance in protecting people from depression following a severe life event, whereas other forms of social support may be of considerable importance on a longer-term basis (p. 261).

It seems as if reliable close relationships act as a buffer against the stress experienced when we are confronted with threatening life events (Cohen and Hoberman, 1983). Oatley (1988) points out that many of these threatening life events involve loss of a major role or social identity and so deprive people of an important aspect of their self-representation (see Chapter 3, Sections 3 and 4). He argues that depression results when the person is unable to identify an alternative role in which they can reconstruct their sense of self-worth. Thus the protective power of close relationships may be that they enable people to appreciate that others value them and to experiment with new ways of thinking about themselves after losing important everyday elements of their 'self'.

These studies suggest that maintenance of a person's well-being may be strongly influenced by the social support she receives. Mumford, et al., (1982), for example, found recovery to a state of well-beings also affected by social support. Their findings demonstrated that the average length of stay in hospital was two days shorter for patients receiving social support than for those without support. Similarly, Gruen (1975) found that, after their first heart attack, patients who were given supportive psychotherapy, that is shown attention, reassurance, positive feedback and encouragement, spent fewer days in intensive care and were discharged from hospital earlier. These patients also showed less evidence of congestive heart failure and supra-venticular arrythmia and were rated as having less anxiety and less retarded activity at a four-month follow-up. Other studies report that such supportive interventions lessen the likelihood of mental distress in those recovering from physical illness (Spiegel, et al., 1981) and injury (Bordow and Porritt, 1979).

Sosa, et al., (1980) examined the effect of support on women giving birth to their first child (primigravidae). One group had an untrained, lay woman attend them from admission to delivery, while a second group had no such support. The lay woman talked to the mothers and offered physical contact, for example rubbing the mother's back. Standard practice in this Mexican hospital had been to exclude relatives and family members to avoid overcrowding. Thus women in the second group had no regular social contact during labour. The study showed that those attended by lay women had shorter average labours (8.8 hours compared to 19.3), were more likely to be awake after delivery and stroked, smiled at and talked to their babies more often than the unattended women. The unattended women were also more likely to suffer problems, for example requiring a caesarian or becoming depressed after birth than the attended women. Overall, support appeared to promote unproblematic births.

The kind of social support most helpful to patients may depend upon their health problem and their role relationship with others. In studying cancer patients, for example, Dunkell-Schetter (1982) found that informational and emotional support was seen as most helpful. In patients undergoing radiation therapy more than 80% of the sample regretted that they were not provided with sufficient information and the opportunity to discuss the situation more fully (see Chapter 5, Section 3). Role relationships may also be crucial (see Chapter 4, Section 2). Advice from a doctor may be viewed as very helpful even when the same advice is seen as unhelpful when offered by relatives or friends.

Overall, it is clear that, whatever the social psychological mechanisms involved, social support promotes well-being. Nevertheless, further research is required to clarify how different types of social support have different effects on our well-being at different times. Currently different measures are included under the general heading of 'social support'. Some studies have used 'objective' measures of support such as number of friends, number of group memberships, attendance at meetings, number of visits to/from others and so on, while others have focused upon the person's perception of potential support. Moreover, few studies have examined how our need for social support and its impact may change across different states of health and during different stages of recovery.

Unhelpful Relationships

Despite the evident importance of social support people who fall ill may actually receive less support from family members and friends (Wortman and Conway 1985). In a study of breast cancer patients, 75% reported that they were treated differently by members of their social network. Of these, over half stated they were avoided or feared and almost three quarters felt they were misunderstood by others (Peters-Golden, 1982). Similarly, O'Brien (1980) found that haemodialysis patients' feelings of social alienation and estrangement increased over time.

Potential helpers' misunderstandings of others' needs may result in unhelpful responses. Helpers' may, for example, believe that they should remain cheerful and optimistic in their dealings with an ill person (Dunkell-Schetter and Wortman, 1982). However, if they feel they cannot live up to this expectation they may shun open discussion of illness and feel uncomfortable in interaction with the sufferer. This may lead to various forms of withdrawal. The ill person is likely to perceive this as rejection, and instead of the social network providing support at a time of crisis, the behaviour of its members may become an additional source of stress (Wortman and Conway, 1985), Peters-Golden (1982), for example, found that the majority of cancer patients regarded 'unrelenting optimism' as false and disturbing and that cancer patients who wanted to discuss their illness were considered less well-adjusted to their situation than those who avoided talking about it. The same study also illustrated how we can misunderstand other people's anxieties. Respondents felt that the most important worries of women after a mastectomy were the psychological and social implications of breast loss whereas in fact many women were more concerned about recurrence of cancer, death and treatment side effects (see Chapter 3, Section 2).

Misunderstanding may be based in misattribution. We noted in Chapter 4, Section 4 that our perceptions of others' need for help is affected by attributional processes. If we attribute people's predicaments to their own characteristics and activities we may retain our 'belief in a just world' and feel no obligation to help. This will undermine helping and may lead to insensitive and uncaring behaviour such as blaming the sufferer (Wills, 1985).   We have also also noted that helping is inhibited by the perceived costs to the helper. Relating to others who are disabled or in pain may be stressful to helpers, particularly if their efforts seem to have little effect. Thus potentially helpful relationships may cease to be helpful if a carer becomes demoralized and begins to count the cost of caring (Dunkell-Schetter and Wortman 1982). This may be particularly important to voluntary caring relationships in the community. If such relationships are to remain viable carers must acknowledge positive interpersonal benefits and limit the costs of caring. Orbell, et al., (1991) have suggested that this depends, not only on the actual demands of caring, but also on the degree of freedom carers feel they have in relation to caring demands. These findings emphasize the importance of supportive community services (such as day care and respite care provision). Such services enable people to *choose to care* rather than feeling trapped into caring obligations which may be seen as increasingly demanding and thereby gradually undermine helping relationships.

Social distance may be created by those who might benefit from help because they believe that their condition is disapproved of. Indeed many diseases and disabilities do elicit negative stereotypes from others including nurses (Chapter 3, Section 1). People with such 'stigmatizing' conditions conceal them, or minimize their apparent severity. Epilepsy is such a condition and Schneider and Conrad (1981) found that the most sufferers strictly controlled who knew about their condition. Such information control requires vigilant self presentation, voluntary exclusion from situations where exposure is threatened and may lead to self doubt due to lack of social validation. This control also eliminates potential sources of social support because fewer people are aware of the sufferer's needs. Health care workers, including nurses, may be excluded from sufferer's confidence limiting their helping role. By developing non-judgemental relationships we are more likely to invite others to disclose their troubles with us and so find ourselves in a position to offer social support (see counselling – Chapter 7, Section 2).

We have considered how social networks can have unhelpful effects on compliance and help seeking (Chapter 2, Section 2). This is illustrated by McKinlay's (1972) study of the uptake of maternity services by working class mothers. He divided a sample of 87 women into utilizers and under-utilizers on the basis of whether they attended ante-natal clinics before the seventeenth week of pregnancy and consequently became regular attenders. Under-utilizers were found to have more family and relatives living locally and to visit friends more frequently. They also reported having more non-professionals to consult about potential problems and tended to make more use of mothers and relatives than under-utilizers.

Family relationships can also be unhelpful and even damage the mental health of family members Critical psychiatrists such as Cooper (1967) and Laing (1967) have portrayed the family as inhibiting individual independence and self-expression. It has been suggested that the apparently bizarre and meaningless aspects of schizophrenic behaviour is an understandable response to the oppressive environment of the family (Laing, 1959; Laing and Esterson 1970). The management of family relationships is

therefore likely to have a crucial impact on the success of rehabilitation programmes in which patients return to their families. Brown,
et al., (1972) studied the family environment of schizophrenic patients discharged from hospital. They categorized families using five indicators of
expressed emotion; (1) the frequency of critical comments made about other
family members, (2) the presence or absence of hostility, (3) expressions
of dissatisfaction (4) warmth demonstrated towards the patient and (5)
emotional over-involvement with the patient. The researchers found that
a high level of expressed emotion in the family made it more likely that
the patients would relapse. This feature of family relationships was found
to be a much better indicator of likely prognosis than the patient's own
characteristics such as age, sex, previous occupational record, length of
clinical history or diagnosis.

4 Caring Relationships in Nursing

Social Support and Nursing

There are a number of reasons for regarding social support as central
to effective nursing practice. First, there is a considerable body of evidence suggesting that social support affects a person's physical and
psychological well-being. Secondly, social and medical changes have
increased the life expectancy of older and physically impaired people
resulting in a larger proportion of disabled members of society. These
groups are at risk of social isolation which in turn threatens their physical
and psychological well-being. Thirdly, nurses are in a position to intervene
successfully in the area of social support by providing direct support
or facilitating the growth and maintenance of patients' social networks.
Finally, nurses own performance may be enhanced by acknowledging the
importance of social support in dealing with stress in nursing (see Chapter
9, Section 2).

Direct Nursing Intervention.

Nurses may use their relationship with a patient to provide social support.
Such direct intervention is often aimed at helping the patient cope with an
immediate problem. In the longer term the nurse may promote independence by helping the patient to develop other separate relationships.

Wills (1985) discusses the various ways in which social support may
contribute to well-being. Consideration of these mechanisms can help in
planning nursing interventions. Relationship-based nursing interventions
include informational care (see Chapter 5, Section 3) and the provision of psychological support aimed at enhancing patients' self-esteem,
increasing perceived self-efficacy or reducing the perceived threat of

potentially stressful events (see Chapter 9, Section 1). Providing information includes primary prevention in which nurses' warn patients of the negative consequences of their lifestyle and help them plan change. It can also involve preparation for anticipated stressors (such as certain treatment procedures) so that the patient knows what to expect and has been able to rehearse a method of dealing with the experience (see Chapter 5, Section 3). Finally, discussion of how a stressful experience affected the patient and how she coped with it may facilitate recovery and readjustment (see Chapter 7).

Another important aspect of social support is the perception that others will provide help if necessary. This faith in the helpfulness of our social networks appears to result in better physical and mental health (Kessler and McLeod 1985). It is therefore important for nurses not only to be helpful but to be perceived by the patient as willing to help. Considerable benefit, including higher self-esteem and increased perceived self-efficacy may result from perceived supportiveness. High perceived self-efficacy and a belief that one is held in high esteem promote positive emotions, help-seeking behaviour, willingness to accept help and more successful coping (Wills, 1985). Enhancing patients well-being through such independence-enhancing relationships is the opposite of the dependency-promoting role relationships we discussed in Chapter 4 (Section 2). The way in which nurses define their roles will dramatically affect patients experience of the nurse–patient relationship which may, in turn, affect their physical and psychological recovery.

Relationships also enable us to compare ourselves with others, either directly or through our discussion about them (see Chapter 3, Section 1). Festinger's (1954) *social comparison theory* suggests that we validate our understanding of social reality through such comparisons and that they have an important impact on our self-representations. Taylor (1983) has proposed that these comparisons help us to maintain a positive, sense of self which assists in coping with stress and adjusting to threatening events. Acknowledging that others are coping with similar problems and that we are as successful or more successful than they are allows us to maintain self-efficacy and self-esteem, even when facing serious threats. Nurses may be able to help patients make relevant social comparisons through discussion or by arranging meetings with fellow sufferers (see – self-help groups, Chapter 8, Section 5).

Indirect Nursing Interventions.

In Chapter 2 (Section 2) we noted the importance of 'subjective norms' to the adoption of health-promoting behaviours. Our social networks provide the bases for such subjective norms and nurses' may wish to promote patient compliance or increase patients' social support by acting upon key members of this network (in addition to working with the patient herself). Patients who have strong, dense networks are more likely to be influenced by them and nurses' may need to take account of these powerful relationships when planning interventions. Those closest to the patient may need to be educated about the patient's problem, her treatment and its consequences. If members of the patient's social network believe that the proposed treatment (for example, a particular medication) is ineffective or that a suggested behaviour change is unacceptable (for example, a dietary change) the patient is less likely to comply. We noted in Chapter 5 (Section 2) that the undermining effect of others may also be reduced by *inoculating* patients against others' potential objections to health behaviours.

In a project described by Dean (1986) nurses directed their intervention towards patients and a network member whose opinion were valued by the patient. The project focused on families 'at risk' of giving birth to premature and low-birth weight infants. In the first two trimesters (the first six months of pregnancy) the nurse dealt with diet, the use of alcohol and cigarettes, physiology, labour and delivery. In the last trimester the nurse prepared the mother and the network member for labour, delivery and care of the baby. Throughout the project, nurses paid attention to the influence of network members on the mothers' behaviour. They included network members who were close to the mother in the home visits and emphasized the importance of at least one person who would be available in times of stress. They also put the mother in contact with community services and self-help groups. By including network members in teaching sessions, eliciting and attending to their opinions and helping mothers to seek help within their social networks nurses were able to harness the influence of mothers' networks in promoting well-being and health behaviour.

Social networks can also be used to the patient's benefit in hospital settings. Rather than seeing a crowd of visitors around a patient's bed as a nuisance and the demands for information by relatives or friends as needless distraction from their 'real' work, nurses may regard visitors as sources of social support. Cooperating with the patient in communicating appreciation of visits and emphasizing the continuing need for contact after discharge can increase the social resources available to promote recovery. Visitors may also be involved in caring for the patient where this is appropriate and welcomed by the patient. Nurses should also be concerned if a patient does not receive visitors. In such cases, the nurse may help the patient identify potentially supportive relationships and encourage their development, thereby extending or strengthening the patient's social network. While this network is being developed, the nurse may herself offer a supportive relationship and arrange for other professional support.

Recognizing the influence of networks on patients' behaviour can also help nurses to understand and accept behaviour which might otherwise be condemned. Dean (1986) illustrates this point by discussing the reaction of hospital staff to a family who brought their child to the hospital after an appendix had ruptured and caused peritonitis. Family members were criticized because they 'should have known better' and this disapproval was reflected in the staff's dealings with the family. However, the history of relationships within this social network revealed that the decision to delay seeking help had been reasonable. The child had often pretended to be ill to gain attention and to avoid going to school. The response by the parents and by members of a close dense network was to ignore such behaviour because they believed that involving health-care professionals would encourage similar future behaviour. Thus the parents had acted out of concern for their child's development and earlier help-seeking would have risked the disapproval of network members' regarding their parenting skills.

Another indirect approach to increasing patients' social support is encouragement of social involvement through participation in clubs and organizations designed to cater for the patient's specific needs. The development of such groups supplements support provided by family, friends and the health service (see Chapter 8, Section 5). Setting up patients' groups may, however, be difficult and patients' may need to be persuaded to attend. Powell (1981) emphasized that staff should spend time interacting with potential group members and discussing the need for a self-help group before attempting to organize one. Again exploring the views of members of the patient's social network may be vital to success.

CORE IDEAS IN CHAPTER 6

- Maintaining a positive, helping relationship with patients is vital to encouraging patient compliance and well-being across nursing specialties.

- Changes in work and social organization may create instability in traditional relationship networks and leave people at risk of social isolation.

- Our management of relationships is strongly influenced by our self-concept (including self-esteem and perceived self-efficacy). Our self concept is in turn affected by others' approval (or disapproval).

- Patients' self-concept may be threatened by illness, injury or treatment and their reconstruction of self may be facilitated by supportive nurse–patient relationships.

- Relationships inherently involve impression management. However, some impression management strategies may inhibit relationship development.

- Relationship development may be understood as a series of filters which may lead to further closeness or withdrawal. Filters include proximity, correspondence to stereotypes (including physical attractiveness) perceived similarity of beliefs and attitudes and matching expectations in relation to role performances.

- Filter models assume that people are free to continue or terminate relationships. However, nurses' are obliged by their professional role to persist with patients from whom they would otherwise have withdrawn.

- The size, density and supportiveness of our social networks can have important implications for our physical and psychological well-being. As well as material assistance and interpersonal support the knowledge that we have potentially helpful relationships can enhance our self-concept. Such relationships seem to act as a buffer, protecting us from the worst effects of threatening life events.

- Nurses can actively and systematically assess patients' social support.

- Misunderstandings and self-protective attributions may inhibit relationship development and helping during illness, resulting in withdrawal and loss of social support. Relationships can also be unhelpful when they discourage help-seeking or compliance.

- Nurses can intervene directly to enhance patients' social support by developing caring nurse-patient relationships and indirectly by encouraging patients to seek and maintain supportive relationships with others.

7

Facilitating psychological and behavioural change

1 Nursing, Personal Change and Therapeutic Relationships

Promoting health -promoting change

Changes in patients' health understanding or their health-related behaviour is often crucial to preventing illness or ensuring appropriate treatment (see Chapter 2, Sections 2 and 3). When such change is simple and short term, as in the case of applying a dressing daily for a week, then compliance will depend primarily upon clear and memorable instructions (see Chapter 5, Section 5). However, where the required change involves giving up a favourite activity, especially where this activity has powerful personal or social rewards – as in the case of smoking or drinking – then even when communication is effective the patient may find it difficult to change their behaviour. Helping people change is therefore an important part of general health promotion.

Facilitating personal change is even more important in mental health. Here illness itself may take the form of psychological or behavioural problems and interventions are evaluated in terms of behaviour change. Indeed as we noted in Chapter 4 (Section 2) some psychiatrists have rejected the idea of 'mental illness' and sought instead to define a series of psychological and behavioural problems to be approached through therapy. Thus in psychiatric nursing facilitating change may be the primary mode of nursing intervention and the acquisition of therapeutic skills of vital importance in nurse training. Similarly nursing people with mental handicaps relies heavily upon facilitating learning and change. People with mental handicaps have difficulties in learning and specialized techniques may be required to promote learning which may be taken for granted by other people.

This emphasis on facilitating change may lead to a redefinition of the nurse role as *nurse therapists* (Barker, 1982; Barker and Fraser, 1985). This may mean adopting role obligations which have traditionally defined the roles of psychiatrists and clinical psychologists. Such an expansion of the nurse role could lead to more equal multidiciplinary team work between nurses, doctors and psychologists but it may also threaten valued social identities and create conflicts which will only be resolved through careful negotiation of professional role relations (see Chapter 3, Sections 3 and 4; Chapter 4, Sections 1 and 2).

Therapeutic relationships and techniques

A person may wish to change their behaviour because it threatens their physical health or because it undermines their ability to function in a socially acceptable manner. In either case, however, the involvement of a professional therapist implies a loss of behavioural control. People regularly change their behaviour without therapeutic interventions. They may take up a new sport, change jobs or start a new relationship. However, this is not always easy or unproblematic. We have noted that our everyday social competence depends upon stable representations of reality. This in turn means that change is often stressful and creates a need for increased social support (see Chapter 1, Section 2; Chapter 2, Section 4; Chapter 6, Section 3). This recognition that changing ourselves is difficult has led psychologists to study methods by which we can help one another achieve desirable changes.

We noted in Chapter 6 (Section 3) how important personal relationships were to psychological well being and physical health. Relationships can inhibit personal change because others discourage change which threatens their social identities. However, personal relationships can also promote and support long-term personal change. Professional therapists must develop relationships which support change without having to do everything else involved in everyday personal relationships. A therapist needs to relate to clients[1] in a friendly manner but cannot become personal friends with all her clients! Thus a therapeutic relationship is one in which one member deliberately uses interactive skills to encourage and support changes in the other. In such a relationship we utilize our interacting *self* in order to influence another's self (see Chapter 6, Section 2).

Facilitating change in others often goes beyond the provision of a supportive relationship. Since we rely on stable representations and routine sequences of behaviour therapists must utilize techniques which break down old routines and habits and establish – or 'routinize' – new behaviours through practice. We shall look at techniques which involve exploring and challenging client's world, changing their experience of their environment and changing their beliefs though talk therapy or 'conversational reprogramming'.

Ethical issues in therapy

When we decide to change our behaviour it is often because we feel others disapprove of us. We may go on a diet, for example, in order achieve a more acceptable body shape. However, changes which please others may not always be best for ourselves. Socially accepted body-shape stereotypes may encourage unhealthy eating and serious eating disorders such as anorexia or bulimia. This raises questions about how we decide that someone needs to change their behaviour. We often wish others would behave differently but we do not assume the right to force people to change unless they endanger us or society. However, if psychological knowledge *can* be used to promote long-term change which persists across different contexts then it is possible that it could be used to change others' behaviour without their consent. Indeed psychological knowledge is applied in torture when isolation, sensory deprivation or punishment are employed to change people's behaviour against their will.

Such ethical concerns oblige would-be therapists to address some important preliminary questions. First, if a behaviour is seen as a problem, who's problem is it? If a hospital patient becomes disruptive is the disruptive behaviour primarily a problem for the staff or for the patient? This can be a difficult question because a person's behaviour may create problems for them because of others' reactions. Secondly, is the client's participation in the therapy voluntary; do they actively want to change themselves? This can also be a tricky question especially when the client is a child or a person with a mental handicap who may have an incomplete understanding of their behaviour or the therapeutic relationship. Thirdly, is the therapeutic relationship operating primarily for the client's benefit? The therapist must be careful not to allow her needs (for acceptance, reputation or financial reward) to affect her therapeutic relationships with clients. There are no simple answers to these questions but they must be addressed in order to avoid the inappropriate use of psychological therapies. The guiding principal here as in the use of other treatments is to seek informed consent and to evaluate the therapy in consultation with the client. We refer to *facilitating change* to emphasize our view that such interventions are only viable or justifiable when the client is committed to change.

2 Counselling: Facilitating Change through Interpersonal Skills

What is counselling?

In everyday conversation 'counselling' is used to describe many types of meetings but this lay use does not always correspond to its psychological definition. We can approach a definition by identifying interactions which are sometimes referred to as 'counselling' but which do not involve psychological counselling. For example, when a student or patient is not living up to others' expectations they are sometimes said to require 'counselling'. In practice this may mean that someone should tell them what other important members of their role-set expect (see Chapter 4, Section 1). It may also mean that they should be given some sound advice on how to meet these expectations or warned of the consequences of failing to do so. 'Counselling' may even be thought of as a 'telling off' for causing others unnecessary trouble. In all these instances the aim of the so-called 'counselling' would be to bring someone's behaviour into line with others' expectations. This is *not* the aim of psychological counselling and none of the above interventions are examples of psychological counselling.

Counselling cannot be imposed and it is fundamentally concerned with helping people to make their own decisions and to act effectively in relation to their own self-representations. It involves providing a caring and respectful relationship within which a client can consider some aspect of her life and deal with it to her own satisfaction. The counsellor may be professional or voluntary but in either case she must be able to establish a suitable relationship with her client and to use particular communication skills to facilitate the client's development. Interactions which deviate from these basic principles are inappropriately referred to as 'counselling'. Thus although leading, teaching, advising, diagnosing, and providing treatments can all be helpful none are appropriate within a counselling relationship (cf. Wilson-Barnett, 1988).

The counselling relationship

Social relationships are vital to our well being and are regulated through implicit rules which ensure that participants meet each others social needs (see Chapter 6, Section 2). However, the counselling relationship is unusual in that it is not reciprocal. It is devoted to meeting the needs of the client. Of course the counsellor may have self-esteem and role-related reputation needs met through offering an effective counselling service but the relationship must exclude the counsellor's other needs if it is to be effective. If the relationship operates to meet the counsellor's needs then the primary function of facilitating the client's self-development is undermined. A relationship which, for example, fulfilled a counsellor's desire for affection or admiration might promote self-limiting dependence in a client. Thus if a counselling relationship becomes distorted by the counsellor's needs it ceases to serve counselling aims and if this is not recognized the relationship may become unprofessional, unethical and exploitative.

Carl Rogers has been an influential figure in the development of counselling practice. He argued that the quality of the relationship between counsellor and client was not only crucial to facilitating change but sufficient in itself to promote such change (Rogers, 1957). He specified three characteristics of such a therapeutic relationship; *empathy, genuineness and unconditional positive regard*. Empathy refers to the ability to understand the client's experiences and feelings in the same way as she does. It involves adopting the client's own meanings and values when considering her experiences and communicating this so that the client is assured that the counsellor has an accurate understanding of her experiences. The client must also be assured that the counsellor is honest and genuine in her concern. This implies the abandonment of professional facades and role-related rights which protect us from becoming personally involved with others' emotions and feelings. The counsellor must be open to involving her*self* with the client's self including the client's perceptions, fears, and hopes. Such genuine involvement promotes trust and confidence in the relationship. Finally, unconditional positive regard refers to an unselfish love for the client that does not depend upon her behaving in a manner approved of by the counsellor. This unconditional care provides a non-threatening context in which the client can explore herself as she really is. This is vital if the client is to disclose and explore aspects of herself which she thinks others' may disapprove of.

An important feature of the counselling relationship which is not addressed by Rogers' list of three prerequisites is the management of *responsibility*. Counselling aims to enable clients to help themselves by changing their thoughts, behaviours or lifestyles. This involves establishing realistic options for the client and encouraging her to acknowledge that she *can* make choices about her life. Counsellors cannot change their clients lives but they can support them in gaining the confidence and self-efficacy required to make new choices and try out new actions. Thus promoting client responsibility is inherent to the counselling process.

The type of relationship outlined above may be vital to all therapeutic interventions. Indeed research into the way in which therapists relate to their clients and the effect they have on these clients suggests that the ability to establish such a relationship may be prerequisite to effective helping (for example, Truax and Mitchell, 1971; Patterson, 1985). However, this does not necessarily mean that if one is able to offer such a relationship one is automatically a good counsellor or that counselling practice is not skill based. It is also necessary to have a model of the counselling process which allows one to plan out what is happening in any particular counselling encounter and to identify progress and difficulties. Part of such a model is an understanding of how change takes place and what skills are useful in promoting progress towards the client's goals. Indeed Egan (1990) points out that an understanding of applied psychology such as that conveyed by this book can be regarded as part of the expertise and competence involved in offering therapeutic help. We shall consider some of the skills a counsellor might draw upon below.

The Counselling Process - five tasks

We noted in Chapter 5 (Section 5) that open communication between nurses and patients may be undermined by nurses' legitimate concerns about responsibility and control over role-related demands. In the extreme this results in a depersonalized patient role and the practice of what Nichols' calls ESO medicine (see Chapter 4, Section 2). In order to adopt a counsellor role, or more generally a therapist role, nurse must *take responsibility* for being able to help clients and acknowledge that this help relies on an inter*personal* relationship regulated by means of *communication skills* which extend well beyond those involved in everyday conversation. This means abandoning role-related defences which protect nurses from others' anxiety and pain through depersonalization. Counselling is founded upon personalized relating.

We cannot provide the reader with a course in counselling skills and those wishing to develop such skills are referred to Egan's (1990) *The Skilled Helper: A Systematic Approach to Effective Helping* or Nelson-Jones' (1990) *Counselling and Helping Skills*. However, we can introduce the counselling process by mapping out some of the tasks which may be undertaken and indicating the type of communication skills involved.

Counselling skills may be divided into two types. First creating an overview. The counsellor must be involved in mapping out the development of the counselling relationship and what it is achieving. She must monitor what is happening in the relationship and guide it towards an outcome which is beneficial to the client. Secondly, interaction management. At a more immediate level the counsellor must know how to respond to particular remarks and disclosures. She must be able to use appropriate responses to further the overall aims of the relationship, moving flexibly between non-verbal encouragement, information provision, summarizing, probing, challenging, self-disclosure and recommendations for action. This not only requires the kind of selfless commitment to the client's concerns discussed above but also depends upon a well-developed repertoire of communication responses.

Drawing upon Egan's multi-stage model of helping and Nelson-Jones' overview of the counselling process we shall consider five tasks which may be accomplished within a counselling relationship. These are described in terms of what the client achieves through the counsellor's help:

1. communicating a clear picture of her concerns;
2. constructing a more useful representation of her situation;
3. defining goals and planing action which effect change;
4. maintaining motivation and abilities to sustain change;
5. becoming independent of the counselling relationship.

Of course not all of these tasks will be achieved or given equal time in any particular counselling relationship. Moreover a single counselling meeting may focus on one or more of these tasks.

The knowledge that someone else has a a clear understanding of one's concerns is a considerable comfort even when that person does not intervene directly. Thus the first task of the counsellor is to develop such an understanding and to communicate her understanding to her client. In linking the stages of the nursing process to the development of counsellor–client relationships Faulkner (1985a) refers to this first task as assessment and certainly some of the skills involved may be regarded as assessment skills. The counsellor must attend closely to the client's verbal and non-verbal communication. Listening is of primary importance and non-verbal encouragement can prompt clients to continue telling their stories without interruption. Listening is an active process in which the listener guides the speaker towards clarification and specification while continually confirming that she is following their story. Summarizing key points and repeating important statements (using 'reflection') serves to clarify what is being said and communicate understanding. Open questions allow the client to offer their own interpretations and to broaden the context of their concerns.

At this stage the counsellor is engaged in a reconnaissance exercise in which she is building up a picture of the client, the client's difficulties and the kind of relationship which she can develop with the client. The counsellor will want to explore the client's feelings and emotional responses to events she describes. It may also be important to establish whether present difficulties are linked to past experiences and to discover how relationships with other people may be shaping the client's feelings. Such exploratory discussion may reveal client strengths which can be drawn upon later and deficiencies in the client's coping skills which may become a target for change. It may also emerge that the client has more pressing problems than those they initially presented. As the client comes to trust the counsellor she can disclose more of her feelings and anxieties and the focus of the problems may change as a result. The client may also evade the counsellors questions and the counsellor must be aware of such resistance.

During this exploration the counsellor may become aware of ways in which the client's representation of her world is inhibiting her development and achievement. The counsellor may then help the client change her view of reality. This may involve identifying gaps in the client's knowledge and providing information which enables the client to change her intentions or think about a problem differently. However, it may also involve challenging the client's self-representation or her understandings of her relationships with others. In this case a more subtle interpersonal influence process begins.

The counsellor may challenge the client by reflecting on the way the client–counsellor relationship is progressing. This may be useful when the client is reluctant to talk about something which seems to be an important aspect of her difficulties. It may also be useful when the client's interaction with the counsellor seems to resemble the client's description of the way other relationships proceed. For example, the client may feel she cannot call upon others for support and the counsellor may be able to point to ways in which she is preventing the counsellor from offering such support. In the process of such reflection on the client–counsellor relationship the counsellor may be able to help by using *feedback*, that is by telling the client how the client's behaviour makes her feel. In our example, the counsellor may have begun to feel frustrated or powerless to help and it may be useful for the client to focus on how she may be evoking similar feelings in others who care for her.

Egan and Nelson-Jones consider a number of ways in which the counsellor can begin to challenge the client's understanding in a helpful and accepting manner. The counsellor may, for example, bring up a feature of the client's experience which the client has not disclosed. By listening carefully the counsellor will have developed theories about how the client acts and relates to others. The counsellor may offer an interpretation of the client's experience using one of these theories, for example, she might suggest that the client feels angry towards someone although the client has not said so. This is part of empathizing with the client and has been called *advanced empathy*. If the counsellor's interpretation is right it may help the client think about a relationship differently and perhaps promote a change of feeling or new plans.

These challenges represent a change in focus from understanding the client's feelings and problems to an analysis of the *thinking and representations* which underpin those feelings. There are many different aspects of clients' thinking which a counsellor may wish to challenge. Clients may be failing to acknowledge some important aspect of their situation, that is, using *denial*; they may be *stereotyping* others or misunderstanding their motives (see Chapter 3, Section 1) they may be *projecting* their own feelings onto others, for example assuming that someone else is angry with them when they feel anger towards that person, they may be setting themselves *impossible goals* or *misattributing* their own failure or success (see Chapter 2 Section 3). Counsellors concern with clients' thinking overlaps with the work of cognitive therapists which we shall consider below. Indeed some counsellors may be cognitive therapists. In general, however, counsellors tend to focus on specific aspects of the client's representation of a problem and challenge these through questions, suggestions and use of advanced empathy. Cognitive therapists, on the other hand, may be involved in challenging more general beliefs and representations and may adopt a more confrontational approach.

The point of challenging clients' thinking is to help them develop an understanding of themselves and their difficulties which can be used to plan improvements in their situation. In nursing terms the next stage of the counselling process focuses upon helping the client plan her intervention. Such intervention should be aimed initially at the problem causing the client most distress. Helping clients identify their *needs and priorities* is a key part of planning for change. Knowing what one wants is prerequisite to knowing how to get it but competing needs and demands may make it difficult to decide what to do. Counselling can help clients to identify and order their needs. However, in order pursue these needs they must also feel that we can act effectively. The counsellor may therefore help the client to consider *realistic opportunities* for change. By exploring strengths and supports available to the client the counsellor may enhance the clients perceived self-efficacy (see Chapter 2, Section 3). Effective planning also requires the identification of barriers to action and consideration of strategies for coping with such problems. Egan points out that explicitly weighing up the costs and gains for ourselves and those around us using balance sheets is a useful way of evaluating goals and ways to achieve them.

Having helped the client to plan realistic ways of coping with her difficulties the forth counselling task is to support the client in maintaining motivation and taking action. Here the focus changes from decision-making to action and change maintenance. We shall consider methods of maintaining behaviour change in more detail below but it is worth noting that aspects of clients' social and physical environment may prompt old behaviours which give rise to old problems while at the same time inhibiting implementation of their resolutions. When this happens the counsellor may help the client to reconsider the planned action and develop strategies to overcome the barriers to change. This may involve focusing upon successes in order to regain confidence, planning new approaches to the same goal, learning new ways of interacting with people who are blocking the client's plans, and finding ways to increase motivation. The counsellor may help the client focus on new sub-goals, practice role-play interaction-sequences which will help the client overcome social barriers or consider the use of rewards for different degrees of success. Nelson-Jones, for example, points out that clients can identify what is rewarding for them by the using the 'pleasant events schedule' (MacPhillamy and Lewinsohn, 1982). Thus, despite initial setbacks, the counsellor may help the client towards effective implementation through reconsideration of earlier resolutions and exploration of new ways of translating goals into achievements.

Counselling is directed towards encouraging clients to take responsibility for their problems and acting independently to deal with them. Termination may therefore occur naturally when the client feels they have made progress with the difficulties which originally prompted them to seek counselling. However, it may be helpful to discuss termination in order to explicitly challenge dependency in the counselling relationship. It may also be important to consider how the client may gain support and help from other relationships. In this way the counsellor can help client towards independence.

Counselling in nursing

Interaction with patients in hospital on a 24-hours-a-day basis gives nurses greater contact with hospital patients than other health care workers. They are also often the strongest health care link with patients and relatives in the community. This close relationship offers nurses an opportunity to apply counselling skills in helping patients and relatives. However, as we have noted institutional barriers may prevent this. Wilson-Barnett (1988), for example, notes that although district nurses may have much to offer by way of counselling and support they only spend a small proportion of their time on such therapeutic relating. On the other hand more counselling courses for nurses are being developed and a number of important applications of counselling skills have been identified.

Naismith, et al., (1979), for example, report how certain myocardial infarction patients may benefit substantially from nurse counselling. They found that patients predisposed to anxiety who had received counselling had considerably better outcomes at six months than similar patients who had not. They also emphasized the importance of the nurse counsellor as a link person who maintains a relationship with the patient across various hospital units and into the community. Kelly (1986) indicates how counselling might be used to overcome problematic denial in patients suffering from chronic ulcerative colitis. Kelly distinguishes 'healthy denial' which forms a part of the patient's attempts to live a near-normal life within the constraints of the disease from 'problematic denial' which may threaten the patient's commitment to disease management or treatment. Problematic denial in which the patient refuses to acknowledge her own health needs can be challenged during counselling. However, the subtlety of judging when to challenge clients' perspectives is emphasized by Kelly's distinction. Drawing upon Parkes (1972) study of grief Kelly notes how initial denial of the loss of health or a relationship may assist us in gradually coming to terms with a new and threatening reality but that prolonged denial may lead to a failure to adjust. Empathy with the client's development and coping competence can enable a counsellor to appreciate the function of healthy denial and to judge when it is appropriate to challenge problematic denial.

Adjustment to loss of a close companion is a stressful process which may be facilitated by counselling. Loss of affection, everyday practical assistance, established role relations and social validation requires substantial psychological readjustment. It is not surprising therefore that comparisons of widows and widowers with similarly aged married people show an increased mortality rate. Recently bereaved individuals are more likely to suffer from a deterioration in health and are especially susceptible to health problems which can be traced to a failure to take care of oneself (Stroebe et al, 1982). Thus here as in many other cases counselling serves a preventative function as well as alleviating current distress.

Parkes and Weiss (1983) and Worden (1982) note that successful readjustment to bereavement depends upon the accomplishment of certain psychological tasks and that the manner in which grieving progresses may be crucial to the maintenance of psychological and physical well being. Expressing loss, establishing alternative sources of social support and beginning to construct new social identities are all important elements of readjustment. Thus those who did not anticipate their loss, who had a problematic relationship with the deceased, who cannot express their loss, who have few alternative social relationships or who have limited opportunities to develop new social identities may be especially prone to readjustment problems (Parkes and Weiss, 1983; Stroebe, et al., 1982). Jones (1989) uses Worden's (1982) work to present an outline of how counselling skills might be used to facilitate grieving. The counsellor can enable the client to admit her loss, help her to express the range of feelings this gives rise to, encourage her to explore the prospect of life without her companion, help her anticipate and understand her feelings over time, challenge withdrawal and destructive coping strategies and offer support while encouraging the establishment of alternative social supports. Such grief counselling facilitates adjustment. Worden distinguished this from *grief therapy* in which cognitive and behavioural techniques may be used because the usual grieving process has broken down and psychological readjustment is disrupted.

The risk of depression resulting from bereavement illustrates how the counselling roles of the general and psychiatric nurse may overlap. A social psychiatric model which acknowledges that psychological disorders may be the result of relationship difficulties supports the view that interaction with health care workers may resolve some of the patient's problems. Thus time spent in hospital between specific treatments is of therapeutic value and nurse–patient interaction is integral part of the therapeutic process. This view was expressed in one of the first World Health Organization (1956) reports which regarded the provision of 'experience in living' (including the formation of relationships which would enhance patients' relationship-building abilities) as an 'essential part' of the psychiatric nurse role. This perspective was shared by Henderson and Gillespie (1964) who concluded that psychiatric nurses as had 'a more important and potentially effective therapeutic role than doctors' (p. 285). However, this potential can only be realized if nurses are able to develop therapeutic relationships with their patients. This will involve encouragement of an active and responsible 'client' role for 'patients' (see Chapter 4, Section 2). Rapoport (1960) advocated a *democratization of the nurse–patient relationship* so that patients are actively involved in everyday decision-making and an emphasis on *reality confrontation* in which nurses offer patients *feed-back* on others' understanding of their behaviour. Creating such a social environment requires a high level of honesty and commitment from nursing staff and involves relinquishing the security of role-related rights which have allowed nurses authority over a wide range of patient communication and behaviour (see Chapter 5, Section 5).

Although the adoption of such a counselling role constitutes a radical departure from the custodial or medical models within which psychiatric nursing has been practised (Towell, 1975) there are optimistic signs for the future. Shanley (1984) found that almost 90%of nurse–patient relationships in psychiatric hospitals were characterized by Rogers' prerequisite conditions, that is, empathy, genuineness and unconditional positive regard and since then the Psychiatric Nurses Association in Scotland has declared that these Rogerian prerequisites should form the basis of all interventions in psychiatric nursing (Shanley and Murray, 1986).

3 Changing People Through Their Environment

Classical conditioning-learning through association

The operation of environmental factors in prompting and maintaining changes in behaviour was highlighted by a group of psychologists known as *learning theorists*. They proposed that we learn about the world by forming *associations* between elements of our experience which occur in quick succession. This associative learning is known as *conditioning* and is used to explain behavioural responses to subsequent perception of the same environmental features. This approach to understanding learning and behaviour change has given rise to debate and controversy within psychology and had widespread implications for disciplines drawing upon applied psychology. It emphasizes environment-behaviour links and focuses attention away from the role of feeling and understanding in personal change. We shall discuss key theoretical ideas derived from learning theory and their application to therapy. A more comprehensive overview of learning theory is provided by Walker's (1984) *Learning Theory and Behaviour Modification*.

The work of Ivan Pavlov is well known and foundational to learning theory. Pavlov (1927) showed how important perception was to dogs' gastric activity. Hungry dogs salivate and begin the digestive process when they are presented with food but unseen food inserted directly into the stomach does not trigger digestion. Established links between perception of an environmental feature (called a *stimulus*) and a predictable response are described in learning theory terms as the link between an *unconditioned stimulus* (the food) and an *unconditioned response* (the salivation). The process of 'classical conditioning' which Pavlov demonstrated essentially transfers such a response to a new stimulus (a *conditioned stimulus*) through associative learning.

By consistently pairing the unconditioned stimulus with some other aspect of the environment, for example the sound of a buzzer immediately before the presentation of food, it is possible to link the unconditioned response to this stimulus. Over time a dog will learn to associate the sound of the buzzer the delivery of food and therefore salivate when it hears the buzzer. Classical conditioning has occurred. The unconditioned stimulus (the buzzer) which did not previously elicit the target behaviour now prompts the *conditioned response* (salivation). The conditioned and unconditioned response are essentially the same although the conditioned version may be somewhat weaker. Such conditioning seems to suggest that the way in which behaviour is linked to our perceptions of the environment is potentially very flexible. Our present behaviour being due to past associations and our future behaviour open to change through new associations.

In associating perceived stimuli dogs and people are sensitive to similarities and differences between them. Having learnt that a buzzer indicates the arrival of food, for example, a dog will salivate when it hears a similar but different buzzer. This is called *generalization*. The more similar two stimuli are the more generalization will occur. This is an important aspect of conditioning because it accounts for the way in which learning affects us in new situations. However, we can also distinguish between stimuli even when they are very similar. If a buzzer of higher pitch than the conditioned stimulus is presented continuously without being followed by food then the dog will quickly learn that one buzzer signals food while the other does not. This is called *discrimination* because the dog is discriminating between two stimuli. We can see this process in operation when our pets respond to our voices but those of other people.

What happens if, after a conditioned reflex is established, the conditioned stimulus (buzzer) is presented repeatedly without being followed by the unconditioned stimulus (food)? Predictably the dog learns that the buzzer no longer signals food and will stop salivating over time. The learned association is weakened by the dislocation of the conditioned and unconditioned stimulus so that the conditioned stimulus no longer supports the conditioned response. This 'unlearning' process is called *extinction* and helps explain why some learnt behaviours eventually disappear.

Operant conditioning and behaviourism

Pavlov's classical conditioning transfers an already established response to a new stimulus through stimuli pairing. The animal or person involved is fairly passive and learns a new way to exhibit an already learnt response rather than a new behaviour. *Operant conditioning* attempts to explain how an animal's own activity can lead to novel sequences of behaviour through associative learning. The idea behind operant conditioning is based on is Thorndike's (1911) *law of effect*. Thorndike studied the behaviour of hungry cats in cages from which they could see fish. The cats could escape and get to the fish by pressing a latch which opened an escape door. Thorndike noticed that when the cats were first placed in the cage they scrambled about randomly but after they happened upon the escape latch they would take less time to escape when placed in the cage again. Indeed, escape times decreased from minutes to seconds over relatively few attempts. Thorndike's law of effect therefore states that out of the many different responses we may make in a particular situation those which lead to rewarding consequences will be more strongly associated with that situation. Similarly, those which lead to unrewarding consequences will be less strongly associated with that situation. In other wards *the consequences of our actions serve to strengthen or weaken the association between our actions and the circumstances in which we make them*. The association here is between a stimulus (the cage) and a voluntary response (pressing the latch).

Building on this work Watson (1913) proposed that learning theory could provide a new basis for psychology. Behaviour could be explained in terms of previous conditioning and psychology could concentrate on investigating how behaviour is linked to particular environmental stimuli. There would be no need to consider what went on inside animals or people. Ideas like 'mind' and 'thought' could be discarded in favour of a new scientific approach relying upon stimuli and response measures which could be made through direct observation of external factors. Watson called himself a 'behaviourist' and we refer to his approach to psychology as *behaviourism*.

It has been clear since the first few pages of this book that it is not written by behaviourists (see Chapter 2, Section 1) and below we explain why behaviourism offers an inadequate basis for the study of personal change. It must be noted, however, that Watson was arguing against a psychology which had tended to ignore behaviour. The the main rival to Watson's behaviourist approach was Freud's psychoanalysis. This approach emphasized unconscious processes which were only accessible though detailed analysis of our response to symbols and by interpretation of dreams. Moreover, it suggested that experiences in the first few years of life established a basic personality which was difficult to change in later life. This was a relatively unscientific approach to studying psychology which was very pessimistic about the possibility of personal change.

Behaviourism was popularized by Burrhus Frederic Skinner (1938) who, inspired by Pavlov and Watson, extended Thorndike's law of effect into a general theory of operant conditioning. He described this as an ABC model of behaviour change. The 'A' standing for antecedent environmental features which prompt a behaviour (for Thorndike's cats, finding themselves in the cage) the 'B' stands for the behaviour we are interested in (pressing the latch) and the 'C' for the consequence that follow this behaviour (escape and tasty fish). By changing the consequences of behaviour in certain situations (that is when specific antecedents are present) Skinner argued that we could gradually change the way an animal or person responds.

Two obvious consequences of a behaviour are *rewards* and *punishments*. Skinner and other learning theorists have argued that, while punishment may decrease the frequency of a behaviour in the situation in which it is punished, punishment may also give rise to generalized fear responses so that the animal or person reacts fearfully to other aspects of the situation. Punishment may therefore have unintended and damaging side effects on behaviour. Operant conditioning is therefore primarily based on the reorganization of environmental rewards. However, Skinner did not use the term 'reward' as it implies inner pleasure and such internal events were not part of the behaviourist view of psychology. The operation of environmental consequences to increase the frequency of a behaviour was therefore referred to as *reinforcement* rather than reward.

By presenting reinforcement immediately after a desired behaviour Skinner found that, just as Thorndike's cats had learned to press latches, his rats and pigeons could learn complex bar-pressing sequences and circular turns. Skinner showed how a desired behaviour such as a circular turn in a clockwise direction could be gradually encouraged by reinforcing behaviours which approximated to it. Initially a pigeon might receive food for any slight movement in a clockwise direction. Then once such movements had become frequent reinforcement would be withheld until the bird produced a more pronounced turning movement. Quarter turns would then be reinforced until they became frequent and so on until the bird would only receive reinforcement for a complete turn. This process is called *shaping* and it allowed operant conditioning to account for the appearance of new behavioural sequences through reinforcement of parts of a sequence over time. In this way operant conditioning goes beyond the transfer of behaviours from one stimulus to another.

Skinner applied his ideas to social behaviour by noting that much of our interaction with one another can be regarded as reinforcement. We have noted, for example, that interviewers' responses affect interviewers' performances (Chapter 3, Section 2). Such responses can be regarded as reinforcers. Greenspoon (1955), for example, showed how non-verbal paralinguistic responses (see Chapter 5, Section 6) to particular words can increase the frequency with which others' use them. Similarly Verplack (1955) showed that statements of agreement following others' expressions of opinion increased the likelihood that they would express further opinions. Thus lecturers who want their students to participate in class discussions might try reinforcing students' views with agreement (or qualified agreement) in the hope of establishing a discussion norm within their class (see Chapter 8, Section 1). Regarding non-verbal and verbal communication as reinforcement led Skinner to view language usage in the same way as other behaviours and therefore to explain language acquisition in terms of conditioning. Operant conditioning principles are certainly useful in encouraging social behaviour in infants. Weisberg (1963), for example, showed that offering social attention to pre-verbal infants for babbling increased babbling. However, as we shall see below Skinner's views on language have been harshly criticized.

Breaking habits through new associations

Watson was one of the first psychologists to apply learning theory to personal behaviour change. Ironically, however, one of the first applications seemed to create rather than resolve a problem. Watson and Rayner's (1920) work with the 11 month-old infant Albert has become a psychology classic. They observed that loud and unexpected sounds startled and frightened Albert (an unconditioned stimulus – unconditioned response link) and that Albert enjoyed playing with a white rat. By persistently banging a metal bar behind Albert when he playfully approached his rodent friend Watson was able to 'transfer' the fear response from the noise to the rat so that Albert cried and crawled away when his old playmate appeared. Indeed Albert went on to generalize this fear response to other white furry things including Watson's hair.

The importance of Albert's traumatic learning experiences was that, by applying classical conditioning principles, Watson and Rayner had artificially created a conditioned fear response. Albert had become frightened of things he had previously been relaxed and happy with.

This served as an illustration of how people might become frightened of things which presented no real threat.

It seemed plausible to think that people's fears and phobias concerning pigeons, spiders, telephones, dentists or even public speaking could be the result of some unfortunate pairing that had lead to rapid conditioning of a fear response. Such behaviour can be categorized as *maladaptive* in that it does not help the person deal effectively with her environment. Watson argued that, since the development of maladaptive behaviour could be explained by conditioning, associative learning could be used to establish new *adaptive* behaviours.

Watson's approach to Albert's liking for his white rat can be seen as a forerunner of 'aversion therapy' as applied to alcohol dependence. People who want to stop drinking may learn to dislike drinking if it is paired with a stimulus which induces a powerful negative reaction. When the drug antabase is taken orally with alcohol it produces nausea and vomiting. Antabase and vomiting can therefore be seen as an unconditioned stimulus – unconditioned response pair. If the person continues to take antabase when they drink alcohol becomes associated with antabase and may over time give rise to feelings of nausea by itself thereby reducing alcohol dependence (Franks, 1966).

More recent work on drug use has applied classical conditioning principles to the development and maintenance of dependence. It had been thought that addiction could be explained as a fulfillment of a need to avoid withdrawal effects once the body had become tolerant of a drug. However, doubts have been cast on this view. In certain circumstances it seems relatively easy to break drug dependence while in others it is very difficult. Robbins (1974), for example, reports how United States' soldiers seemed able to give up heroin relatively easily upon return from VietNam. On the other hand ex-users who have completely detoxified during a period in prison may experience strong cravings once they return to the places in which they had previously used drugs. Stewart, et al., (1984) argue this and other biochemical evidence is best explained by a classical conditioning account of dependence. They argue that a drug such as heroin gives rise to a an unconditioned brain response involving dopamine release. By repeatedly pairing the drug (the unconditioned stimulus) with unconditioned stimuli such as needles, injecting and places where injecting is performed, these unconditioned stimuli come to trigger a conditioned response similar to the drug itself. In other words *classical conditioning results in the contexts of drug taking giving rise to a 'conditioned high' which is similar to, but weaker than, that induced by the drug.* This then motivates the user to seek a drug-induced high and reduces cognitive control over behaviour. Thus perception of the conditioned stimuli prompts a neural response which motivates drug seeking behaviour.

Recalling our discussion of representations of reality in earlier Chapters, it appears that the representational processes shown in Figure 2b (Chapter 2, Section 1) are short circuited by such conditioning. In the case of drug-induced conditioning then we must modify or diagram as shown in Figure 7. This explains why changing beliefs and intentions is often not enough to break drug dependence. It also explains why those, like the VietNam soldiers, who are no longer exposed to stimuli prompting a conditioned high may find it relatively easy to give up but even those who are completely detoxified may experience difficulties when returning to previous drug-taking contexts.

This classical conditioning account of drug dependence suggests that *induced extinction* may be the more appropriate treatment. Just as Pavlov's dogs stopped salivating so ex-users should gradually cease to experience their conditioned high if the unconditioned stimulus (the drug) ceases to follow the conditioned stimulus (for example, injecting). Extinction could therefore remove the conditioned high and enable the person's beliefs, intentions and representations to direct their behavioural responses to situations in which they had previously used drugs. This would change Figure 7 back into Figure 2b. Such extinction could therefore pave the way for further therapeutic work on the beliefs and intentions sustaining drug use (see below). The equivalent of ringing the bell without presenting food might be going through previously used injecting procedure repeatedly, including handling the drug but not actually injecting it, or actually injecting but using saline solution (O'Brien, et al., 1974). Applying the same principle to alcohol dependence suggests that supporting drinkers to consistently drink non-alcohol substitutes in their usual bars with their usual company would be an effective way of breaking old associations and regaining control over their drinking.

This application of extinction uses controlled exposure to a conditioned stimulus to break down conditioned associations. Watson also used controlled exposure to form new associations with that stimulus which might overcome previous conditioning. One might, for example, arrange to repeatedly encounter a feared stimulus in the presence of something which made one laugh. This is aversion therapy in reverse and is known as to as *counter-conditioning*. Watson worked with Jones in applying counter-conditioning to the kind of fear he had induced in Albert (Jones, 1924).

In one famous case Watson and Jones observed a marked fear of animals

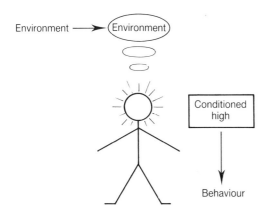

Figure 7 'Conditioned high' links perception directly to drug seeking behaviour.

(including rats and rabbits) in a child called Peter. Watson reasoned that if such feared stimuli were presented together with a stimulus which induced pleasure, contentment and relaxation then the fear association might be broken. In Peter's case a rabbit was gradually but repeatedly presented while he was enjoying his lunch. Initially the rabbit was merely in the room in a cage while Peter ate but it was gradually brought closer and when Peter learnt to enjoy lunch with the rabbit's cage close to him the rabbit was allowed to run about during lunch. Over time, such repeated pairings of eating with ever closer encounters with the previously feared rabbit, enabled Peter to enjoy lunch while stroking the rabbit! It seems as if eating had produced new positive associations with the rabbit which overcome the previous conditioned fear. Jones also emphasized the role of Peter's relationships with people who were handling the rabbit and encouraging him to do so.

Change through selective reinforcement

We have discussed a number of applications of classical conditioning but, in fact, operant conditioning has probably been more widely applied to behaviour change. These applications seek to control the reinforcement which follows a behaviour and therefore increase or decrease its frequency. In the case of a problematic behaviour eliminating reinforcement is crucial. This may include the use of *time out* procedures when the person is removed from sources of reinforcement by, for example, sending them out of a room in which social reinforcement may be available. In the case of desirable behaviours reinforcement is provided immediately after the target behaviour in order to increase its frequency. This may include the removal of unpleasant environmental aspects when the behaviour occurs. This is called *negative reinforcement* and may be thought of as an escape from punishment. More commonly, however, rewards or *positive reinforcement* are used to increase the frequency of desired behaviours.

Interventions based on the principles of operant conditioning are referred to as 'behaviour modification' programmes. They begin with baseline observations in which the 'natural' frequency of the target behaviour is recorded and any usual antecedents and consequences noted. This provides a picture of how the behaviour is currently triggered and reinforced and helps define goals for the programme. It also allows subsequent evaluation of a programme through comparison of baseline and post-programme behavioural frequencies.

Problems with young children's sleep patterns, for example, have been shown to be effectively treated using behaviour modification programmes by health visitors and psychologists (Sanger, et al., 1981; Richman, et al., 1985). In such cases a parent may be asked to keep a 'sleep diary' recording how the child settles and wakes each night for a week or two.

This might include where, with whom, and at what time the child settles to sleep as well as how often the child wakes and what happens as a result. In practice such baseline observation can sometimes have a therapeutic effect on adults because they themselves gain insight into the nature of the problem and begin to alter their behaviour. However, the primary use of baseline observation is to design an appropriate intervention.

The intervention programme in such cases will involve identification of social reinforcement for night waking. Parents may be responding immediately to the child's waking with interaction, holding or taking the child into their own bed. Removal of such reinforcers will encourage the child to resettle upon waking and hopefully lead to extinction of the waking and crying behaviour. Thus the parents may, for example, be asked to leave the child to cry for longer and if crying persists to comfort the child at timed intervals rather then responding immediately and consistently to crying. At the same time reinforces for settling at night may be explored. The child may be allowed to take toys to bed and play for a period before being settled to sleep, a story may be read before settling or a surprise left under the child's pillow. With such behaviour modification advice parents can alter their reinforcement of their child's settling and waking behaviour and thereby improve sleeping behaviour.

In a similar manner to parents' unintentional reinforcement of undesirable behaviour nurse's attention may reinforce patient dependency (see Chapter 4, Section 2). The power of nurses' behaviour to reinforce and shape patients' behaviour was noted by Ayllon and Michael (1962) who described psychiatric nurses as 'behavioural engineers'. Implementation of behaviour modification programmes which identify the social reinforcers delivered by nurses can have powerful effects on patient behaviour in institutional settings and can play an important part in the rehabilitation of patients who are moving from an institution into the community. An extension of this idea led to the establishment of *token economies* in some psychiatric wards (Ayllon and Azrin, 1968). In these programmes patients would receive tokens (such as plastic disks) for performing particular behaviours agreed in advance. They could then use these tokens to 'buy' privileges such a chocolates or visits outside the hospital. Token economies appeared to be quite successful in encouraging psychiatric and mentally handicapped patients to adopt self care and other socially acceptable behaviours (Barker, et al., 1978; Barker 1982). However they do raise ethical problems as staff must decide what counts as a privilege which must be earned through behaviour change and what counts as a basic right which cannot be withheld. This can be especially difficult if the patient is unable to discuss and negotiate an agreed behaviour modification programme.

Token economies also highlight a more general issue in behaviour modification, namely the maintenance of desirable behaviours. Success depends upon these behaviours continuing after artificial reinforces, such as tokens, have been removed. This can be done by gradually reducing the artificial reinforcers (a process referred to as *fading*) and at the same time increasing social reinforcers such as praise so that the behaviour is rewarded through everyday social interaction. In this way common social reinforcers replace the artificial reinforcers in maintaining the desired behaviours.

Systematic desensitization – internal representations and behavioural control

Leaving applied operant conditioning for a moment and returning to classical conditioning we shall briefly consider the work of Joseph Wolpe. Wolpe was a psychiatrist who was influenced by both Freud and Pavlov. He reached the same conclusion as Watson concerning the presentation of two stimuli which prompt opposite responses, that is that one could be used to overcome a learnt maladaptive response to the other. Wolpe (1958) called this effect *reciprocal inhibition* and it is exactly the same principle which Watson and Jones applied when using counter conditioning to treat Peter's fear of rabbits. However, instead of eating lunch Wolpe used relaxation to inhibit anxiety responses. He also found that the social events which made his clients anxious could not easily be put in a box and brought gradually closer during therapy. He therefore used his client's imagination and paired relaxation with the client's image of the anxiety-provoking experience. The resulting technique is known as *systematic desensitization.*

Systematic desensitization begins with an exploration of the client's anxiety. The therapist helps the client identify experiences which would provoke the anxiety they want to reduce. In the case of a person who fears public speaking, for example, proposing a toast at a small dinner party for her friends might represent the least problematic instance of her difficulties. By thinking of progressively more anxiety provoking situations the client can create a graded sequence of situations which would make her more and more anxious. In our example, giving a talk about work practices to a large audience of better qualified members of her profession might be her most feared experience. In this way the client constructs an *anxiety hierarchy*. The client is also taught how to relax by deliberately taking slow, deep breaths and by tensing and then relaxing different parts of her body in turn. This will increase oxygen in the blood, decrease heart rate, decrease blood pressure and reduce muscle tension. In other words induce the opposite physiological responses to those usually produced by anxiety. Clients practice such relaxation until they are able to deliberately induce a relaxed state.

The desensitization procedure involves deliberate relaxation while imagining anxiety provoking experiences. The client begins with the least anxiety provoking experience in the hierarchy and only moves on to the next most anxiety provoking experience when she is able to remain fully relaxed while actively imagining herself in the situation. The technique has been widely applied and shown to be effective in helping clients to overcome a range of fears from public speaking anxieties to pigeon phobias. Confronting and overcoming anxiety in one's imagination appears to provide clients with new ways of coping with previously frightening experiences.

An important element of Wolpe's technique is its reliance on the clients' internal representations of situations. The client attempts to change the meaning of a remembered or imagined situation by concentrating upon it while feeling relaxed. This is certainly not an example of Watson's behaviourism. It relies on seeking to to change the client's behaviour through changing her understanding or representation of the world (Chapter 2, Section 2). The same issue arises in operant conditioning. In identifying reinforces we must explore the individual's understanding of events. A disruptive child may experience a 'telling off' as rewarding and some clients may experience humiliation when offered gold stars or tokens. The therapist must explore what is rewarding for her client how those experiences could help her overcome other difficulties. As we noted above MacPhillamy and Lewinsohn's (1982) pleasant events schedule lists occurrences which many people find rewarding and can be used to assess client's personal rewards and the extent to which they have recently been rewarded. Reinforcement is therefore defined in terms of internal representations of rewarding experiences.

Behaviourists have referred to techniques involving internal representations as 'covert conditioning' involving 'private stimuli' but this is a misleading portrayal. Internal representations are the basis of meaningful perception. They allow environmental features (stimuli) to be perceived as meaningful events by relating them to personal memories and beliefs. Even the basic associations involved in classical conditioning rely upon such *internal expectations*. Associations between unconditioned and conditioned stimuli do not depend solely upon the pairing of stimuli. The conditioned stimulus must also act as a good predictor of the unconditioned stimulus over time. If the stimuli are paired but the unconditioned stimulus also appears without being preceded by the conditioned stimulus then little or no associative learning may occur (Rescorla, 1968). Thus stimuli and reinforces as they affect individuals are *created inside* the person's representation of reality. In this sense *all stimuli are private* but because we share many representations of the world we can anticipate what events mean to others (see Chapter 1, Section 3). We have, for example, already seen how beliefs about our own competence and control can change the meaning of environmental stimuli and therefore the way in which we respond to them (see Chapter 2, Section 4) and how our perceptions of others rely upon our implicit personality theories (see Chapter 3, Section 1).

Acknowledgement of the dependence of our perceptions of physical and social reality upon personal internal representation is foundational to therapy. This is the essence of Rogers' emphasis on *empathy*. Unless we can understand what environmental events mean to our clients by exploring their beliefs and understandings we will be of little help to them. The implication of this theoretical point is that the effective application operant and classical conditioning depends upon a rejection of behaviourism.

The inadequacy of behaviourism

Tolman presented one of the earliest and most straightforward criticisms of behaviourism. He was committed to an empirical psychology involving the measurement of behaviour and behaviour change but he rejected an exclusively associationist account of learning because he thought it underestimated the complexity of behavioural control. He argued that rats behave purposively and form representations of their environment which go well beyond simple associations between consequences and behaviours (Tolman, 1925). Tolman and Honzik (1930) demonstrated the power of this critique in a well-known experiment involving the reinforcement of three groups of rats running through a maze. One group were always rewarded with food at the end of the maze while another group received no reinforcement. As operant conditioning theory would predict the reinforced group made fewer and fewer errors on successive runs while the rats which were not reinforced continued to make frequent errors. It seemed then that positive reinforcement was accelerating maze-learning. However, a third group were allowed to run through the maze without rewards ten times but were then rewarded with food on future attempts. Tolman and Honzik found that this group made as many errors as the unrewarded group for the first ten trials (neither group received rewards and so errors remained high). However, once they had been rewarded they were able to run through the maze with as few errors as the rats which had been rewarded on every trial. This group were able to immediately catch up with the performance of the reinforced group as if they too had been receiving reinforcement on the first ten attempts. They did not show the same gradual decrease in errors as the group receiving rewards from the beginning. The importance of this result is that the rats had clearly been learning the maze before they received rewards. Moreover it appears that they had learnt a map of the maze which they could use when motivated to do so.

Tolman's work demonstrated that although reinforcement may exert a powerful influence on the performance of behaviour it does not determine learning. Like Tolman's rats we learn about our environment without reinforcement. Bandura (1965), for example, has demonstrated that when children observe an adult being punished for aggressive behaviour they are less likely to spontaneously imitate the behaviour than children who observe the same behaviour being rewarded. However, this difference disappears when the children themselves are offered incentives to repeat the aggressive behaviour. Children who saw the aggression being punished are just as able to copy it as those who saw it rewarded. In this case observational learning of aggressive behaviour occurs regardless of reinforcement. *Reinforcement directs the performance, not the acquisition of the behavioural sequence.* This ability to learn behavioural sequences by observing others model them corresponds to Jones' observation of the importance of others' example to Peter's treatment. It is the basis of 'social learning theory' which offers a more social and cognitive explanation of learning (Bandura, 1977a; see too Bandura, 1986)

Chomsky's (1959) critique of Skinner's (1957) attempt to explain language acquisition in conditioning terms also empathized learning through the development of internal representations and the performance of behaviour. Chomsky argued that in order to account for the creativity of infants' language, that is the great variety of things they learn to say, we must explain their underlying competence in terms of stored rules about language. The flexibility of their performances cannot be explained by behavioural extensions such as those produced by shaping. Thus Tolman, Bandura and Chomsky all argue that we must seek to describe internal representations in order to account for the complexity of behaviour.

We have noted above that discovering what counts as a reinforcer for any particular individual is always a matter of investigation. However the work of Deci (1975) suggests that people's motivation and therefore their behaviour may be much more complex than is suggested by operant conditioning. A series of studies has demonstrated that when people find a task interesting they are more likely to choose to spend time on it if they believe they are doing it for its own sake than if they believe they are doing it for payment. In other words their *intrinsic motivation* is undermined by the idea that they are working for an external reward. It is not the appearance of the reward that undermines motivation. Surprise rewards do not have this effect (Lepper, et al., 1973). It is the knowledge that one is working for a reward rather than one's own interest. Close association with payment may therefore act more like a punishment than a reinforcer for interesting activities. This is not easily explained in operant conditioning terms. Deci's work highlights the importance of self-representation in motivation. If we view ourselves as working at something *because it is interesting or enjoyable* this in itself is a powerful reward which is removed when we begin to see ourselves as working for payment. By ignoring internal representations an operant conditioning perspective is unable to take account of the way in which such beliefs about ourselves affect motivation. We shall return to this distinction between intrinsic and extrinsic motivation in relation to nursing in Chapter 9 (Section 2).

By ignoring the internal representations which direct everyday behaviour behaviourism takes psychology out of psychology and fails
to provide an adequate theoretical framework within which to model
behavioural change. In Chapter 1 (Sections 2 and 3) we began by
emphasizing how our responsiveness to the environment depends upon
shared representations learnt through socialization. To understand personal change we must return to this psychological perspective and
acknowledge the reality of beliefs and emotions based on person perception, self-awareness, a search for social validation and attempts to enhance
imagined reputation.

Legacy of the learning theorists

While the behaviourist position of Watson and Skinner proved inadequate the work the learning theorists led to important psychological
advances. An understanding of how environmental factors can become
powerful threats or incentives through association with memorable
physiological changes such as those underlying fear, pain or drug-
induced states has helped psychologists understand phobias and drug
dependence. The idea behind 'reinforcement', that rewards may sometimes encourage and routinize desirable performances can be effectively
applied outside a behaviourist framework. By exploring what people enjoy
and find rewarding we may help them understand their motivation and
assist them in practicing skills which offer no immediate intrinsic reward
but have long-term payoffs.

An operant conditioning approach to shaping behaviour through
changes in environmental rewards is especially useful when it is
difficult to discuss the client's beliefs and understandings. When the
client has limited abilities to represent herself and her social world,
communication through external rewards may be the most effective
way of encouraging socially acceptable behaviour. This was already
evident in Watson's work with infants and young children. Similarly
in the case of people with severe mental handicaps we may be unable
to discuss the social meaning of different behavioural responses or how
the client's needs can be met through alternative behaviours. In such
cases behaviour modification may be the most effective method available.
Certainly, behaviour modification regimes have proved to be effective with
infants (for example, Richman, et al., 1985) and those with severe mental
handicaps (for example, Barton, 1975).

Behaviour modification is also a very practical and common sense
approach to promoting change. It is therefore fairly easy to teach non-
psychologists, clients and relatives how to apply it. Many professional
groups including psychiatric nurses and health visitors have adopted

such techniques (Barker, et al., 1978; Sanger, et al., 1981). Indeed Barker's *Behaviour Therapy Nursing* (1982) describes an approach to promoting change which is based almost exclusively upon learning theory principles. Clients can also take an active part in therapy by monitoring and controlling their own rewards. Parents, for example, can change their children's behaviour by modifying the rewards they deliver (O'Dell, 1974; Cunningham, 1975). Thus behaviour modification can be presented in a do-it-yourself manner which empowers clients and saves scarce professional resources. We shall see how this idea has been adapted by cognitive therapists below.

In addition to particular theoretical insights and behaviour-change techniques learning theorists have given psychology an optimistic view of change. The idea that new learning can counteract past experience to engender change emphasizes people's capacity for development and argues against the pessimistic view that one cannot teach old dogs new tricks. Learning theorists offer an alternative to giving up on people as lost causes and inspire us to think that *we can facilitate change*.

Learning theorists also established a more scientific approach to evaluating therapeutic interventions. The idea that we can *measure behaviour changes* from baseline to post-intervention levels allows us to demonstrate whether or not our therapy has been successful. Thus the value of particular approaches to facilitating change can be examined using experimental designs. Comparing people with similar problems who do and do not receive therapy allows definition of an independent variable (see Chapter 1, Section 4). This can be done ethically by operating a waiting list and making baseline observations on people before they receive therapy. The degree to which the therapy successfully changes the targeted behaviour from clients' baseline levels (the dependent variable) can then be compared to any behaviour changes in those not receiving therapy to provide a rigorous test of effectiveness.

4 Beliefs Emotions and Behaviour: A Cognitive Approach to Change

Challenging Irrational Beliefs – cognitive behaviour therapy

Cognitive therapists have studied ways in which we can promote change in clients' beliefs and, as we have noted above, these techniques may be used in some forms of counselling. Most cognitive therapists acknowledge the importance of behavioural evaluations of their interventions and the usefulness of operant and classical conditioning. However they also recognize that that effective behaviour change is most likely when a client's representations of reality also change. In practice therefore this cognitive focus results in cognitive behaviour therapy which is concerned with behaviour change through cognitive change.

Albert Ellis' (1962) rational emotive therapy is a good example of a cognitive behaviour therapy. Ellis adopts the view of the Greek philosopher Epictetus as a central assumption in his therapeutic approach. Epictetus proposed that, 'man is disturbed not by things but by the views he takes of them'. Ellis therefore regards emotions and behaviours as the products of beliefs rather than direct responses to the environment. Thus instead of trying to change the environment, emotional disturbance may be alleviated and maladaptive behaviour eliminated by changing people's internal representations. Anxiety about failing an examination, for example, is not caused by the examination itself but by our beliefs about how awful it would be if we failed and what others might think about this. It follows that we can reduce such anxiety by acknowledging this 'catastrophizing' and trying to reconceptualize the situation. We might begin by telling ourselves that even if we fail there will be other opportunities to gain the qualifications we want and that our friends and relations will not stop valuing us because we have failed an examination. Challenging irrational beliefs and replacing them with more realistic and adaptive ones is the basis of *'cognitive restructuring'*. This is a process of reprogramming or re-socializing by which the therapist involves the client in an examination and rejection beliefs which are maintaining maladaptive behaviour.

Ellis has identified a series of common irrational beliefs which may underpin emotional disturbance and maladaptive behaviour. These include the beliefs that we must be approved of by everyone, that to lose someone's approval is awful, that we must always perform well and that making mistakes is catastrophic. It is interesting to note how these beliefs relate to our everyday understanding of impression management and role obligations (see Chapter 3 and 4). We are socialized into a world of other's perceptions and expectations and if we are unable to develop standards of performance which allow us to value our own efforts or if we are unable to prioritize the approval of various role-set members then everyday living can become a fearful nightmare of failure and disapproval leading to stress and depression. The belief that mistakes are terrible, for example, is especially detrimental to those learning a new skill and can prevent students from experimenting and inhibit learning. Of course there are many other types of irrational belief. People may, for example, come to believe that they are extremely susceptible to to illness or contamination, that they are perpetually in danger, that they lack basic motor abilities or that they are repulsive to others.

Challenging irrational beliefs is a difficult undertaking. If a person is able to change an erroneous belief when it is pointed out to them that it is irrational then they do not need therapy. A conversation with a friend or colleague is enough to dispel their misunderstanding. Irrational beliefs which have been sustained over time and underpin established emotional and behavioural patterns are more enduring. Clients do not experience these beliefs as irrational but see them as representative of reality. Indeed clients may not be conscious of the psychological operation of these beliefs. Such beliefs may lead automatically to emotional responses such as fear which the client experiences as entirely appropriate to the situation. Thus the process of helping the client will involve raising their awareness of the importance and operation of irrational beliefs, identifying specific beliefs involved in their problem and attempting to undermine and change these beliefs.

Cognitive restructuring: self-theories, self-instruction, and behavioural practice

Ellis' (1962) *rational emotive therapy*, Meichenbaum's (1977) *self-instructional therapy* and Beck's (1976) *cognitive therapy* have many common features and in this section we shall draw upon all three to develop a better understanding of the techniques involved in bringing about emotional and behavioural change through cognitive restructuring.

The initial approach of a cognitive therapist will be similar to that of a counsellor. The therapist will explore what is problematic in the client's life, in what contexts problems occur and what kind of resolution the client hopes for. During this clarification stage the therapist may be identifying beliefs which she regards as irrational and sustaining destructive emotional responses or maladaptive behaviour.

Like most therapies cognitive therapy needs to educate the client about how change might be brought about and to engage their commitment to the activities involved. Ellis, for example, shares the basic assumptions of rational emotive theory with his clients in order to persuade than of the importance of irrational beliefs in maintaining problematic emotions and behaviours. Clients who accept this psychological explanation have already made a very important change in their representation of themselves. Remembering our reference to Harré's work in Chapter 1 (Section 3) we can say that they have begun to develop a new theory of self. This is consolidated when they accept that they themselves can contribute to changing the beliefs which underpin their undesirable emotions and behaviours. In attribution theory terms they cease to explain their experience in terms of external uncontrollable factors and acknowledge that internal controllable factors may shape their future behaviour (see Chapter 2, Section 3). Thus instead of viewing fear as a physiological reaction which can only be controlled by avoiding certain situations a client sees her own representations of those situations as an important control factor. Mathews (1988), for example, discusses how a nurse therapist employed rational emotive therapy to help a woman recognize the way in which her beliefs and horrific thoughts maintained an irrational fear of becoming infected by human immunodeficiency virus. By accepting the assumptions behind rational emotive theory and learning to challenge her beliefs this woman was able to resume social and sexual activities which she had been avoiding because of her fear. This acceptance of the self as an agent which can operate on her own representations in order to change behavioural control mechanisms is an important first step in the cognitive restructuring process.

The client can then be involved in a process of questioning the validity of relevant beliefs and exploring their contribution to problematic emotions and behaviours. Beck, for example, encourages clients to become aware of distortions in their belief system such as over-generalizations, inferences which are not justified, selective memory which emphasizes negative aspects of the past and viewing events in oversimplified black and white terms. Similarly, Ellis argues with clients and asks them to provide evidence to substantiate their beliefs. For example, a client might be asked to show how she is to blame for her husband's affair, or why God should wish to punish her or to support the view that she is a terrible person who people do not care for. Such debate will involve proposing alternative versions of the client's experience and other people's perceptions of her. Much of this is likely to focus upon persuading the client to accept herself as valuable and worthwhile despite her difficulties and at the same time convincing her that she will be able to overcome some of these difficulties in time. In this way the therapist and client work together to identify and change beliefs which undermine her sense of self-esteem and self-efficacy (see Chapter 2, Section 3).

Over time the client can learn to challenge her own beliefs. She may monitor the appearance of negative and self-defeating thoughts, identify how they prevent her doing what she wants to and begin to challenge them.

Dodd (1988) discusses how a nurse therapist can measure the extent to which a client accepts destructive beliefs. The client might, for example, record how convinced she was of a self-defeating belief about their abilities on a scale of 1–100 and then repeat this over time to show changes in the their belief structure. Noticing and questioning destructive and self-defeating thoughts which have been identified in therapy sessions allows the client to continue the cognitive restructuring process by herself. Dodd describes such self-challenging to clients as 'talking back to one's thoughts'.

This is very similar to the processes used in Meichenbaum's self-instructional therapy. Here the client is taught to reassure herself and guide her behaviour using self-talk which can be internalized to become silent self-instruction over time. A client who is trying to control anger, for example, might be helped to identify upsetting situations and talk herself thought them, 'I know this is going to upset me, I'm not going to take it too seriously, I should avoid argument here, I don't have to take this personally, Remember to relax. . .' (Novaco, 1978). Such training could, for example, contribute to a programme designed to reduce type A behaviour amongst myocardial infarction patients (see Chapter 2, Section 4). Similarly a client fearful of contamination might use the following self-statements, 'I've just touched that door handle but I know it won't do me any harm, I feel a bit anxious but not very anxious, I'm managing very well, I don't need to dwell on it, I'll just get on with my work and forget about it. . .'. Meichenbaum (1977) also discusses how clients can use self-encouragement by promising themselves valued rewards while instructing themselves through difficult situations. Thus cognitive therapy can be seen as a re-socialization process using inter-nalization to achieve a kind of reprogramming (see Chapter 1, Section 3). However, because therapy involves *re*programming a much higher level of self-consciousness and self-monitoring is required. The client becomes her own cognitive psychologist by adopting a self-representation in which a stimulus-response account of her behaviour is rejected in favour of one based on cognitive behavioural control. This view of the self as composed of modifiable beliefs, provides an opportunity to drive a wedge between events in the environment and automatic thoughts and responses. Such self-conscious escape from automatic reaction by means of challenging intervening beliefs is the key to cognitive therapy.

Cognitive therapists have combined these methods with reinforce-ment programmes. Ellis (1976) for example, recommends that clients are given self-challenging homework assignments and a reinforcement programme which enables them to reward themselves for challenging and surrendering destructive beliefs. Meichenbaum (1976) also discusses how clients can encourage themselves to instruct themselves through difficult situations by the promise of valuable rewards. Planned rewards can encourage clients to persist with cognitive challenges to their pre-vious beliefs and assumptions and also motivate them to practice new behavioural routines which may be difficult at first.

Behavioural control depends upon practice as well as cognitive change. Initially practice in pretend or role-play situations may be easiest. Such role-play allows clients to anticipate and develop ways of dealing with role-related and situational barriers to the planned behavioural change (see Chapter 4, Section 1). It can be used to experiment with ways of handling difficulties without the having to suffer the real social consequences of making mistakes. A client can practice a new behaviour in an experi-mental way while the therapist acts out the part of someone who may present difficulties for the client. Over time much practice may be required to establish a new behavioural sequence as routine. *Routinization* is important because of the effort involved in conscious self-monitoring and self-talk. Through practice the client not only establishes new beliefs and thoughts as 'natural' but develops the motor skills involved in enacting new behaviours. As these skills are developed through practice the effort of willing oneself to persist with appropriate action is reduced. The desired behavioural sequences become routine responses requiring less and less self-instruction.

The mix of techniques which are applied in such therapies must of course be tailored to the needs of the client. This means that the problem must be carefully assessed taking account of cognitive, emotional, physiological and behavioural aspects. Lazarus (1976) has described such assessment as 'multimodal' and has highlighted the importance of understanding how these different aspects of a person's functioning can combine to create psychological problems.

Integrating therapeutic approaches – pain management

We have seen how beliefs about ourselves can affect our perception of situational threats and our ability to cope with such threat. Meichenbaum (1977) illustrates the point in relation to public speaking. A confident speaker may regard departing members of the audience as an event prompted by outside demands which does not necessarily reflect on her speech but a speaker with low self-esteem may begin to worry that the audience is negatively evaluating her performance. Such threat perceptions activate the sympathetic nervous system, the hypothalamus and the pituitary gland. This leads to changes in heart rate, blood circulation pattern, and the conversion of fats into usable energy sources. As the person becomes aware of such physiological changes they may become worried that their concern is visible to others or that bodily reactions will interfere with their ability to cope. This increased anxiety will have further physiological effects. Anxiety and embarrassment may disrupt cognitive functioning and the person's ability to deliver a fluent and interesting speech may be undermined. This interaction between impression management, attributional processes, perceived self-efficacy and physiological responses in our experience of stress and ability to cope with potential stressors emphasizes the need to include cognitive, behavioural and physiological considerations in our stress-related interventions.

Pain is an important stressor in illness and its control has illustrated how an understanding of the relationship between physiological and psychological factors can facilitate treatment. While pain is clearly physiological there is no one-to-one correspondence between physical injury and pain experience. Pain may be experienced long after a wound has healed and amputees may experience phantom limb pain, suggesting that the body is able to reproduce pain through memory-like processes. Moreover, in certain circumstances people may not feel pain even when they sustain injuries (Melzack and Wall, 1988). Our experience of pain is also affected by our understanding of the consequences of our injuries, for example soldiers who believe that their suffering will lead to removal from a battle zone appear to suffer less discomfort than civilians who have undergone surgery and anticipate a more uncomfortable and disruptive period in their lives (Beecher, 1956). Pain expression is also variable and affected by our socialization history. Thus members of different cultures exhibit different behaviour in response to similar pain experiences (Zborowski, 1952; Sternbach and Tursky, 1965).

The work of Melzack and Wall (1965) on gate control mechanisms has helped us understand the relationship between various aspects of pain. The essence of the theory is that nervous signals which alert the brain to pain-inducing physical states pass through the grey matter in the spinal cord and may be modified as they do so. The physical processes operating in the dorsal horns of the spinal cord form a neural gate which when closed inhibits pain signals from passing upwards to the brain, thereby reducing pain experience. Nervous signals from other physical stimulation and messages from the brain can therefore inhibit pain (see Melzack and Wall, 1988 for a more detailed description). Such downward signals from the brain provide a physiological pathway by which mood, emotion and concentration can affect pain experience. This also helps to explain placebo effects in which medicines that have no active ingredient can reduce pain through patients' anticipation of relief.

Pain is therefore an area in which we require what Engel (1977) called a *biopsychosocial* model. Engel, a psychiatrist, argued that psychiatry must retain a biochemical perspective but move beyond a purely physiological perspective. He rejected both the traditional medical model and the radical departure from it proposed by critical psychiatry (see Chapter 4, Section 2). He traces the divide between the biological and the psychological to religious distinctions between body and soul, and proposes that modern health care should abandon Decartes' seventeen century division of persons into separate minds and bodies. Using the example of grief he shows how psychiatry and medicine as a whole can assess and treat problems more effectively by taking account of their physiological, psychological and social aspects. This biopsychosocial approach corresponds to nursing models which emphasize holistic care.

Approaching pain in this way allows for a combination of physical, behavioural and cognitive interventions which have various effects on the subtle neural mechanisms controlling pain experience. Physical interventions include surgery and drugs which directly block pain transmission as well as massage, heat and electrical stimulation which activate nerves that inhibit transmission (Melzack and Wall, 1988). Psychological interventions include counselling, relaxation training, biofeedback, hypnosis, operant programmes and cognitive therapies.

One psychological approach has been to focus upon behavioural responses to pain rather than the experience itself. Fordyce (1976) adopted a behaviourist perspective, arguing that a range of pain behaviours including inactivity are maintained by social reinforcement and can therefore be decreased by removing this reinforcement. These reinforcements are likely to be social attention, pain-relieving medication or the removal of role-related obligations. Patients suffering from chronic pain may receive such reinforcement for maladaptive behaviors such as complaining, physical inactivity, social withdrawal and negative emotional expression (see Turk, et al., 1985; 1987 for analyses of what is meant by 'pain behaviour'). Fordyce trained ward staff to offer medication and attention for adaptive behaviour such as physical activity, social interaction or acknowledging a reduction in pain and, at the same time, to ignore complaints, inactivity and withdrawal. Observation of patients with chronic pain showed dramatic decreases in pain behavior from baseline levels during this intervention. Flor, et al., (1987) have noted how the same effect may operate between pain sufferers and their spouses. Referring to spouses who offered reinforcement for pain behaviour as 'solicitous', they found that patients with solicitous spouses were less active and showed more pain-related behavior. In Chapter 4 (Section 2) we noted how encouraging patients to adopt 'sick role' behavior can lead to dependency and loss of self-efficacy and thereby undermine good health. Here again we see that caring which is not directed towards the promotion of an independent patient may accelerate disability.

Fordyce has also shown how reliance on medication may be reduced by removing its reinforcement function. Medication can be delivered at set time intervals rather than in response to pain behaviour. When pain is well controlled the time intervals between medication can be very gradually increased to discover whether less frequent medication maintains pain control. Dosages can also be gradually decreased by giving medication in a sweet cocktail so that patients are unaware of how much they are receiving. In this way the minimum dose which achieves pain control can be identified. Such operant interventions focus upon pain behaviour rather than pain but for patients who have become disabled by chronic pain they may greatly enhance life by extending their activities and enabling them to distract themselves from pain through greater social involvement. Reduced pain behavior and increased social activity will also change others' perception of the patient and may lead to increased social support because others find relating to her more rewarding (see Chapter 6, Sections 2 and 3).

Beliefs shape emotions and our psychological state of mind affects the gating control of pain messages. Therefore pain experience and emotional responses to pain will depend upon how people represent their pain. Turk and Kerns (1983), for example, report a study showing that participants with lower pain tolerance had lower self-efficacy regarding tolerance and engaged in self-defeating thoughts and 'catastrophizing' during pain. Other people's thoughts and beliefs may also be important. Solicitous behaviour promoting dependency and disability may be based on erroneous beliefs held by spouses, friends or nurses (Turk, et al., 1983).

Thus cognitive methods designed to change the way sufferers or their carers represent pain may be applied in a similar manner to their use with stress or anger.

Turk has designed a 'stress inoculation training' approach designed to change pain experience and increase tolerance (Meichenbaum 1977; Turk, et al., 1983). The intervention was tested using the muscle-ischemia procedure in which pain is induced by inflating the cuff of a sphygmoma- nometer (blood pressure gauge) to a high level. This can be safely endured for about three-quarters of an hour and participants recover within five minutes. Participants were informed about the implications of the gate control theory of pain for psychological control of pain experiences and taught various coping skills. They were trained to relax by attending to their breathing and muscle tension. They were also encouraged to use cognitive strategies in which they tried to think about their pain experi- ence in a way which minimized suffering. First, diverting their attention by, for example, engaging in mental arithmetic or focusing upon some detailed feature of their environment. Secondly, somatization in which the participant concentrates on analysing and describing their physical responses to pain in a detached way as if they belonged to someone else. Thirdly, imaginative inattention in which the participant imagines they are doing something pain-free such as lying on a beach. Fourthly, imaginative transformation in which the participant imagines they are someone else in a different situation in which pain tolerance is very important, for example, a spy who has been shot but must escape from enemy agents. Participants were also taught self-instructional statements with which they could encourage themselves during the pain experience, for exam- ple, 'Don't worry you have lots of strategies to draw upon, just relax, use your coping skills, well done you knew you could cope. . .'. They were then given time to review and rehearse their coping strategies by imagining themselves tolerating pain using these strategies and imagining themselves explaining the whole procedure to another person. Participants who had been through this training were able to endure ischemic pain for 15 min- utes longer and reported less intense pain experiences than those who had not had the training. This suggests that cognitive coping strategies may be useful in helping patients cope with pain.

The interplay of physiological, cognitive, behavioural and social pro- cesses we have discussed implies that pain assessment must go beyond a description of location, intensity and clinical history. Turk and Kerns (1983) point out that we must explore the meaning of the pain for the sufferer, the impact it has on various aspects of her life, the responses and coping methods she has developed and the manner in which others treat her. Turk, et al., (1983) point out that interviews with important people in the patient's social network can provide vital assessment information (see Chapter 6, Section 3). They discuss how such people may be involved in observing the client and completing a behavioural diary recording the

patient's pain behaviour and their response to it. Standardized questionnaires may also be employed to measure aspects of the individual's pain
perception. Melzack's (1975) McGill Pain Questionnaire is well known
and attempts to record sensory, emotional and evaluative aspects of a
person's pain experience by asking them to choose adjectives to describe
their pain. However, some of the distinctions between the adjectives
provided may not be salient to people with limited vocabularies and
it may have limited use across different cultural groupings (Chapman
et al., 1985). Finally, nurses' observation of pain behaviour provides
useful information and may be used as a baseline comparison if operant
interventions are implemented.

An appreciation of the biopsychosocial nature of pain has led to the
establishment of *pain clinics* in which multidiciplinary professional teams
employ a mixture of methods focusing upon physiological, cognitive and
behaviour change in chronic pain sufferers. Such clinics may involve
those close to the sufferer and may employ therapeutic group work to
help patients develop better control and coping strategies (see Chapter 8,
Section 4).

CORE IDEAS IN CHAPTER 7

- Helping others change is an important aspect of health promotion.

- However, the use of psychological knowledge to encourage
  change raises ethical questions.

- Effective psychological counselling involves relating in an empa-
  thetic and genuine manner, offering clients unconditional positive
  regard and managing responsibility.

- Counselling is directed towards enabling clients to make their own
  decisions and act effectively in relation to their personal goals. It
  may support clients in communicating their concerns, changing
  the way they view reality, defining new behavioural targets, maintaining motivation and becoming independent.

- Classical conditioning can result in drug users experiencing conditioned highs in situations associated with previous drug use.
  This may undermine cognitive behavioural control. Repeated
  exposure to these situations without drug use should lead to
  extinction.

- Skinner's operant conditioning can be used to shape behaviour
  and increase the frequency of desired responses. Initially artificial

reinforces (such as tokens) may be used but these must be faded out and replaced by social reinforces (such as approval) if new behaviour is to be maintained.

- Reinforcement may shape performance but learning may take place in the absence of reinforcement.

- Systematic desensitization involves generating responses incompatible with fear or anxiety. Relaxation is combined with the client's representation of increasingly fearful encounters.

- Watson's behaviourism focused upon observable stimuli and behaviours. However, in order to establish which stimuli are important to clients or what counts as a reward we must explore their representations of reality. For example, extrinsic rewards may sometimes undermine intrinsic motivation. This leads us back to a consideration of internal representation in behavioural control.

- When we cannot discuss goals with clients, for example in the case of infants, changing the consequences of their behaviour may be the most effective way of encouraging adaptive behaviour.

- Cognitive restructuring involves persuading clients that their perceptions and emotions are based on their own representations of reality and these can be changed.

- Challenging one's assumptions about others and one's situation and practicing new ways of responding can gradually establish new behavioural routines.

- Our representations of reality, our physiological responses and habitual behaviour patterns can all be involved in maladaptive behaviour which undermines our personal goals. Therapeutic approaches should therefore be biopsychosocial and take each of these factors into account. Pain management provides a good illustration.

Note

1. The term 'patient' has unfortunately passive connotations when applied to those engaged in therapy. We shall therefore refer to these people as 'clients' (see Chapter 4, Section 2 for further discussion of the two terms).

8

Working and changing in groups

1 Interaction and Influence in Groups
The nature of groups

In previous chapters we emphasized how individual behaviour is shaped
by shared representations and interaction with others. We examined

interaction in relation to its social context, looking at the way in which role definition, perceived reputation and relationships with others affect everyday behaviour. In this chapter we shall explore interaction *within* groups. Such interaction is common in work and leisure and offers an additional approach to facilitating psychological change (see Chapter 7).

When two people meet both are closely involved in all interaction. However, once one or more people join this pair the pattern of interaction changes. Some members of the group will now be observing while others interact. Separate interactions between pairs may occur simultaneously and individuals may form liaisons and pacts which do not include all members. It is these changes in the pattern of interaction and their effects on group members which makes group dynamics interesting.

Research into group dynamics began in the 1940s and was prompted by two main interests. First, an interest in the processes by which democratic decisions are made. Countries and organizations which attempt to implement a collective or democratic approach to decision-making inevitably employ groups of people to discuss and evaluate proposals and then recommend action. It is therefore interesting to ask whether the nature of these groups lead to different decisions to those which would be made by lone individuals. Secondly, groups are seen to affect their members' behaviour. Indeed many countries have employed small group meetings to persuade populations of particular political views. We can therefore ask how groups change their members and whether such change processes can be employed to promote positive personal change (see Zander, 1979 for a useful review).

A *group* has been defined as three or more persons who interact in the context of shared norms and goals. Shared norms are sets of rules which group members follow (see Chapter 4, Section 1) while shared goals refer to common purposes within the group. The crucial element is, however, the interaction. Seven people on a platform waiting for a train may have the same goal and may be behaving according to shared rules, that is, social rules relevant to 'waiting for a train'. However, they are not necessarily interacting. If they are told their train has been cancelled and they must walk a mile down the road to catch a coach they may begin to interact in a manner which leads to the development of role relations and social influence processes typical of more established groups. In particular they may begin to develop a shared social identity (see Chapter 3, Section 3).

Groups have traditionally been divided according to size. Groups of 20 or more have been regarded as 'large groups' while those with fewer than 20 members are thought of as 'small groups', with the typical small group having around seven members. Most of the decision-making, teamwork, and change processes we are interested in occur within small groups. Most nursing groups and multidisciplinary teams, for example, are small groups in this sense.

We can also categorize groups according to their central tasks and functions. In particular we distinguish between task-oriented groups, social or friendship groups and personal growth or therapeutic groups. *Task oriented groups* attempt to act upon and change their external environment. Groups that fit into this category include clinical teams, management teams and other work groups. *Social or friendship groups* exist primarily to provide pleasurable interaction for members, for example social clubs. *Personal growth or therapeutic groups* attempt to change aspects of the members' thoughts, emotions or behaviours. These include self-help groups in which individuals with a particular problem meet with others to offer mutual support.

Group influence – norms, conformity and polarization

Sherif (1935) was one of the first people to study the way in which shared rules develop within groups and affect individual members' representations of reality. He set up experiments in which participants were presented with a small stationary light about 5 metres away from them in a dark room. In these circumstances we tend to see a stationary light as wandering erratically because the darkness removes reference points. This is an illusion, known as the *autokinetic effect*. Sherif did not inform his participants about the effect and asked them to estimate how far the light was moving. Since the perception of movement is an illusion different individuals tend to make different estimates of the magnitude of movement.

Half Sherif's participants made their initial judgements alone and were then asked to announce their decisions in groups of two or three. The other half began by making judgements in groups and then later estimated the distance moved alone. Sherif found that participants who first made their judgements alone quickly developed an individual average around which they grouped their estimates. Although these individual averages differed, participants asked to announce their judgements aloud in a group gradually converged towards a shared group average. Moreover, participants who had estimated in group continued to make judgements based on the group average even when making judgements alone.

Sherif had demonstrated that when we find ourselves in an ambiguous situation we tend to create a stable internal frame of reference against which to view reality. If we find that this viewpoint conflicts with that of other group members we tend to modify it so as to achieve greater agreement. This allows us to develop shared representations of reality through common frames of reference within groups. These group agreements about the world are referred to as *group norms*. Such norms simultaneously enable us to share our world and constrain our individual freedom and decision-making.

Work on how we are influenced by others in groups was continued by Asch (1951; 1956). Asch was interested in what effect group influence would have on more straightforward judgements than those arising from the autokinetic effect. He invited students to say which of three lines was equal in length to a another standard line and found that, over a series of such judgements, his participants choose the correct matching line more than 99% of the time. This provided a fairly unambiguous judgement task which could be used to explore the influence of group norms on public decision-making.

Using six confederates Asch led participants to believe that they were making judgements in the presence of six other students recruited in the same way as themselves. Each group member, in turn, judged which line matched the standard and made their judgement aloud so other members could hear. It is worth noting that this was one of the first instances in which a social psychologist used confederates or actors to investigate the impact of a social situation on individuals' behaviour. This method of investigating social influence through the creation of artificial social situations has since become widespread (see Chapter 4, Sections 3 and 4).

Asch's confederates gave predetermined answers. In a series of 18 matching judgements they chose the correct line on the first two judgements and on four others distributed over the remaining 16 line-matching judgements. On the 12 other trials all the confederates gave the same incorrect answer. This must have been quite disconcerting to the real participants who could clearly see which of the three lines matched the standard but also heard other students agreeing on the wrong line! Asch found that they made wrong judgements 37% of the time. Thus, although participants who made their judgements alone were correct more than 99% of the time, participants subjected to a group who regularly agreed on the wrong answer were only correct 63% of the time. The majority of participants made correct judgements most of the time and a quarter were entirely independent (Harris, 1985). Nevertheless, three-quarters of the real participants made at least one mistake demonstrating that, even in unambiguous situations, we can be affected by others' judgements in group discussions. Nicholson, et al., (1985) replicated the Asch study with students from Britain and the United States and found that although students in the 1980s were more independent, group influence continues to prompt unexpected errors amongst a minority who were influenced by confederates' erroneous choices.

Deutsch and Gerard (1955) considered how our susceptibility to such group influence follows from our concerns about expressing our judgements in front of others. We are concerned to be right so that further checks and measurements will validate our expressed view. However, we are also sensitive to others' perceptions of us and want them to think of us as a competent and sensible person (see Chapter 3, Section 2). We use two sources of information in making such judgements, our own experience and the expressed views of other group members. Where these concur we have no problems. Others validate our perceptions and a stable representation of reality is established. However, when these conflict, as they did for Asch's real participants, we have to decide which is the most reliable source of information. In many cases we may decide to accept others' views because we trust their judgement more than our own. This type of group influence is known as *informational influence* because we are using others as an extra source of information. We may, however, also accept others' views even when we do not trust their judgement and suspect that they are wrong. In order to be accepted by others as someone who shares their social norms and is sensible in their terms we may go along with the group regardless of our private thoughts. This type of group influence is known as *normative influence* because we are agreeing with others in order to fit into an established group norm. Thus remaining independent in the face of expressed opposition within a group we want to belong to requires robust self-confidence.

Insko and colleagues (1983) examined both normative and informational influence by comparing group participants who made judgements publicly (so others knew their choices) and privately (so that their choices were hidden from others). They found that the influence of other group members was greater in the public condition. This shows that although group discussions exert informational influence on members the impact of normative influence may be reduced by asking members to make private written decisions in advance of public discussion. In the case of selection panels, for example, if members record their candidate choice on a piece of paper which is collected before the group discussion a more comprehensive view of members' impressions is likely to result than when decisions are made simply on the basis of the public discussion (see Chapter 3, Section 2).

The degree to which we are influenced by group members is also affected by our perception of the judgement task itself. Insko et al., used a second independent variable, namely whether participants thought there was only one right answer or many potentially correct viewpoints. They discovered that when participants thought there was only one answer they conformed more often, showing that our desire to be right leaves us more susceptible to informational influence when we think that there is only one correct view of reality.

Group decision-making is therefore more than simply averaging the views of members in order to reach a consensus. Imagine a meeting in which nurses on a ward discuss their reactions to proposals for a new system of patient care. It becomes clear that the new proposals are unpopular but that individuals vary in the strength of their opposition. Will those who are more favourably disposed to the proposals be influenced by those most opposed or vica versa. Social psychological research suggests such a meeting is more likely to strengthen opposition to the proposed changes.

Studies in the 1960s suggested that when groups considered decisions involving risk they tended to reach riskier conclusions than individuals (Stoner, 1961). However, later studies cast doubt on the conclusion that groups generally produce a 'risky shift'. Indeed some groups were shown to make more cautious decisions than the average opinion of their members (Knox and Stafford, 1976). Overall then it seemed that group discussion tended to lead to a conclusion which was somewhat more extreme than the average of the individual members' views. If the members were positively disposed group discussion tended to lead to further acceptance but if members generally disliked a proposal opposition would grow during group discussion. This tendency is called *group polarization*. It was clearly demonstrated in the realm of political judgement by Moscovici and Zavalloni (1969) and Lamm and Myers (1978) discuss its operation in relation to various types of group discussion.

Both normative and informational influence may contribute to group polarization. As members compare others' judgements to their own, their desire for social acceptance, and participation encourages them to express their views in a corresponding manner. In a group where members already hold negative views of a proposal then normative influence continually operates to encourage somewhat more negative expressions of opinion. Listening to such negative views may provide members with new information and arguments which suggest that the proposal should be rejected. This is informational influence. Thus normative and informational influence are likely to lead our group of nurses to emerge from their meeting more strongly opposed to the proposed changes.

Group polarization is a worrying phenomenon because it suggests that group dynamics may stifle debate and lead to more extreme decisions. This could clearly result in poor decisions and the acceptance of group norms even when they have become inappropriate in changed circumstances. This is exactly the process which Janis (1972) described as *groupthink*. Janis argued that social influence processes can lead to poor decision making when a group of people with strongly held views lose the ability to critically reflect on their group's norms and operation. The most famous example considered by Janis was the Bay of Pigs invasion of Cuba in 1961. President Kennedy and a small group of advisers planned the operation in which a group of Cuban exiles invaded the island. The attack went disastrously wrong for the Americans and retrospective commentators (including the president) agreed that the decisions taken by the group were based on extremely poor logic.

If group discussion is to generate thoughtful decision-making then we must identify and eliminate factors which encourage acceptance of extreme and unconsidered opinion for the sake of social acceptance. Janis argued that several factors encourage groupthink. First, when a group is highly cohesive, that is, members hold similar views and value one another's social support. Secondly, when it is isolated from alternative sources of information, for example when members deliberately avoid exposure to other viewpoints. Thirdly, when the group does not devote time to evaluating its decisions. Fourthly, when a leader with power and authority expresses her views strongly thereby increasing normative pressure and encouraging conformity and obedience (see Chapter 4, Section 3). Finally, groupthink is more likely when the group is under pressure, with little time to consider complex problems. In such circumstances simplistic solutions which strongly affirm key group values may seem attractive. Collectively these factors promote a faith in the group's correctness and moral superiority. This may strengthen members' sense of identity with the group and lead to negative out-group stereotyping (see Chapter 3, Sections 3 and 4). This will result in further censorship of alternative viewpoints, greater isolation and increased normative influence. Such a group becomes incapable of openly discussing alternatives, considering potential negative consequences of planned action or questioning basic assumptions. Inevitably poor decisions which are not tailored to reality result.

It is therefore naive to assume that by bringing together knowledgeable and experienced individuals we guarantee rational and thoughtful group decisions. An awareness of how social influence processes can inhibit debate and evaluation is crucial to high quality democratic decision-making at either ward or government level. Establishing discussion norms which allow the acknowledgement of alternative viewpoints and the questioning basic assumptions is crucial if a group is to remain adaptable. This has important implications for the definition of role relations within groups and in particular the performance of leadership roles.

Fostering, innovation and careful discussion of new ideas is especially important in multidisciplinary teams where the aim is to benefit from a range of expertise based upon different competencies and experiences. If group norms stifle members' views then the idea of sharing different professional perspectives is undermined so that the team may represent little more than the views of its most powerful member. Thus minimizing group influence (for example, by tabling individually prepared reports) may be important in order to benefit from the diversity of experience within the group.

This is the aim of *nominal group* meetings. Such meetings begin with members writing down their ideas on an issue without discussion. These ideas are then publicly recorded (for example, on a board) with each member offering one idea in turn until all ideas are listed. The group then discusses the ideas in relation to their clarity, applicability and practicality. Finally each member silently rank orders the ideas and the group's decision is to select the idea which gets the highest rankings. In such nominal groups the generation of ideas is protected from group influence in order to ensure a diverse input of ideas.

On a wider scale it is also important that professions encourage internal diversity and evaluation if they are to promote development and adaption to changing circumstances. Within nursing various specialist groups may hold different views on nurse management and nurse role definition. These different perspectives were denounced as 'tribalism' by the management consultants Peat Marwick McLintock (1989) in their review of the structure and function of the statutory bodies governing nursing in the United Kingdom. However, opposing views and positions may also lead to necessary evaluation and reconsideration of nurse role definition and create a climate encouraging debate, change and development.

Offering members security within the group and encouraging them to comment on and evaluate group activities and performance are likely to foster independence and thereby protect the group from the worst excesses of social influence. Individuals' confidence also affects independence. Members with high perceived self-efficacy (see Chapter 2, Section 3) who believe that there may be more than one right answer to the challenges facing the group are most likely to share their perspectives. This of course means that the way roles are defined within a group will affect who is able to influence group discussions. If members feel that their role-related obligations include reporting assessments and offering advice they are likely to contribute but if they feel their obligation is to listen to higher-status group members they are unlikely to contribute. This takes us back to the question of nurse-role definition within multidisciplinary teams (see Chapter 4, Sections 2 and 3).

Role-related rights within a group can minimize normative influence on certain members (Chapter 4, Section 1). Dittes and Kelly (1956) found that medium status group members were more likely to be influenced than either high or low status members. High status members may be allowed to step outside group norms as part of their role-related rights while low status individuals may feel they have little to lose within the group and so be less subject to normative influence. Medium status individuals, on the other hand, may lack the right to deviate and also feel they cannot risk losing support within the group.

In this section we have considered public discussion and acceptance of views and judgements within groups. We have seen that normative influence may lead us to accept group decisions which we do not agree with. This type of public acceptance is known as 'compliance'. When informational influence leads to a change in our private views we say that 'conversion' has occurred. Conformity includes both compliance and conversion. These may be indistinguishable within the group but individuals who are merely conforming to group norms are unlikely to do so when out of sight of other group members. Those who are converted, by contrast, will like Sherif's participants continue to act in accordance with the group norm in other contexts.

Resisting the majority – social support and minority influence

Asch also investigated the way in which social support within groups can minimize social influence. He found that if one of his confederates gave the correct answer (while the others continued to give incorrect responses) conformity amongst real participants dropped dramatically. With a supporter in the group the error rate for real participants dropped from 37% to less than 6%. Realizing that someone else has a different view to that of the majority punctures the majority's informational influence. It raises the possibility that there may be more than one way to look at an issue and validates the individual's own perspective. This frees the individual from much of the normative and informational influence which operates when no one else expresses dissent. This effect is similar to the way in which social support allows people to resist the views of authority figures (see Rank and Jacobson's work, Chapter 4, Section 3). Remarkably, social support seems to reduce conformity in groups even when it is provided by dubious sources, for example someone who has very poor eyesight in the case of a visual comparison (Allen and Levine, 1971). Thus encouraging the expression of alternative views fosters further diversity of opinion because members who may have conformed in the presence of a unanimous majority will express their dissent once support is forthcoming. This also means that small minorities are much more likely to resist majority influence than lone individuals.

Nurses in a team of health workers will sometimes need to rely on the views of others when making decisions. It is therefore important to remain aware of our susceptibility to normative and informational influence and check with others when one's own view differs from that of the majority. Questioning a majority view may lead other members to reconsider which may in turn lead to a better group decision and a better service for clients. Conforming without questioning decisions or discouraging discussion may lead to inappropriate service delivery.

If social support allows individual members to question majorities in groups then it must be possible for small minorities to undermine a majority view. Moscovici (1976, 1980) has emphasized that processes minority influence are vital to change and innovation. The expression of a minority view forces those in the majority to recognize that there are other ways to view the issue. This exerts informational influence on behalf of the minority position.

Moscovici and colleagues have examined factors which determine whether or not a minority can influence the majority and found minority consistency to be important. Moscovici, et al., (1969) set up an Asch-like experiment involving groups of six people making colour judgements. The groups were shown a series of blue slides of different shades and asked to say aloud what colour they were. Some groups included two confederates who either judged all slides to be green (instead of blue) or alternatively judged two-thirds of the slides to be green. Results showed that the naive participants who were not subjected to the minority viewpoint were almost universally agreed that all slides were blue (99.75% of judgements were blue). However, when the minority judged two thirds of the slides to be green a few majority members also began to make green judgements (1.25% of non-confederate judgements were green). This effect was greatly strengthened when the minority was entirely consistent (with green judgements increasing to 8.42%) and almost a third of non-confederates making at least one green judgement. Thus the consistent minority were almost seven times as influential as the inconsistent one.

It seems that majority members only begin to question their position and consider the feasibility of the minority position if the minority members agree with one another and maintain their position over time. However, once minority influence begins to take effect it is likely to gather momentum because established majority members may be even more susceptible to persuasion once their old allies begin to advocate the minority position.

Moscovici has argued that this persuasion process is likely to challenge majority member's views so that they ask themselves why minority members think as they do. Moreover, because of the normative influence of the majority people may initially be discouraged from expressing support for a minority view. This means the private agreement is likely to precede public support for minority views. By contrast the normative influence of a majority may lead to public acceptance without private agreement (that is, compliance). Thus while minority influence may require consistent argument over a long period of time it may be more likely to lead to conversion rather than compliance and therefore have longer lasting effects (Moscovici and Personnaz, 1980).

This research into social support and minority influence in groups has important practical implications for group decision-making. It strongly emphasizes the importance of participation and the value of hearing and considering different views in group discussions. Such openness not only ensures a democratic decision-making process but also avoids the pitfalls of groupthink. Involvement, participation and debate are essential ingredients of effective decision-making which is sensitive to change and external reaction. This emphasis is important when planning and leading multidisciplinary meetings – all perspectives and reports including those of the client or client advocate should be regarded as potentially influential contributions. This of course means that one of the chairperson's role obligations should be to facilitate participation and to invite discussion of alternative perspectives. Thus the definition of leadership roles is also important to group decision-making.

2 Leadership and Group Dynamics

Leader characteristics or leadership behaviour

We often think of leadership as being provided by special people. In everyday conversation we may describe someone as a 'born leader' when we observe them making useful contributions to the a group's interaction. This of course implies that leadership is an aspect of personality and furthermore that it is genetically determined. If this was the case and we could devise tests to identify individuals who had more of these personality characteristics then we could ensure that the most appropriate people were appointed to influential positions and thereby ensure better organizational functioning and government. Psychologists have therefore devoted some effort to tracking down leader characteristics.

Unfortunately this proved to be a fairly unproductive search and in 1954 Gibb concluded that attempts to identify leader characteristics had failed. Yet in everyday life we continue to think of particular people as having leadership qualities. Attribution theory can help us understand this (see Chapter 2, Section 3). Since we tend to see people in similar situations and over-attribute their behaviour to themselves rather than the situation (an example of the 'fundamental attribution error', see Chapter 3, Section 1) we see leadership behaviour as an expression of individual personality. We do not usually observe leaders we know in different types of group. Would the senior nurse whose leadership qualities we admire in intensive care make an equally good play-group leader, insurance manager, facilitator in a therapeutic group and commando officer? Different types of group need special contributions to enhance their functioning. Thus the ability to successfully lead one group does not necessarily imply leadership skills relevant to groups in general.

Psychologists have therefore turned their attention to the way in which leadership behaviour contributes to necessary *group functions* within particular kinds of group (Cartwright and Zander, 1968). This is an example of social psychological research challenging first-order, common sense views about interaction (see Chapter 1, Section 1) and again questioning the power of personality theories to explain social behaviour (see Chapter 4, Section 3).

This focus on the functions which leaders perform does not mean that there are no common elements to leadership across groups. There are similarities between leaders in different groups but in order to select the most effective leader for any particular group we must consider its special needs. Leaders have to be able to understand what is happening within their group. They need to be able to communicate with other members and they need to have enough self-confidence to be able to take the initiative. However, specialist expertise may be required to understand interaction and manage communication effectively within different types of groups (for example, a therapeutic group and a commando assault group). Thus Stogdill (1974) reports that leaders are likely to have higher intelligence, self confidence and energy levels than their followers but that task-specific knowledge and expertise are also also key factors in distinguishing leaders from other group members.

Establishing leadership credentials

Since communication and expertise are important to effective group functioning social psychologists have examined members reactions to those who talk a lot in groups and those whose contributions are seen to be well informed. Sorrentino and Boutillier (1975), designed an experiment in which they manipulated two independent variables (see Chapter 1, Section 4), the quantity and quality of talk a confederate contributed to a group. The groups had four other participants and the confederate's contribution was preplanned to be seen as high in participation and quality, high in participation but of low quality, low in participation and quality or low in participation but of high quality. After group discussions members recorded judgements about one another, including their perception of others as potential leaders. This judgement was Sorrentino and Boutilliers' dependent variable and they found that the level of participation had more influence on members' perception of leadership potential than the quality of this participation. This suggests that in the early stages of group formation participation may be a more important contribution than specific knowledge. Once the group's aims and objectives are clarified expertise may become important. Those with relevant skills and knowledge may be able to provide leadership without being especially active. However, those lacking such expertise have to persuade others of their leadership potential through high levels of participation. Thus without expertise one must persuade others of one's leadership potential through high levels of participation but as an expert one may be perceived as a leader without high participation.

The implication of these findings for nurses working in clinical or management teams is that they can maximize their acceptance as group leaders by taking an active part in the discussions. Such participation may be especially helpful in the first few team meetings. If nurses also have expertise relevant to the group's aims they will further strengthen their claim to a leadership role.

Multidisciplinary teams are, however, different to the laboratory groups discussed above. Members of such teams already have professional roles which shape their perceptions of, and responses to, other professionals (see Chapter 4, Section 2). Thus nurses' claim to leadership potential in multidisciplinary teams may be adversely affected by other professionals' stereotypes of nurses as followers rather than leaders and by nurses' own stereotypes of other professionals as higher status or more expert. Stereotypes can become self-fulfilling prophecies (see Chapter 3, Section 1) so that nurses who regard accountants, doctors or administrators as higher status may feel obligated to refrain from leadership contributions and may even de-skill themselves by taking on non-expert tasks such as making and serving tea for the team. By consciously recognizing the operation of these stereotypes nurses can avoid limiting themselves to follower roles and channel skills into leadership contributions.

Gender and Leadership

Gender stereotypes and socialization are also likely to be important to the adoption of leadership roles by nurses. We have considered Gilligan's (1982) proposal that girls' feminine socialization may prepare them better for intimate relationships than boys but prepare them less well for competitive relationships (see Chapter 4, Section 5). Evidence for such differences can be found in the different patterns of play developed by girls and boys. Lever (1976) noted that primary school boys tended to be more competitive and play in larger groups than girls. Boys were seen to quarrel much of the time but they rarely abandoned a game because of a dispute. Girls' games, on the other hand, were frequently ended by disputes, seemingly because it was was more important for girls to maintain good relations than pursue their games. Moreover boys' liking for one another tends to be based on the amount of fun they have playing together while girls value closeness achieved through mutual self-disclosure.

These findings suggest that while girls are learning person-orientated social skills which enable them to develop and maintain intimate relationships, boys are learning how to deal with competition in a fairly assertive manner within complex rule-bound interaction. To highlight this distinction we might say that girls are learning skills prerequisite to therapeutic relating while boys learn how to relate within competitive bureaucracies. We have noted that overcoming gender differentiation by assimilating typically masculine and feminine social skills (that is, becoming psychologically androgynous) enables people to be more adaptable and mature in their approach to relationship formation and work-role performance. Nevertheless gender socialization typically provides men and women with different leadership skills. Many women may have more to learn than their male peers about power and authority role relationships while many men may have more to learn about empathy and consideration for other group members.

Buhrmester and Furman (1983) found that men and women college students experienced leadership roles differently. Men in leadership roles tended to be less lonely, less emotionally isolated and a have higher levels of self-esteem than men who were not leaders. However, women leaders had the opposite experience, tending to be more emotionally isolated, more lonely and having lower self-esteem. Women may not reap the social benefits of leadership because its role-related obligations are less consistent with their feminine self-representations than those of their male colleagues (see Horner's work – Chapter 4, Section 5). However, leadership may also be more difficult for women because of stereotyping by the men and women they lead. Gender stereotyping may make it more difficult for women to establish leadership credentials and to retain their authority within leadership roles. This may mean that they experience more conflict and less acceptance than their male counterparts, making their job simultaneously more difficult and less socially rewarding.

Leadership styles

We have noted that disillusionment with the search for personality characteristics which would predict leader effectiveness led to a focus on leader behaviour. Kurt Lewin (1948), who played a leading role in establishing social psychological research into group dynamics (see too Section 4, below), was one of those who began to investigate the effects of different styles of leadership on group members. In a very famous study he and his colleagues compared the effects of three different approaches to fulfilling the role-related obligations of a leadership role, namely, authoritarian, democratic and laissez-faire styles (White and Lippit, 1968). They systematically varied the behaviour of leaders of small groups of ten year old boys and examined the boys work output and reactions. Authoritarian or autocratic leaders dictated group policies and plans, assigned work tasks and workmates, tended to be personal in their praise and criticism and did not become involved in group activities. Democratic leaders, on the other hand, involved the groups in discussion of all policies and plans, encouraged members to choose work tasks and work companions, tried to be objective in their praise and criticism and joined in group activity without doing too much of the work. Finally, laissez-faire group leaders simply provided work materials and refrained from contributing unless approached for information.

The researchers found somewhat greater work output in groups with autocratic leaders than those with democratic leaders. However, they also found greater dependence, aggression and scapegoating in these groups. Members of democratic groups were most content, motivated, self-reliant and original. Laissez-faire groups produced less and poorer work and members expressed a preference for a more democratic style. The democratic style offered members most personal involvement and self-esteem and was therefore most popular. Although work output was somewhat lower than in autocratic groups, destructive behaviour was also minimized.

Using a similar perspective on leader behaviour Tannenbaum and Schmidt (1957) outlined a range of behaviours which span the autocratic-democratic continuum. At one end the truly autocratic leader makes all decisions and allows members little freedom, while at the other end the committed democratic leader allows members a great deal of initiative within agreed limits. Between these extremes leaders may present members with decisions but invite discussion, they may present proposals and invite critical comment or present problems and ask members to provide solutions. Research into these styles has consistently shown that members prefer greater participation and democratic leadership and that interaction within such groups is more positive than in groups with autocratic leaders. There is, however, some inconsistency in findings regarding productivity levels achieved by the two styles (Hamner and Organ, 1978).

The negative effects of autocratic leadership may well outweigh any benefits in productivity. We have noted that low levels of member participation may lead to greater compliance and in the extreme groupthink. This then results in stagnation and poor decision-making. Flowers (1977) found that leaders who refused new ideas and imposed their own opinions on group members was more likely to generate groupthink. Moreover, the dissatisfied, dependent, and aggressive climate which can result from members feelings of powerlessness may threaten commitment to the group, leading to absenteeism and high member turnover. Thus in the longer term the social climate of the group may affect its productivity. This may be especially true in nursing where work effectiveness depends crucially on positive and constructive relationships with patients and other staff. Orton (1981; 1984), and Ogier (1984), for example, noted the powerful effect that charge nurses have upon nurse students and how an authoritarian approach leads to a poor learning climate. A democratic leadership style which nurtures initiative-taking and participation seems crucial to the socialization of responsible, independent nurses who can critically assess their own competence and therefore rely on their own judgement.

Despite the benefits of a democratic style of leadership there may be circumstances in which a more directive style is more appropriate. For example, when a group is under pressure, has few resources and members are suffering from stress a directive leader may be welcomed because she relieves members from the responsibility of decision-making. This is often used to explain Winston Churchill's popularity as a strong prime minister of the United Kingdom during the second world war and his subsequent failure to be re-elected after the war. Different styles of leadership may be effective and popular in different situations. Thus as a group's circumstances alter a successful leader will adapt her approach. Similarly different styles of leadership may be appropriate in different nursing contexts. If the demands of an intensive care unit are different to those of a community mental handicap team, different leadership styles may be required.

Group needs and leadership functions

Recognition of the importance of *matching* leadership style to the needs of the group prompted research into the various social functions performed by leaders. Leaders may, for example, develop group aims, plan work schedules, assign work tasks (thereby defining members' roles), offer advice on how to tackle problems and represent the group's interests at meetings with other groups. These functions are all directly concerned with the management of the group's work. Another set of functions concern the management of interpersonal relations within the group and include, encouraging and evaluating members, relieving tension, resolving disputes between members, arranging for recreational group experiences and offering personal counselling where appropriate. This division between *task-related* and *relationship-related* functions has emerged in a number of studies (Cartwright and Zander, 1968).

Bales and Slater (1955), found that high participators quickly emerged in leaderless laboratory groups. These high participators tended to contribute to task-related functions and helped their groups to establish norms and role structures. Again emphasizing the importance of participation as a means of establishing leadership credentials in initial group meetings. High participators were liked by members at first but as groups developed members turned increasingly towards another member who performed relationship-related functions (such as encouraging others). It seemed that members were initially concerned to understand the group's structure and learn how to perform their roles effectively (see Chapter 1, Section 3; Chapter 4, Section 1). However, once this early socialization had occurred the leader's focus on performance and productivity could become oppressive if it ignored members' social and emotional needs. At this point a ('socio-emotional') leader who identifies and attends to members' relationship-related needs is welcomed.

A very similar distinction emerged from the work of a group of psychologists at Ohio University. They also identified two broad categories of leadership contribution which facilitated effective group functioning, namely the provision of 'structure' and 'consideration' (Korman, 1967). These two types of leadership contribution are not expressions of particular leaders' skills or personalities. Individual's prior experience may enable them to offer leadership in task-related or relationship-related areas but every group needs to manage its work and its internal relationships if it is to achieve its aims. Thus in our exploration of leadership we have moved from a search for *leader* characteristics to an identification of social tasks which are essential to effective *group* functioning. Bales and Slater observed a separation of task-related and relationship-related leadership functions. However, such separation may be unusual. Most leaders may offer some leadership in both task and relationship related areas. Indeed,

Stogdill (1974) maintained that leaders needed to do so in order create effective and cohesive groups.

Focusing upon leadership functions highlights the fact that many members may make leadership contributions. Although groups depend upon their official leaders to fulfill many of their leadership needs they may also rely on non-leader members to provide leadership in some areas. Indeed when incompetent official leaders are appointed many of the leader's role-related obligations may be assumed by other members for the good of the group. Ideally an official leader should complement the skills and talents available amongst group members. Thus leadership selection should be based a on a careful consideration of group membership and particular group needs and problems.

There is therefore *no best leadership style*. A charge nurse will make most impact on her team if she is able to adapt her style of leadership over time. For example, if there are a number of inexperienced nurses on the team then task-related leadership may be a priority but when her team becomes more experienced a focus on relationships and team support may be the best way of promoting good patient care. Thus being able to assess group needs and change one's leadership style is crucial to effective leadership over time. Developing such social sensitivity may require specialized training. Skills in a particular type of nursing are not, in themselves, an adequate basis for leadership responsibility. Nursing skills may indicate a potential for task-related leadership but this may be of limited use in a group composed of competent nurses who already provide a good service and resent interference.

Bales and Slater (1955) suggested that individual's characteristics may limit their leadership flexibility so they are only able to offer leadership in certain areas of the group's functioning, for example, they may be able to offer task-related leadership but unable to offer relationship-related leadership. Thus personality characteristics may have to be considered in leader selection, not because there are particular 'leader personalities', but because previous experience may limit official leaders' flexibility and it is important to ensure that an individual's leadership potential complements existing group skills. It might be interesting, for example, to consider the way gender socialization affects people's potential to offer task and relationship-related leadership. We might expect psychologically androgynous leaders to be more versatile in their leadership contributions (see chapter 4, Section 5).

Feidler's (1967) contingency theory is based upon investigations of the match between leader and group characteristics. Feidler first characterized leaders according to whether they tended to attach greater importance to task performance or relationships. Using his 'least preferred coworker' (LPC) questionnaire he asked leaders to evaluate the person they found most difficult to work with. Those who saw this person positively (and had a high LPC score) were thought to prioritize interpersonal relationships whereas those who saw this person negatively (low LPC score) were regarded as primarily task orientated. Feidler then characterized aspects of the group's dynamics. In particular the degree to which members got on with the leader, how much power the leader's role-related rights gave her and how clearly members understood their roles within the group (see Chapter 4, Section 1). This enabled him to categorize groups in terms of the degree of leader control (for example where the leader has a great deal of power, gets on well with members and members clearly understand their roles the leader has high control and vica versa). Feidler then examined the relationship between leader characteristics and group performance across different control conditions. His results suggest that in group situations which allow leaders a high degree of control or seriously limit their control a task-related approach may give rise to higher productivity but where control is moderate a focus on relationships will be more productive.

Feidler's 'least preferred coworker' scale relies upon a measure of person perception and a more sensitive measure of typical managerial style would be preferable. Moreover, the dependent variable of group performance is only one aspect of the group's overall well-being and potential. A high-achievement group may still be in jeopardy if working relationships are deteriorating. Nevertheless Feidler's work emphasizes the importance of leader-group match and highlights the danger of inflexible leaders persisting with an inappropriate leadership style. Chemers, et al., (1985) provided some support for Feidler's conclusions. They found that when administrative decision-makers' LPC scores did not match their group-control situation in the manner recommended by Feidler they reported greater work stress. This result suggests that the poorly matched leaders may be suffering stress because they find their management efforts are ineffective. Undoubtedly, other group members will also find this their failed leadership stressful (see Chapter 9, Section 3).

Hersey and Blanchard (1982) have developed another contingency model, taking both leader behaviour and group composition into account. In this model leaders are regarded as capable of both task and relationship-related leadership and their style is described in terms of how *much* of each they provide. A leader who displays high task and low relationship leadership is described as having a *telling* style while a leader who offers high task and relationship leadership has a *selling* style. High relationship but low task leadership is a *participating* style and finally a leader who shows little of either behaviour has adopted a *delegating* style. Hersey and Blanchard also considered group development over time and in particular the way staff groups may mature over time. Figure 8 shows how different leadership styles may be more or less appropriate to different stages of group development. With a group of new recruits who are neither competent or confident a high task-related, telling style may get best results. However, if group members are motivated but not competent then an additional focus on relationships, that is a 'selling' style may be most appropriate. Where members are competent but unwilling to perform a high relationship related leadership style (that is, 'participating') may be most effective and where group members are both competent and motivated a delegating style may be most efficient. As in Feidler's theory attention to interpersonal relations is recommended in mixed group conditions. However, this model emphasizes that group characteristics are unstable because groups evolve and therefore have changing leadership needs.

3 Organizational Context

The importance of organizational context

The aims and priorities of a working group such as a clinical team will be primarily determined by the performance indicators used to assess its work by managers working within a wider organizational context. This means that the meaning of 'effective leadership' or 'productivity' will be determined by criteria which are imposed on the group by other groups or individuals. Thus the way in which large-scale organizations such as hospitals or health boards are managed and the priorities they set can have a critical influence on nurse role definition (see Chapter 4, Section 2).

Despite gathering momentum to shift the emphasis of health care from large hospitals to community based services, in-patient hospital-treatment continues to account for a large part of health-care provision. In the United Kingdom there are almost 3000 hospitals ranging from those with less than 50 beds (over one-third of all hospitals) to those with more than 1000 beds (approximately one-tenth of all hospitals). Psychiatric hospitals, although reducing in size and number, make up one-fifth of all hospitals and contain one-third of all beds in the United Kingdom. It is therefore worth considering the impact that hospital organization can have upon nursing practice.

We often complain about seemingly pointless organizational rules, procedures and meetings which use valuable time and resources but do not

LEADERSHIP ORIENTATION	TELLING (High task, low relationship)	→	SELLING (High task, high relationship)	→ PARTICIPATING→ (Low task high relationship)	DELEGATING (Low task, low relationship)
GROUP COMPOSITION	LOW COMPETENCE LOW MOTIVATION	LOW COMPETENCE HIGH MOTIVATION	HIGH COMPETENCE LOW MOTIVATION	HIGH COMPETENCE HIGH MOTIVATION

Figure 8 Matching leadership style to group needs; the Hersey–Blanchard Model

seem to contribute to what we regard as the important aims of our work. We may, for example, claim that bureaucracy conflicts with patient care. In doing so we are drawing upon the work of Weber (1947) who developed a theory of large-scale organizations. He defined a *bureaucracy* as a hierarchical system of authority figures in which each has clearly defined role-related rights over other workers. Bureaucracies are run on the basis of recorded rules and procedures. Work and non-work activities are strictly separated and each worker performs a specialized function. Management of workers is impersonal so that the worker role is clearly differentiated from the person who performs it. In other words the role should remain the same even if another person fills it and the worker is not held personally responsible for the duties which define her role. Workers are selected and promoted on the basis of technical qualifications and competence and are expected to make the post their main occupation. In return the organization offers them a 'career track' subject to competent role performance.

The problem with such organizations is that they may be resistant to change because rules, procedures and role definitions are retained long after their application has ceased to exist. As well as discouraging organizational innovation bureaucratic structures may also discourage individual participation and initiative which, as we have seen above, may encourage conformity and groupthink. At their worst bureaucracies socialize workers into mindless procedure-following rather than goal-orientated problem solving. Acar and Aupperle (1984) illustrate this 'pathological' procedure-following with the case of a nurse receiving emergency calls to an ambulance service who delayed dispatching an ambulance because the rules required her to speak with the patient despite being informed that the patient had had a heart attack and was unable to speak. The patient died while her stepson negotiated on her behalf, graphically highlighting how inflexible adherence to procedure can undermine the aims of an organization. These drawbacks have led organizational theorists to recommend more flexible organizational structures which give the individual worker greater responsibility and discretion (Burns and Stalker, 1961). However, despite its problems the bureaucratic model provides an efficient way of organizing large numbers of people and allowing an organization to maintain its operations even when it loses key individuals (Perrow, 1972).

Nursing in a bureaucracy?

Hospitals encompass bureaucratic features but are not perfect bureaucracies. Nurses and other health care workers are organized into professional and para-professional groupings which prescribe standards of conduct which take priority over organizational procedure. They also have discretion and are expected to exercise professional judgement in a critical and rational manner rather than adhering strictly to predetermined rules. Thus Bucher and Stelling (1969) portrayed hospitals as a mixture of two lines of organizational authority. A bureaucratic line represented by the hospital administrators and a charismatic-traditional one governed by doctors. Nurses are subject to both lines of authority which can create conflicts of accountability and consequently role strain and role stress (see Chapter 4, Section 1; Chapter 9, Section 2). For example, as a member of a clinical team a nurse will be accountable to the team leader, usually a doctor, but will also remain accountable to nurse managers who may work outside the clinical area.

Since hospitals are not perfect bureaucracies there is room to negotiate and renegotiate the rules and roles which constitute its organization (see Chapter 4, Section 1). This idea of a 'negotiated order' draws upon a symbolic interactionism perspective (see Chapter 1, Section 3) and was applied to hospitals by Strauss, et al. (1963). Since official hospital rules are not specific enough to guide staff activity on a daily or hourly basis, inter-action is organized around a series of bargains and agreements which are made, forgotten and re-negotiated by individuals at different times. Nurses negotiate with patients, managers and other occupational groups. Hall (1977), for example, illustrated how nurses in children's wards 'negotiated' the conditions under which play leaders could work on the wards. The previously agreed play-leader role threatened to disrupt ward routine so, exercising their negotiating power, nurses restricted play leaders to a more marginal position within wards and kept their ward routine intact. As well as negotiating with other professionals nurses and doctors are increasingly involved in negotiating treatments with patients (see Chapter 4, Section 2; Chapter 5, Section 2). Consumer satisfaction and patient compliance are critically affected by these negotiations (see Chapter 2, Section 1; Chapter 5, Section 4).

While this negotiated order perspective explains much of the flexibility and development within hospitals we must also remember that bureau-cratic lines of authority do operate in hospitals and nurses sometimes feel obliged to obey orders rather than negotiate or exercise professional judgement. We have previously noted how destructive obedience can fol-low from the creation of powerful authority figures and how consultation and expertise can maximize the individual's negotiating power in the face of legitimate authority (see Chapter 4, Section 3).

4 Therapeutic Groups

The advantages of group work

In the previous chapter we considered therapeutic interventions involving one-to-one relationships between therapists and clients and in this chapter we have seen how social influence in groups can change member's behaviour. This raises the question of whether such influence could be directed towards changing behaviour in a therapeutic manner. In the next two sections we shall consider how specially created groups can foster self-chosen change amongst their members.

The value of gathering patients with similar problems together to promote discussion and the development of better coping strategies was recognized within medicine at the beginning of the century. Patients with similar problems were invited to relevant lecturers and gathered together to discuss their common difficulties. This tradition has continued and given rise to a flourishing self-help movement which we shall return to below.

A somewhat different use of groups was pioneered by Lewin who was responsible for the development of sensitivity training (or 'T') groups. Here too the emphasis was on sharing but not in relation to any particular common difficulty. These groups focused on sharing everyday thoughts and feelings. The common issue for members was their experience of personhood, that is, the hopes, fears and feelings which everyday interaction creates and the practical issues involved in managing our relations with others in order to achieve mutual satisfaction. 'T' groups provided an early illustration of how personal development could be facilitated through the use of group dynamics (Smith, 1980a). This approach was developed by a number of therapists influenced by Freud's psychoanalysis including Klein and Bion and by those, like Rogers, who focused primarily upon our conscious experiences of who we are and what others think about us (Smith 1980b). The power of groups to facilitate personal change is now widely acknowledged and many distinct groupwork traditions have been established. We shall not focus upon any particular approach but explore the mechanisms by which groups can promote personal change.

From a professional point of view the development of groupwork has important economic implications. It means that a number of clients can simultaneously benefit from a facilitator's time or, in the case of self-help groups, that important therapeutic work can continue without utilizing professional resources. We shall return to the implications of this reduced professional involvement in relation to self-help groups below. However, in the case of therapist or facilitator led groups it is important to remember that the aim is not simply to deliver a service to a number of clients simultaneously but to harness social influence processes to promote beneficial change. This means that the manner in which such groups are set up and managed will determine whether or not they work effectively.

Setting up a therapeutic group

In Chapter 7 (Section 2) we identified a number of important features of counselling relationships. Many of these characteristics must be created amongst group members if the group is to promote change. Just as trust is important in a one-to-one therapeutic relationship so group members must trust one another before they will be able to discuss private concerns and feelings. Facilitators must therefore focus initially on creating an environment in which group members feel that other members are positively disposed towards them and are able to empathize with their experience.

Smith's (1980a) *Group Processes and Personal Change* offers a useful overview of the field and identifies group characteristics which foster change. He notes the importance of establishing the group as a *cultural island*, that is a meeting which separates members from their usual social identities and role relations. We have seen how others exert a powerful influence on our behaviour through our need to manage social reputations and fulfill role-related obligations (see Chapter 3, Sections 2 and 3; Chapter 4, Sections 1, 2 and 3). These everyday relationships encourage stability and predictability in our behaviour and provide few opportunities to experiment with new ways of relating. Separation from these social constraints is therefore crucial if group members are to consider new ways of representing themselves and interacting with others. In practice this may mean that such groups are held away from members' homes and workplaces and are residential so that members do not return to their everyday social world during group meetings.

Of course members must know how long they are to be separated from their everyday lives and this means that a *time contract* is vital. In other words, members commit themselves to a specified time in the group. On the one hand this provides a sense of security in that members know that the group will not disintegrate at the first signs of difficulty and on the other it reassures members that they do not have to give up too much to the therapeutic experiment. Residential groups may last two to three days while others may meet for six to ten weekly or fortnightly sessions.

We have noted that group norms can exert considerable influence over members' behaviour and view of reality. If therapeutic groups are to facilitate change they must develop *norms* which allow interpersonal exploration and experimentation. Smith (1980a) draws on the work of Luke (1972) and Lieberman et al. (1973) to show that this can be achieved. These studies demonstrated the establishment of norms relating to the expression and acceptance of feeling, the development of trust, sharing one's reactions to others, asking others about their impression of oneself and challenging the leader. Such norms emphasize disclosure of one's thoughts, emotions and reactions to others as well as acceptance of others' expression of their views and feelings.

Such an intense focus on interpersonal relations is unusual in everyday meetings. However, because group norms are so influential the establishment of unusual norms will generate unusual behaviour. These norms therefore facilitate members' exploration of new ways of representing themselves and interacting with others. Smith (1980b) points out that one implication of a time-limited, cultural island in which such norms are established is that many of the relationship filters which we discussed in Chapter 6 (Section 2) cease to operate. Members quickly stop judging one another on the basis of superficial appearance and their interaction extends beyond attitudinal validation through discussions of beliefs and values. Moreover, they are not involved in assessing one another in the context of specified role obligations. Thus by encountering one another's feelings, doubts and fears through unusually revealing discussion and being unable to easily withdraw members quickly build up meaningful relationships and develop liking and respect for one another. This in turn fosters further empathy and trust.

Two particularly important norms in therapeutic groups are those concerning *self disclosure* and *feedback*. In everyday interaction we often manage our impressions by withholding information about ourselves which we feel might prompt rejection or disapproval. This results in a hidden areas of our experience which remains unvalidated. In other words we do not know if others' have similar experience or to what extent they would approve or disapprove of our hidden experience. By disclosing such hidden aspects of ourselves we can discover how they relate to others' experience and what others think of us as we really are. This is especially true when those listening to our disclosures tell us honestly what they think about what we have said or how they feel about us as a result, that is when they offer us feedback. We shall see below that this process of revealing oneself and receiving reactions is central to personal change in therapeutic groups.

It is clear that there a number of prerequisites to the creation of a working therapeutic group. In order to achieve these groups must go through a development process in which members adopt particular styles of interaction. We can therefore identify stages of development in the life of a therapeutic group. A simple mapping is provided by Tuckman's (1965) mnemonic – 'forming, storming, norming and performing'. This describes how members struggle towards the establishment of norms after a period of confusion. This period may involve conflict between members about appropriate norms and particularly between the facilitator and other members. However, if the group is able to establish appropriate norms it may enter a phase in which members learn new things about themselves, thereby creating opportunities for personal change.

The central role obligation of the facilitator or leader is to encourage the group to develop norms and relationships which provide opportunities for personal change. Since 'productivity' in such groups can only be measured in terms of members' personal change a task focus means prioritizing interpersonal relationships! Fostering appropriate group norms and setting a good example in showing acceptance of others, demonstrating empathy, making self-disclosures and offering feedback are all important aspects of the facilitator's role. By contrast, adopting an authoritarian or expert stance is unlikely to be effective as only members themselves are able to define what is important for them to explore and perhaps change during the group. Therapeutic group leaders are described as 'facilitators' in order to emphasize the importance of *creating opportunities* for personal development rather than ensuring specified outcomes for particular members.

Self Representation, feedback, feeling and change

How then does personal change occur in therapeutic groups? Oatley (1980) offers an explanation based on the provision of special opportunities for learning about how others see us. We understand ourselves through various representations of who we are (see Chapter 1, Section 3). These include social identities which we wish to maintain (see Chapter 3, Section 3) and roles we occupy (see Chapter 4, Section 1). Much of the time this understanding goes unchallenged in fairly predictable role-specified daily interactions. Even when others do question who we are or how we behave we tend to disregard them and attribute their reactions to ignorance or competitive motivation.

However, in therapeutic groups with established self-disclosure and feedback norms members share these understandings of themselves. Such self-disclosure and reflection on the self is unusual in itself but to hear others reactions or feedback is even more unusual. Moreover, when such feedback is offered at the performing stage of group's development and concerns some aspect of ourselves which we would like to change it can have a very powerful effect. Within the group where we have been accepted and experienced support it is difficult to dismiss such feedback. Thus feedback is most powerful when it is received from those who have also offered us support. Encouraging members to offer both support and feedback is therefore an important aim for facilitators.

Accepted feedback is especially powerful when it contradicts one's established understanding of oneself. Oakley points out that such discrepancies lead to emotional responses. When someone tells us honestly that we are insightful, helpful and caring when we doubt the value of our comments we may feel pleasure and happiness. Similarly, when someone tells us we are domineering and intimidating when we imagine that we are being helpful we may feel remorse or sadness. These emotions might be quickly suppressed in everyday encounters as we distract ourselves from the seeming indulgence of self-reflection and 'get on with it'. However, in a group where there is no competing business and time to reflect on oneself, emotional reactions can be acknowledged. Moreover, because of the supportive social setting emotions can be publicly expressed. In everyday interaction we may conceal feelings of joy or rejection even when we acknowledge them to ourselves but in a group in which empathy and support have been established we may express and experience them in the presence of others. Thus in many respects the supportive group which encourages self disclosure and invites challenging feedback provides members with a very unusual experience.

Emotions arising from the recognition of discrepancies between our understanding of ourselves and others' feedback provide salient and memorable experiences. However, in order to learn from these we must link them to the way in which we typically relate to others. Therapeutic groups can help members discuss how such discrepancies arise from misunderstandings of the way others' perceive them (see Chapter 3, Sections 1 and 2). Such discussion can lay the foundations for more accurate representations of the impact of their behaviour on others. In this way feedback can prompt the development of new (and more realistic) self-representations. Changes in our understanding of how others see us may lead to a desire to manage our impressions differently and alter our social behaviour. For example, having realized that others experience us domineering and intimidating when we are trying to help, we may resolve to listen more carefully to others' perspectives rather than imposing our own solutions. In other words we may acknowledge that we need to adopt a more counselling style when dealing with others' issues (see Chapter 7, Section 2). Overall, this process of disclosure, feedback, emotion, interpretation and intention formation (see Chapter 2, Section 2) provides a powerful learning experience.

It is worth emphasizing that the combination of support and challenge is essential to this process. The supportive nature of such groups prohibits the kind of dismissive external attributions which commonly follow feedback in everyday interaction (see Chapter 2, Section 3). Similarly without challenging feedback the group may encourage compliance but it will not create the discrepancies which prompt members to rethink their personal understandings of themselves. Kolb, et al. (1968) demonstrated this point by comparing groups in which feedback was and was not encouraged. They found that almost nine times as much change was reported in groups where feedback norms were established!

The seeds of change and change maintenance

Having considered the way in which therapeutic groups encourage change we must ask whether they are in fact effective change agents. After reviewing the literature Smith (1980c) offered a positive but qualified answer to this question. Members may have a more favourable self-representation, they may feel better able to offer and receive affection and others may see them displaying greater interpersonal warmth and sensitivity. Lieberman et al. (1973) reported that about two-thirds of participants in the groups they studied experienced such changes at the end of the group and that six months later a third were still reporting such benefits. Smith argues that sufficient empirical studies have been conducted to draw the conclusion that there is: 'A good deal of measurable change . . but a substantial fade-out. . in subsequent months' (p. 46). In other words these groups seem able to provide the seeds of change but change maintenance depends upon the individual member's ongoing use of the experience.

This conclusion raises the question of why some people are able to build on the experience over time while others are not. Smith (1980a) draws on attribution theory to explain this difference (see Chapter 2, Section 3). He categorized group members according to whether they attributed events internally or externally and found that although they did not differ in relation to reported benefit at the end of groups, they *did* show differences in relation to fade-out. Internals tended to have maintained their reported interpersonal benefits at a five month follow-up while externals' had lost benefits experienced at the end of the group. Thus it appears that the tendency to take responsibility for events enables members to internalize the insights and intentions generated during therapeutic group experiences and helps them work towards long term behaviour change. Smith proposes that internal attributions for change are more likely when members receive support and challenges from the same influential person in the group, again emphasizing this crucial balance.

Groupwork in Nursing

Groupwork is relevant to nursing because nurses may lead such groups as part of their contribution to promoting health-related changes amongst their patients and clients. Therapeutic groups may be helpful to those who wish to to change their behaviour in order to maximize physical well-being as well as those who are primarily concerned to improve their interpersonal relations. Wilson-Barnett (1988), for example, discusses Dracup, et al.'s (1984) work on nurse-led group-counselling for couples in which one member had been a myocardial infarction patient. In this case the focus for change was how couples could change their joint lifestyles to minimize the risk of relapse.

The management of therapeutic groups is, however, more common in psychiatric or mental handicap nursing where clients wish to develop new ways of dealing with others. The aim of such groups may be to develop new social identities (see Chapter 3, Section 4) or to increase awareness of others' perceptions and needs as in Lewin's 'T' groups. Nurse facilitators will be involved in encouraging group development so that opportunities for personal reflection and change occur.

The importance of such groups was highlighted by those involved in the setting up of *therapeutic communities* (Jones, 1953). Such communities can be regarded as the fullest expression of treatment based on the social psychiatric model in which client participation in group decision-making and group therapy provide the basis for personal development. In this context interpersonal relationships and groupwork are the medium through which treatment and care are delivered. ESO medicine is banished (see Chapter 4, Section 2) and democratization of the nurse-patient relationship is built into patient and staff roles (see Chapter 7, Section 2). Nurses working in this context avoid some of the problems of a bureaucracy (see above) but may well face other stresses due to the high level of personal commitment and involvement required (see Chapter 9, Section 2). Though there are few operational therapeutic communities, the movement has had some influence on mainstream psychiatry by emphasizing the key role of interpersonal relations in the process of personal change and development.

As well as leading and organizing groupwork nurses may also benefit from participating in such groups. Nurses may benefit from opportunities to reflect on their own interpersonal relations and how these affect their work. Smith (1980c), for example, reports a study by Geitgey (1966) which demonstrated that student nurses were perceived more positively by their nurse tutors and their patients after attending a 'T' group. Therapeutic groups may also be used to help nurses develop more effective ways of coping with stress at work (see Chapter 9, Section 3).

5 Self Help Groups

Towards a self-help culture?

We have seen how interaction in therapeutic groups can provide powerful learning experiences which enable people to change their behaviour. This raises the question of whether such groups could operate successfully without professional leadership. Could groups undergo appropriate development without a paid group facilitator? Just as importantly, can groups be beneficial to members even if they do not follow the pattern of development described above. The answer to these questions must surely be 'yes' since so many people give up their time and energy to attend groups which are not necessarily led by professional facilitators. In 1979 Robinson and Robinson estimated that there were 233 different health-related self-help groups in Britain. The proliferation of 'self help' in Europe and the United States may be due to cultural changes emphasizing personal responsibility for health-care and the fallibility of health-care workers.

Self-help groups may serve an important function for individuals who feel neglected by traditional health-care systems or discriminated against by wider society. They can provide forms of assistance which may not be available from professional services and enable participants to reflect upon and change social identities which lead to low self-esteem. For example, those suffering from obesity, alcoholism, or chronic health problems may feel that they are not legitimate health service consumers or that help is unavailable once an acute phase had passed. Similarly those who feel alienated from everyday social networks may find an alternative source of social support in self-help groups (see Chapter 6, Section 3). For example, people who suffer as a result of stereotyping and discrimination, such as single parents or people with physical disabilities may use self-help groups to provide mutual support (see Chapter 3, Section 1).

Self-help groups are inexpensive and allow participants to access help without having to compete for scarce professional time. In the United Kingdom changes in the philosophy and organization of health care outlined in the White Papers *Working for Patients* (Department of Health,1989) and the National Health Service and Community Care Act (1990) emphasize the responsibility of the individual and her community for health care. Self-help groups offer participants an opportunity to take responsibility for their problems and to take control of the way in which they should be managed. In this way they simultaneously complement and challenge the expertise of health-care workers.

What is a self-help group?

Self-help groups support people with a diverse range of problems. Levy (1976) points out that these include problematic behaviour such as drug addiction and gambling, shared stressful situations such as single parenthood or divorce and shared stigma or discrimination such as that experienced by ex-prisoners or gay men. They may offer information, social support, material help and promote the adoption of new identities. They are orientated towards promoting change in participants and may aim to enhance perceived self-efficacy and actual coping skills. They are, by definition, organized by members rather than professionals but many employ non-members and professionals to provide administrative support, counselling or professional advice. Thus while we can identify common features we must recognize that the term 'self-help group' refers to a range of groups, organizations and activities.

Killilea (1976) listed features which have been used to identify and characterize self-help groups. These included, the common experience of members, the mutual provision of help and the operation of a 'helper principle'. This refers to the benefits and therapy derived by helpers from helping others who share their problem. Sharing information, developing shared goals, offering social validation of other members' beliefs and values and associating with others who do not employ negative stereotypes or discriminate on the basis of the shared problem are also key elements of the self-help group experience. The sharing of experiences and identification of common needs and aims may facilitate the development of change-orientated norms within self-help groups (see Section 4, above). Moreover, recognition of peers' shared beliefs and experiences may increase the social influence of such group's over their members (Deutsch and Gerard, 1955; Emrick et al, 1977).

Robinson (1980) describes how this sharing of experiences can lead to an analysis or 'de-construction' of the individual's view of her problem, herself and her coping methods. This prepares the way for a 're-construction' of the problem in which the participant adopts new perspectives on her life and new approaches to managing her problem. Emrick et al. (1977) have compared this change process to that occurring in one-to-one cognitive therapy (see Chapter 7, Section 4). Deconstruction involves participants in a process of acknowledging their problem and recognizing that they need help to deal with it effectively. For example, in Alcoholics Anonymous (AA), one of the most established self-help organizations, members initially categorize themselves as 'alcoholics' and publicly acknowledge that they cannot control their drinking. Although this appears to involve external attributions and a reduction in perceived self-efficacy (see Chapter 2, Section 3) it is, in fact, an acknowledgement that the person has been unable to develop effective ways of managing her problem. Such de-construction of previous perceptions of the problem has much in common with the challenge to self-representations provided by feedback in therapeutic groups and the construction of more useful representations of one's situation encouraged through counselling (see Chapter 7, Section 2). Having accepted the need for change the participant is ready to embark on a reconstruction of her situation.

This reconstruction process occurs through participation in group projects which incorporate self-examination and practicing new skills. The group may involve members in setting personal behaviour-change targets (such as abstaining from alcohol) and organize collective activities which express a positive identification with their shared problem (for example campaigning for better services). As in cognitive therapy participants are encouraged to believe that change and improvement are possible and that *they themselves can effect such change*. Feedback from other group members may play an important part in helping participants adopt new self representations and new approaches to managing their behaviour. Internalization of new representations is important to successful change (see Smith, 1980a, Section 4, above) and Emrick et al. (1977) propose that internalization is inherent to the reconstruction process used in AA. They suggest that those who do not learn to take personal responsibility for emotional and behavioural control tend not to join or to leave in the early stages. In many respects then the individual change processes sustained within self-help groups resemble those occurring in therapeutic groups.

As well as promoting personal change self-help groups often seek to change the wider societal context in which members' problems arise. Groups which focus upon problems created by discrimination against their members may be primarily involved in consciousness raising (see Taylor and Mckirnan's work – Chapter 3, Section 4). Women's groups and gay groups, for example, have sought to establish a higher status social identity for members inside and outside group meetings. Such consciousness raising processes act directly on the individual's social identity and at the same time involve political action designed to change the perceptions of non-members. A woman's refuge, for example, provides material help and accommodation for battered women and their children, helps women cope with emotional and practical problems arising from assault and persecution and provides a focus for political protest against women's low status position in society (Pahl, 1979).

Development and impact of self-help organizations

Self-help groups may develop differently and operate differently at different times. However, Katz (1970) proposed an idealized sequence of development followed by many groups. They arise out of the concerns of disadvantaged persons and their relatives and gradually involve a larger proportion of people suffering from the same problem. Leaders emerge within the growing movement and good practice guides, rules and organizational structures are proposed. Finally, in seeking to enhance resources and services for their members those within the growing self-help organization engage with professionals and seek to influence their perceptions and treatment of group members. The danger of such organizational development and professional involvement is that the self-help organization may become absorbed into traditional service delivery systems which it initially sought to challenge. This may result in its aims and practices being shaped by the priorities of professionals, such as health-care workers. On the other hand delayed organizational development may leave the organization vulnerable to collapse if key members leave and there is no structure for new members to rely on. Thus the survival and influence of a self-help movement depends upon steering a path between bureaucratic inertia and organizational collapse.

When self-help movements are successful in providing good quality health services for their members there is a danger that state-run health care services will redirect resources away from this area because an alternative service exists. Thus, if self-help movements do not influence professionals they may inadvertently promote further marginalization of their members from mainstream service provision (Sidel and Sidel, 1976). Self-help movements have tended to be dominated by middle class people and may therefore perpetuate the already evident disparity between uptake of health care services by better off sectors of society. Robinson (1980) points out that, if state-run services rely upon self-help movements composed of predominantly middle class members, then poorer people with the same problems will be left with a deteriorating service. Thus the impact of self-help movements depends upon their ability to negotiate access to professional services for their members and attracting members from all sectors of society.

The effectiveness self-help movements depends, therefore, upon the extent to which they can prioritize members' needs within health-care services and society generally. Although such movements seek to enhance the perceived self-efficacy and competence of their members, an exclusive focus on the individual nature of members' problems may relieve outsiders from an obligation to help. We saw in Chapter 4 (Section 4) that the tendency to attribute responsibility for events to others can inhibit helping. It is therefore important for self-help movements to emphasize that their members are not responsible for their situation and deserve help. If they fail to persuade outsiders of this they may actually discourage economic, social and legislative interventions which could result in greater benefits to their members more than personal therapeutic interventions. Thus an examination of the social context of members' problems and a promotion of societal changes must be a central part of the work of effective self-help movements.

CORE IDEAS IN CHAPTER 8

- Shared rules of behaviour within groups are referred to as group norms. These exert a powerful influence on members' behaviour and, once adopted, may shape behaviour outside the group.

- In his famous studies of conformity Asch was one of the first social psychologists to use confederates to study social interaction.

- In group discussions we may be influenced by others' views both because they provide an extra source of information about the world (informational influence) and because they indicate what is acceptable within the group (normative influence).

- Normative and informational influence tend to produce group polarization, that is a shift towards the majority view. In the extreme this can result in 'groupthink'.

- Private decision-making, after group discussion, decreases normative influence and an acknowledgement that there may be more than one correct viewpoint decreases informational influence.

- The expression of a minority viewpoint may validate other

members' perspectives and lead to further disagreement with the majority view. Minorities within groups can promote change and innovation and are most effective when they are consistent amongst themselves and across time.

- High participation and relevant expertise help to create the perception of leadership potential.

- Gender socialization may typically provide men and women with different sets of social skills which enable them to make different leadership contributions within groups. Gender stereotypes may also make leadership roles more difficult and less rewarding for women.

- Democratic (as opposed to autocratic) leadership is preferred by members, fosters initiative, discourages groupthink and reduces destructive social behaviour.

- Different leadership contributions are required by different types of groups at different stages in their development.

- Two broad categories of leadership functions have been identified, task-related and relationship-related leadership. All groups require both functions to be fulfilled by official or unofficial leaders.

- Task-related leadership may be particularly important in the early stages of group development when roles and norms are being defined.

- In order to maximize their contribution to group functioning leaders need to change their leadership style as their group develops (for example, from a 'telling' to a 'delegating' style).

- Group leadership and decision-making occur within larger organizational contexts which often define group aims.

- Nurses negotiate their roles within wider organizational contexts but are also subject to direct lines of bureaucratic authority. These different sources of role-related obligations may conflict, leading to role strain.

- Therapeutic groups seek to harness social influence processes to promote self-chosen change. Their effectiveness depends upon establishing special social environments including self-disclosure, empathic relating and feedback norms.

- Therapeutic group leaders, or facilitators, must try to promote the development of such norms in initial meetings.

- Self disclosure followed by challenging feedback can highlight discrepancies between self-representations and the way others perceive us. These may generate emotions which can be acknowledged and expressed in an accepting social setting. Interpretation of such discrepancies can lead to a desire to alter one's impression management and therefore change one's social behaviour.

- Those who take personal responsibility for their experiences (through internal attributions) appear to maintain changes for longer after therapeutic groups.

- Leading therapeutic groups may be an important part of nurses' contribution to promoting health behaviour. Nurses may also improve their interpersonal skills by participating in such groups.

- Self-help groups may be attractive to those who feel unable to access professional help or who are discriminated against in society at large.

- Through sharing experiences and developing new ways of thinking about common problems self-help groups may improve members' coping skills, enhance their perceived self efficacy and also address the social context in which members' problems arise.

9

Satisfaction and coping in nursing

1 Understanding Stress

Work stress and well-being

The vast majority of men in developed countries are involved in full-time employment for most of their lives. Most women are also in paid employment and mothers increasingly combine child care with employment. The posts held confer important social identities (see Chapter 3, Section 3) and work experience has a crucial impact on the quality of their everyday lives. For some, work is a rewarding and fulfilling experience but for others it creates stress and unhappiness. This depends upon whether people are able to fulfill intrinsic and extrinsic motivations (see Chapter 7, Section 3) and deal with work-related problems without experiencing excessive stress.

This chapter examines factors which determine whether work and especially nursing is experienced as stressful or satisfying. We shall focus on the nurse's own well-being rather than her effectiveness as a carer. However, all health-care workers' effectiveness is likely to be affected by job satisfaction.

We shall begin by considering three models of stress:

1. stress as a demanding stimulus;
2. stress as the result of our physiological and emotional responses to environmental stimuli;
3. stress as the interaction between the person and her environment.

A Stimulus Model

The stimulus model of stress is based on a simple analogy with one of the laws of physics (see Chapter 1, Section 2). Hooke's Law of Elasticity explains the effects of weights on metals, that is, the heavier the load the greater the stress within the metal. In the same way the greater the pressure on a person the greater the stress she experiences. Studies using this model have tried to identify environment demands which exert such pressure. Holmes and Rahe's (1967) *Social Adjustment Scale* (see Chapter 2, Section 4), for example, quantifies life events in terms of their potential stressfulness.

Despite its simplicity and intuitive appeal there are a number of shortcomings that undermine the usefulness of the stimulus model in accounting for stress-related responses. One problem with the pressure analogy is that, although light loads have little or no effect on the metals, extreme boredom, caused by under-stimulation can be as stressful as high workloads. A second weakness is its failure to take account of the way people's representations of reality shape the environmental stimuli to which they respond (see Chapter 1, Section 3; Chapter 2, Section 4; Chapter 7, Section 4). For example, some people find working with dying patients challenging and rewarding while others experience it as intolerably stressful. Finally, the model does not consider the psychological mechanisms by means of which we cope with environmental demands. It attempts to identify environmental causes but ignores the person's responses.

Despite criticisms of this model, studies employing it have identified many characteristics of the social environment within hospitals which are likely to have a detrimental effect on the well-being of staff and patients. Where people share representations of reality shared sources of stress may be identified. Some of these factors, such as inadequate staffing, are discussed below.

A Response Model

In contrast to the stimulus model, this model defines stress in terms of the individual's responses to perceived stressors. Selye (1974) described stress as a non-specific bodily response to environmental demands. This general response is referred to as the *General Adaptation Syndrome* (GAS) and is divided into three phases; the alarm reaction, the resistance phase and the exhaustion phase. Each stage can be characterized in terms of the person's physical and psychological states.

The alarm reaction is a *fight or flight* response. Physiological changes include the hypothalamus secreting a hormone that causes the adrenal glands to release adrenalin. Adrenalin increases heartbeat and causes breathing to become shallow and rapid. Blood flows to the muscles and brain and away from the skin (resulting in pale complexion and cold hands and feet). The hypothalamus also releases the adrenocorticotrophic hormone (ATCH) which stimulates the adrenal glands to release corticoids. These hormones in turn affect other glands which might otherwise adversely affect the functions such as breathing during times of crisis. The liver releases vitamins B and C which increases the ability of the blood to clot and cholesterol which enhances the supply of energy to the muscles. The spleen is primed to release greater numbers of red blood cells and muscles, particularly those of the neck, shoulders and lower back become tense (the position and size of these muscles making them one of the most obvious stress indicators). This frantic physiological effort leaves us prepared for rapid and perhaps violent action, that is, ready to fight or to run away!

The resistance phase occurs if the adaptive response does not reduce the perception of threat. The person continues to respond as outlined above and many stress-related diseases are thought to occur as a result of the prolonged secretion of these hormones. For example the heart has to work much harder to force the thickened blood through the narrowed arteries and veins with the increased likelihood of blood clotting and the occurrence of cardiovascular disorders such as strokes or coronary diseases. Raised blood pressure can also cause kidney damage.

As well as physical damage the relentless response to threat also has cognitive and emotional consequences (Fontana 1989). The person is likely to experience reduced concentration and attention span, increased distractibility and a deterioration in both short-term and long-term memory. This will result in forgetfulness, more mistakes in problem-solving activities and a reduced ability to plan and organize action. These effects are, of course, likely to create further demands on a person suffering from stress. People in this state are also less able to sustain constructive relationships with others and may become emotionally unpredictable. In their attempts to maximize effort devoted to dealing with perceived stressors they may resent interpersonal demands and become over-sensitive, defensive and hostile. They may also have difficulty in relaxing, feel helpless and depressed and become prone to hypochondria. The stressed individual is locked into an ineffective but unrelenting effort to overcome perceived environmental demand and feelings of incompetence and worthlessness predominate (see Chapter 2, Section 2; Chapter 7, Section 4).

These cognitive and emotional effects contribute to characteristic behavioural changes associated with prolonged stress. These include a decrease in the repertoire of interests and activities; a reduction in energy levels with daily fluctuations; an increase in absenteeism or lateness for work; a tendency to express cynical views about patients and colleagues; a tendency to attribute responsibility for shortcomings to others; an increase in drug use (for example, alcohol, caffeine, nicotine or illegal drugs); problems in getting to sleep and disturbances in sleep patterns.

The final stage of GAS arrives when the person's physical or psychological functioning breaks down as a result of attrition during the resistance phase. Unrelenting reaction without time for recovery leads to disease or breakdown and the person can no longer keep up their attempts to cope with perceived environmental demands. This is the exhaustion phase in which the person may already have seriously damaged their health. Stress management involves identifying the problem before this stage and intervening to change the person's environment or coping strategies during the resistance phase.

The GAS has given us a greater understanding of the physiological, cognitive and emotional responses to stress. Its application has helped identify the processes by which threat perception can undermine health. However, it tends to portray the individual as fairly passive, merely responding to demanding environments. We need to extend this model in order to appreciate the active interpretation of that environment which is involved in threat perception. This is crucial if we are to consider psychological interventions which can interrupt threat perception and thereby prevent the GAS running its course. This deficiency can be addressed by adopting a more social psychological perspective such as that provided by the transactional model.

A Transactional Model

The transactional model or, to give it its full title, the cognitive-phenomenological-transactional model (CPT) offers a more comprehensive view of stress and coping. It is based largely on the work of Lazarus (1966) and, as its name implies, concerns the person's intellectual processes (cognitive), her subjective interpretations (phenomenology) and her interaction with her environment (transactions). Whereas the stimulus and the response models each focuses on one aspect of the phenomenon, the CPT model deals with the whole process. According to this model the individual's ability to deal with problems, that is, whether stress is experienced or coping occurs, depends on the way she interprets or '*appraises* her relationships with environmental events. There are three stages in appraising a potentially stressful situation. *Primary appraisal* concerns the individual's perception of the environment when she evaluates the challenges or demands being made of her. *Secondary appraisal* refers to the person's assessment of her ability or resources to cope with the perceived problems. Finally, *reappraisal* concerns an estimation of the relative effectiveness of coping behaviour in reducing or removing the threat.

Consider a nurse who approaches the bed of a newly admitted patient to find her slumped over and ashen. The nurse quickly assesses whether the patient is dead or alive (primary appraisal) and then decides on her response. Should she spend precious time checking her initial assessment, report her observation to other staff or take immediate action (secondary appraisal)? The outcome of this appraisal process will determine how the nurse responds physiologically, psychologically and whether she delivers appropriate help (see Chapter 4, Section 4). Later reappraisal involves evaluating her response. Similarly if a terminally ill patient asks a charge nurse about her prognosis, the charge nurse must assesses the demands being made on her, including the patient's likely reaction to her reply (primary appraisal). She then assesses whether she has the ability to deal effectively with the patient's response (secondary appraisal). If she decides that she can cope with the process of informing the person of his impending death she may arrange a time to discuss the patient's prognosis, perhaps inquiring whether it would be appropriate to include a spouse or friend in this discussion. Later she assesses whether she met her aim of telling the patient while causing minimum distress and providing appropriate support to her and those close to her (reappraisal).

In this model the individual is not seen as a passive victim of environmental demand. She is portrayed as an active agent whose interpretation of situations determines how she experiences them. This has the crucial consequence of highlighting the individual's power to reduce or avoid stressful experiences (see Chapter 2, Section 4; Chapter 7, Section 4). The perceived threat is the person's own creation in that it is derived from her representation of reality. It may be based on memories of past experiences, present circumstances or anticipated events and can be experienced even when the stressor is not present. This means that, as observers, we may wrongly attribute others' stress-related behaviours to their immediate environment. We may think a colleague's stress is the result of her poor relations with her charge nurse because we observe them in conflict whereas, in fact, she is responding to worries about domestic financial problems. In this case the source of stress is not present in the ward and ward experiences are not directly related to her problem. Nevertheless her behaviour on the ward is affected by her ongoing experience, worries and concerns.

The CPT model also acknowledges that the same threat may elicit different responses at different times from the same individual. The person's experience depends upon her appraisal of demands and the coping resources at a particular moment. This suggests that helping others to cope with stressful situations begins with focusing on the 'here and now', that is, what the person is feeling at that moment. In some cases people perceive what to others is a harmless stimulus as very threatening. Extreme examples are seen in phobias where specific objects (such as animals) are experienced as threatening and sometimes terrifying (see Chapter 7, Section 3). Coping with these threatening situations depends upon the person's ability to change her appraisal or interpretation from a threatening to a non-threatening one (see Chapter 2, Section 4).

The CPT model has been criticized for proposing such an elaborate process when, in many situations, the individual's perception of threat seems almost instantaneous. However, Lazarus (1966) has pointed out that these appraisal process are not necessarily conscious and may occur very quickly because they are the result of automatic perceptual processes. Indeed part of the psychological process of changing appraisals involves bringing these interpretative processes to conscious attention (see Chapter 7, Section 4).

2 Motivation and Stress in Nursing

Motivation in nursing

Historically nursing has been identified with altruistic motives associated with religious principles. For many centuries throughout Europe nursing was carried out mainly by religious orders who were particularly concerned with the plight of the poor. However, in eighteenth century Britain the development of caring provision took a different route when, during the reformation, Henry VIII banned the Catholic Church. This led to the dissolution of many caring establishments and a transfer of responsibility for caring for the sick and destitute to local government bodies. Consequently, people who provided nursing care were no longer expected to be motivated by religious principles and were recruited mainly from women who had been employed as domestic servants and were seeking alternative paid employment (Maggs, 1984). Despite this development the idea of nursing being something of a religious calling persisted. For example in the latter part of the nineteenth century it was suggested that women who might have difficulty sustaining the rigors of monastic life might consider nursing:

Revival in the Church . . . was awakening in the hearts of earnest women the desire for definite religious work ... for those to whom the severe and dedicated life of the religious was not possible [there was a] life devoted to the care of nursing of the sick (*British Medical Journal*, 1897, p. 1645)

The development of nursing in Britain and in the United States has been beset by the conflict between those who regarded it as a vocation and those who viewed it as an occupation. This debate is founded on the question of whether nurses' motivation was primarily intrinsic or extrinsic (see Chapter 7, Section 3). When registration was first considered those opposing it, including Florence Nightingale, argued that nurse registration would attract nurses with less laudable motives and therefore lead to a deterioration in standards of care.

More recently, concern about manpower levels has encouraged research into nurses' motivation with a view to improving recruitment and staff retention. In the United Kingdom, for example, the management consultants Price Waterhouse (1988) found that the main reason given by the 7600 nurses questioned for staying in the nursing was a desire to help others. These nurses did not justify their work in terms of extrinsic rewards valued by the entrepeneural culture, popular in the 1980s in the United Kingdom. This may mean that many nurses' job satisfaction is based on intrinsic rather than extrinsic rewards. It may also imply that many nurses are prepared to sacrifice their need for extrinsic rewards, such as increased salary or status, to avoid distressing patients. This emphasis on intrinsic rewards may undermine motivation to challenge management concerning the extrinsic rewards provided for nursing, making it more difficult to increase the market value of nursing labour. Altruistic motivation may, therefore, conflict with campaigns to improve the material circumstances of nurses and thereby the quality of patient care. Of course it could also be argued that increasing extrinsic rewards, by paying higher salaries, could undermine this intrinsic, altruistic motivation to nurse. Perhaps Nightingale had a point!

It is difficult to quantify the balance of intrinsic and extrinsic motivation within nursing and establish the importance of job satisfaction to recruitment and staff retention. Barrett (1988) examined nurses' motivation to stay in their jobs within a Health Authority in the United Kingdom and identified four work-related reasons; satisfaction with their job, a good working atmosphere, good managerial support and availability of continuing education and professional development. Waite and Hutt (1987) identified more specific work-related factors affecting nurses' decision to return to or to remain in nursing, including realistic staffing levels, better pay and better counselling or support for nurses. Similarly, McDowell (1989) found that job satisfaction, professional development, working conditions and salary levels were important to nurses' decisions to stay in nursing. In the United States Hinshaw, et al., (1987) surveyed 1597 nurses and identified several factors that promote the retention of staff; professional status, general enjoyment of one's position, the ability to deliver quality nursing care, group cohesiveness, recognition of a nurse's uniqueness, the opportunity for professional growth and control of professional practice.

General sources of stress in nursing

Interviewing nurses working in different settings in the United Kingdom McGrath, et al., (1989) found substantial agreement about general sources of stress in nursing; 67% of respondents identified insufficient time to perform duties satisfactorily as the most important source of stress, 54% identified the rationing of scarce services and resources and 46% identified deadlines imposed by others. Similarly, the work of Birch (1979) and Ellis and Lees (1990) suggest stable perceptions of stress in nursing over an 11-year period. Under-staffing was identified as the most stressful aspect of nursing work while specific work demands, such as dealing with dying patients and their relatives, were regarded as less stressful. In the United States Dewe (1989) surveyed a sample of 1801 general nurses and examined stress in terms of the frequency of their experience of tension and tiredness and their methods of dealing with these experiences. Analyses revealed five main sources of work stress which are listed in order of importance below:

1. *work overload,* for example, nursing too many patients, experiencing difficulty in maintaining high standards, feeling unable to give colleagues the support they need and dealing with the problems of staff shortage;
2. *difficulties in relating to other staff,* for example, experiencing conflict with colleagues, recognizing that they do not value one's contribution and failure to establish team work amongst staff;
3. *difficulties involved in nursing critically ill patients,* for example operating unfamiliar equipment, managing new procedures or treatments and working with doctors who demand instant answers and action;
4. *concerns over patient treatment,* for example, working with doctors who do not appear to understand the social or emotional needs of patients, being involved in disagreements concerning treatment, feeling uncertain about how much to tell patients or relatives and nursing difficult or helpless patients;
5. *nursing patients who fail to improve,* for example, elderly patients, chronic pain patients or those who die while being nursed.

This study also emphasized the priority nurses' give to staffing levels and work demands in identifying stress at work. It could be argued that attributing stress to working conditions (such as understaffing), rather than the nature of nursing work, preserves nurses' self esteem by protecting their 'nurse' identity from criticism. However, such consistent reporting of stress due to work overload and under staffing suggests that this is an important aspect of everyday nursing which undermines satisfaction and enjoyment in nursing.

Stress and role definition

McGrath, et al., (1989) also investigated social workers' and teachers' perceptions of stress arising out of interaction with clients and students. They reported that these workers found such contact more stressful than nurses found interaction with patients. These differences reflect the way in which specific work role definitions lead to different perceptions of stress (see Chapter 3, Section 3; Chapter 4, Section 1).

Differences in nurse role definition may also lead to different experiences of stress at work. Dewe (1989), for example, found differences between perceived stress amongst different grades of nursing staff. 'Difficulties in relating to other staff', were more frequently reported by enrolled nurses than staff nurses or charge nurses. 'Difficulties involved in nursing critically ill' were more frequently reported by staff nurses than enrolled nurses or charge nurses and 'concerns over patient treatment' were most frequently reported by charge nurses. As role-related obligations change so the sources of job-related stress also shift. Studies investigating stress amongst nurses in different roles show that while some stressors seem relatively constant across nursing roles (for example, work overload), other role-specific stressors are also important.

In a small study of nurses working in intensive care, Huckabay and Jagla (1979) found that work overload was regarded as the most important source of stress with patient deaths and communication problems with colleagues being the next most important stressors. However, in a larger study of 1794 intensive care nurses Steffen (1980) found that interpersonal conflict was regarded as the most important source of stress with unit management procedures, the nature of patient care and inadequacies in knowledge and skill also being identified as important stressors.

Hingley and Cooper (1986) found work overload to be the most important source of stress amongst their sample of 521 nurse managers. Relationships with senior staff, role strain and ambiguity, interpersonal relationships and dealing with death and dying were also identified as important sources of stress by these nurse managers. Interestingly, 71% of participants complained that decisions which affected their work were often made by superiors without consultation.

Dawkins, et al., (1985) investigated six categories of stressors within psychiatric nursing; negative characteristics of patients, administrative-organizational issues, resource limitations, staff performance, staff conflict and scheduling issues. They found administrative-organizational issues were the most important source of stress. These included not being notified of changes before they occurred, dealing with people in management who were unable to make decisions, lack of support from administration, and having excessive paperwork. The next most stressful aspects of their job concerned staff conflict such as that arising from reassignment to other units against their wishes or shortages of appropriately trained staff in potentially dangerous environments. This study used only a small sample from one hospital, so the results are therefore of questionable generalizability. However other studies such as Cronin-Stubbs and Brophy (1985) and Jones, et al., (1987) support the pre-eminence of administrative issues as a major cause of stress among psychiatric nurses and also confirm the findings of studies cited earlier that direct patient contact was *not* usually regarded as the most important source of work stress.

Role strain revisited

We have previously discussed how ambiguity and contradiction in role-related obligations may lead to role strain (Chapter 4, Section 1). Nurses' basic role-related obligations are outlined in various documents such as employers' job descriptions and relevant legislation (for example in the United Kingdom the Nurses Midwives and Health Visitors Act (Amendments) 1990 and in the UKCC Codes of Conduct). Moreover, nurses' are also held accountable by others including nurse managers who operate within a bureaucratic system (see Chapter 8, Section 3), medical staff who have ultimate responsibility for patients' well-being, and patients who are consumers of nursing services. Nurses' documented, professional obligations may conflict with the expectations of these powerful role set members or with employers' staff policies. For example, nurses who publicly criticize the quality of care caused by staff shortages may be disciplined within some health authorities. Professional role-definition may also conflict with informal expectations developed in particular work settings. Such expectations may define the nature of role-relations with other health-care workers, outline appropriate nurse conduct and even imply acceptance of particular values. The role strain resulting from such competing and conflicting demands upon nurses' time generates perceptions of continual work overload. The consistency with which nurses' identify work overload as a source of stress suggests that such role strain may be common.

When we feel we must fulfill competing expectations in order to be judged competent we are likely to become stressed. Initially we may try to meet competing demands within limited time and become increasingly anxious when this proves impossible. Our primary appraisal of work demands becomes perpetually greater then our secondary appraisal of the ability and time we have to meet those demands. Moreover, by failing to meet these demands we erode our sense of self-efficacy and reduce work-related self-esteem. In this way role strain leads to anxiety, tension, fatigue and eventually impaired performance (House and Rizzo, 1972).

3 Coping with Stress

Organizational factors in nurse stress

Reducing work-related stress may involve changing the organizational context of nursing or changing individual nurses' approaches to work. Improving the work environment may be viewed as a managerial responsibility because failure to eliminate work-related stressors may result in decreased employee performance and deteriorating consumer services. In the case of health services nursing staff who are highly stressed may lose motivation, experience 'burnout' and be absent from work more often (Gray-Toft and Anderson 1981).

Gray-Toft and Anderson (1981;1985) demonstrated that, within nursing, role strain can be generated by supervisory practices (for example, the way work tasks are organized by one's immediate boss) and by relationships with colleagues. Managerial intervention may minimize role strain by changing stress-inducing supervisory practices and work role relations. Rivicki and May (1989), for example, found that nurses were more satisfied and more effective when administrative and supervisory practices encouraged an open expression of views and shared problem-solving. Thus the leadership style advocated by management may have an important impact on the stress of nursing (see Chapter 8, Section 2).

Recently there have important changes in the philosophy of management within the health service operating in the United Kingdom. Decision-making responsibilities previously held by professional groups have been transferred to professional managers and accountability for decision making has been increased (Working for Patients 1989, National Health Service and Community Care Act 1990). It will be important for health service management to monitor the consequences of these changes for organizational climate, the role relations of health-care workers and the stress experienced by those delivering care.

Hawkins (1987) has advocated an ergonomic approach to matching work demands and workers' abilities. Work overload in nursing, for example, could be analysed in a detailed and systematic way (using nursing audit systems) and the results used to develop less stressful work routines. Similarly, involvement in decision-making and relationships with colleagues could be examined in relation to various possible role relations between staff (see Chapter 4, Section 1; Chapter 5, Section 1). Hawkins suggested that team organization in which each member is aware of her personal involvement in decision-making and has some control over the day-to-day organization of her work time could reduce nursing stress.

Nurse role definition and coping strategies

Individuals may adopt different approaches to coping with and reducing work stress. Dewe (1989) surveyed nurses' reported responses to work stress and identified six different coping categories, namely:

1. problem-solving strategies;
2. trying to unwind and put things into perspective;
3. keeping the problem to oneself;
4. throwing oneself into work and working harder for longer;
5. accepting the job as it is and trying not to let it upset you;
6. passive strategies.

Comparing charge nurses, staff nurses and enrolled nurses Dewe found that nurses in different grades tended to use different coping strategies. Charge nurses tended to adopt problem-solving approaches more frequently than staff nurses and enrolled nurses. Passive strategies were more frequently used by staff nurses than charge nurses and most frequently by enrolled nurses. This may be because their different role-related rights give them different levels of control over organizational sources of stress. Enrolled nurses, for example, may not have the authority to attempt problem-solving approaches to reducing work stress.

The categories used by Dewe can be considered in relation to a more general distinction used to understand individual approaches to coping with stress, that is, the distinction between focusing upon the feelings associated with stress (*emotion-focused coping*) or the source of stress itself (*problem-focused coping*).

Emotion-focused coping: changing feelings

Emotion-focused strategies, for example, denying work problems or continually turning to an alternative, enjoyable activity may make us feel better in the short term. However, they are unlikely to alleviate the problem if the source of stress remains unchanged (for example Hawkins, 1987). As soon as we return to work we are confronted with the same demands, stress-related hormones are activated and we continue to suffer the physical and emotional strain of Selye's 'alarm reaction'. Moreover, the distractions (passive strategies) we use to change our feelings may themselves become a health threat, for example excessive eating, drinking or smoking. Thus, as well as the direct (physiological) effects due to alarm in stressful situations, stress may have damaging indirect (behavioural) effects on our health through the strategies we use to escape from stressful circumstances.

Overeating in response to stress, for example, may contribute to obesity which increases the risk of cardio-vascular problems. Excessive alcohol intake is also hazardous. More than three measures of an alcoholic drink per day for men and two for women (one measure = one glass of wine, a measure of spirits or a half pint of beer) can cause physical and psychological damage. Even the apparently harmless practice of drinking tea may damage our health. Fontana (1989) pointed out that the body stores caffeine and that caffeine intake has been associated with heart disease. More than four cups of tea a day can be harmful and coffee, with its higher caffeine content, may be even more damaging.

Smoking is another emotion-focused response to stress. It is associated with lung cancer, other respiratory problems and heart disease. Moreover, it also affects those who smoke passively around smokers. Nurses smoke more cigarettes than most other occupational groups with different specialties being differentially associated with smoking. Hawkins et al (1982) found that 42.5% of nurses in psychiatry smoked while only 21.2% of community nurses smoked. They explained this in terms of differences in role definition, proposing that community nurses are less stressed because they have more day-to-day control and more autonomy over their overall workload. However, other factors, such as organizational policy and work patterns may affect smoking amongst nurses. For example, periods of relative inactivity broken by episodes of intensive social interaction with disturbed clients (as frequently experienced by psychiatric nurses) may encourage smoking. Therefore a direct causal relationship between autonomy at work and smoking habits cannot be assumed without further supporting evidence.

Making increasingly greater efforts at work appears superficially to tackle the source of stress. However, it does not focus upon the cause of excessive, threatening or contradictory work demands. It may therefore merely address work anxiety without changing our perception of work demands or our approach to dealing with them. Indeed it may lead to a frantic but impossible struggle to gain control through greater and greater work commitment. This may result in generalized type A behaviour (see Chapter 2, Section 4). Extending work beyond the end of the shift, into the evenings and weekends may result in reduced contact with family and friends, creating role conflict and further anxiety (see Chapter 4, Section 1).

Emotion-focused strategies are therefore generally ineffective at removing work stress. When a stressor is short term and likely to disappear without further intervention such temporary distraction may be effective. However, for longer term sources of stress something more than temporary escape is required.

Problem-focused coping: tackling the source of stress.

Problem-focused strategies may involve attempts to change the work environment, for example, dealing with interpersonal problems or changing work routines. However, since stress derives from our primary and secondary appraisals changing the way we view demands or abilities may also lead to stress reduction (see Chapter 2, Section 4; Chapter 7, section 4).

We noted in Chapter 6, (Section 3), that our well-being is heavily dependent on our interpersonal relationships. Adopting different styles of communication and interaction may lead to more positive relationships at work but, as we noted above, nurses with fewer role-related rights may be less able to change working relationships. We noted in Chapter 7, (Section 2), how those in leadership positions may adopt the degree of person and task orientated leadership they offer to match the needs of the group. Changes in leadership style may enhance relationships between leaders and group members and between group members thereby minimizing an important source of stress at work. In particular delegation which allows responsible and competent workers greater control over their work, encourages initiative and facilitates participative decision-making enhances self-efficacy, and increases trust. This can and reduce stress while simultaneously enhancing the quality of work output.

We noted above that believing there is too little time or too few resources to fulfill role-related obligations is a common source of stress in nursing. Therefore reducing perceived demands or increasing perceived ability to meet these demands is likely to be an important element of stress management in nursing. Four main approaches may be identified:

1. *using time more effectively* so that new work routines result in greater output and thereby match job demands;
2. *attempting to change work demands or available resources* by presenting arguments to superiors highlighting the impossibility of meeting current demand. Individuals and professional or political groups may attempt to change work role definitions in this way;
3. *altering one's perception of what can be achieved* at work given present resources and constraints, for example, lowering expectations regarding the quality of care which may be provided. This may allow the nurse to retain her level of self efficacy within a redefined set of role obligations;
4. *changing employment*. If we believe that we cannot bring about change either in others' expectations or our own appraisals then the only escape from work stress may be an escape from the job itself.

The first of these, effective time management, is worth considering in further detail. Time at work like money earned are finite resources which can be managed in similar ways. As with money management it is important to identify how much time you have and how you spend it. Unfortunately assessing how time is spent is more difficult than checking your bank statement. Creating a reasonably accurate 'time statement' itself involves time and a commitment to this extra investment is required. As with other assessments, honest and accurate record-keeping is also essential. Although there are several ways of recording how long you spend on work tasks, the simplest is to record each task performed in a set time period (for example a week) and note when it was begun and finished.

The list of timed tasks can then be used to reconsider work routines. We can begin by comparing the profile of tasks to our job description to check that the tasks carried out are those we are employed to perform. Secondly, tasks can be divided into (a) essential tasks, (b) tasks we should carry out and (c) tasks we would like to carry out. These categories enable us to prioritize work tasks so that essential tasks are completed before we respond to other demands. Thirdly, tasks may be classified into whether they are self-initiated or responses to others' demands. Managing work so that we initiate our own activity enhances self-efficacy and reduces stress. Finally, we must use our time statement and analysis to plan a reorganization of work time. This may involve drawing up a list of work to be done with short (days), medium (weeks) and long-term (months) deadlines. Nurses working in multi-disciplinary teams or sharing responsibility with others may wish to involve their colleagues in such time-management exercises or confer with them about time-management decisions.

Attempting to change perceptions of role-related obligations by reconsidering the standards of care which can be reliably achieved within available resources is an example of a problem-focused response which targets our own appraisal processes. We have already considered a number of approaches to changing our perceptions of threat (see Chapter 2, Sections 3 and 4; Chapter 7, Section 4). For example, attributing failure to external factors (such as staffing levels), whether justified or not, can lead to maintained self-efficacy in the face of performance pressures. Similarly, reassessing the consequences of loss of others' approval may alleviate stress by reducing threat perception. Having considered such cognitive change in previous chapters we shall now focus upon the role of relaxation and in particular meditation in individual, problem-focused coping.

We have already noted the importance of relaxation in reducing anxiety (see Chapter 7, Section 3). Meditation may be regarded as a special form of relaxation which it is claimed can enhance general everyday performance and reduce stress (Benson, 1976). The earliest records of meditation have been found in Hindu literature and it was practised within the early Christian Church. It is still practised in the Greek and Russian Orthodox

Catholic Churches but it is popularly associated with Buddhism.

Meditation is practised in many forms but all are centred on one apparently simple theme. This theme involves focusing attention on a single object, sound or experience. Other thoughts that impinge on our awareness are denied attention. The idea is to gradually train attentional processes to overcome distractions and maintain concentration on this object of meditation. Distracting thoughts are not actively denied or stopped. They are allowed to pass into and out of consciousness but attention remains focused upon the object of meditation. This attention control can induce physiological changes such as a decrease in; metabolic rate, oxygen consumption, blood lactate levels, noradrenaline levels, blood pressure, heart rate and alpha brain waves. By learning to control attentional processes and change physiological functioning we may alter both our perception of threat and our responses to it.

The point of attentional focus can be a mandala which is a geometric design the person concentrates on either in reality or in her mind's eye or a mantra which is a single word or phrase repeated continuously during meditation. An alternative point of focus which is also used in relaxation exercises is the rhythm of breathing. The major muscle of respiration is the diaphragm which increases the capacity of the lungs by moving down into the abdominal area. However when we become conscious of breathing we tend to use our chest muscles to increase the capacity of the lungs. In deep breathing the idea is to refrain from using these muscles and concentrate solely on the movement of the diaphragm.

Regular meditation requires an initial commitment to creating time when we can be unavailable to others and finding a time and place where we will be free from interruptions. Success will depend on ensuring that this short time (10 minutes to 20 minutes) is strictly guarded and not to be postponed till later. A typical procedure might involve sitting upright in a kitchen chair, back firmly against the chair, legs uncrossed, feet squarely on the ground and hands resting on one's legs. Typical instructions might advise you to close your eyes and become aware of your abdomen moving during breathing. Concentrate on its movements, you become aware of it moving into your abdomen then returning to its 'resting' position pushing the air out of the lungs and moving downwards to fill the lungs again. Count 10 exhalations in a slow unhurried manner. On reaching the tenth begin counting backwards from ten to one and continue the exercise by counting each exhalation up to ten and then back to one. When thoughts intrude into consciousness, perhaps causing you to lose count, you either recommence at the last remembered number or calmly start at the beginning of the sequence. Distracting thoughts will lessen or disappear by refocusing attention on abdominal movement. Success in holding your concentration may vary from session to session but becomes easier with practise. When stressed it may take longer to focus and intrusions may be more frequent. However, learning to control concentration in this way may develop a useful stress management skill and allow us to return to our problems refreshed. Sticking to a daily routine of meditating regardless of whether we are feeling stressed or relatively stress-free develops these skills.

In our day-to-day experiences we spend most of our time preoccupied with our own thoughts, going over past events in our heads, evaluating their implications, considering future events and being largely oblivious of the immediate experiences of our senses and of the 'here and now'. Relaxation and meditation offers a respite from these preoccupations and helps us to become more aware of the present. Sporting or recreational activities may also focus our attention on the present but by focusing upon the self meditation encourages us to change our perspective on ourselves and our situation. In deeper meditation a person becomes detached from her immediate emotions and can reflect upon her emotions and behaviour in a more detached manner. This detached self reflection may be prerequisite to controlled personal change (see Chapter 8, section 4).

Conclusion

An assumption underpinning this and previous chapters is that the application of social psychological theories in nursing can improve the quality of nurses' lives and those of their patients. Nursing is primarily about relationships with others, and to help people achieve greater well-being, nurses require a good understanding of the 'hows and whys' of social interaction and interpersonal relationships. Much of our discussion has concerned the application of social psychological ideas to develop nurses' therapeutic effectiveness. However, as we have seen in this chapter nurses' own experience of work may also be enhanced through change based on social psychological insight. This is an important point because nurses' dedication to caring may mean that they and their colleagues underestimate their needs for social support, counselling and personal fulfillment.

We have considered:

- stress in nursing and methods of coping with it;
- the benefits and problems of working in groups;
- the way in which we can facilitate psychological change and development;
- the nature of relationship development and the importance of social support to well-being;
- the foundations of effective communication;
- the way in which everyday social behaviour is regulated within social rules and roles;
- the processes by which we understand ourselves and others;

- the structure of our understanding of health and illness;
- the nature of scientific investigation in these areas.

We hope that by developing a more detailed understanding of these aspects of social life nurses may be able to view their experiences from a slightly altered perspective and become better able to organize and change their thoughts and behaviours to enhance judgement, problem-solving, motivation, relationship development, social support and satisfaction in their professional and personal lives.

CORE IDEAS IN CHAPTER 9

- Employees devote much time and energy to work. It confers identity and status and structures daily life. Work stress and satisfaction are therefore important determinants of quality of life.

- The stimulus model of stress focuses upon environmental factors which many people find stressful.

- The response model of stress, illustrated by the general adaptation syndrome, concentrates on the person's reactions to stressful situations and in particular the alarm (fight or flight) response, resistance during prolonged stress and exhaustion fails to reduce perceived threats.

- The transactional model takes account of our interpretations of environmental stimuli in the perception of threat and highlights the importance of primary (demand) and secondary (resource) appraisals.

- Studies of nurse motivation suggest that the desire to help others and the intrinsic rewards of caring may be more important to nurses' than extrinsic rewards.

- Work overload, problems in professional relationships and difficulties in nursing certain types of patient have been identified as common sources of stress in nursing. However, patient contact appears to be the least important of these. Self-protective attributional processes may encourage such perceptions of nursing stress.

- While common stressors can be identified, different nursing roles (with their own rights and obligations) generate their own particular stressors.

- Role strain is a major source of nursing stress. Contradictory and ambiguous expectations lead to high perceived work demands (primary appraisals) and reduce perceived competence (secondary appraisals). This can reduce nurses' ability to deliver high quality care.

- Managerial intervention in defining work roles, organizing work tasks or recommending particular leadership styles can alleviate such stress and enhance nursing care.

- Individual coping responses to stress can be classed as emotion-focused or problem-focused.

- Emotion-focused coping is unlikely to be effective unless the threat is short term and diminishes of its own accord. It may also involve gratifying behaviour which itself threatens health.

- Problem-focused coping includes attempts to change threatening aspects of our environment (including our relationships with others), changing our approach to environmental threats and changing our perceptions (appraisals) of these threats and their consequences.

- Time-management strategies and meditation are two problem-solving coping strategies which appear to help many people cope effectively with their daily demands.

References

Abraham, S. C. S. (1988) Seeing the connections in lay causal comprehension: a return to Heider. In D. J. Hilton (ed.) *Contemporary Science and Natural Explanation: Commonsense Conceptions of Causality.* Harvester Press, Brighton.

Abraham, S. C. S. (1989) Supporting people with a mental handicap in the community: a social psychological perspective. *Disability, Handicap and Society.* **4**, 121–30.

Abraham, S. C. S., Sheeran, P., Abrams, W. D. J., Spears, R. and Marks, D. (1991) Young people learning about AIDS: a study of beliefs and information sources. *Health Education Research: Theory and Practice,* **6**, 19–27.

Abrams, W. D. J., Abraham, S. C. S., Spears, R. and Marks, D. (1990) AIDS invulnerability: relationships, sexual behavior and attitudes amongs 16–19 year olds. In P. Aggleton, P. Davies and G. Hart (eds) *AIDS: Individual, Cultural and Policy Dimensions.* The Falmer Press, Basingstoke, Hampshire.

Abramson, L. Y., Seligman, M. E. P., and Teasdale, J. (1978) Learned helplessness in humans; critique and reformulation. *Journal of Abnormal Psychology,* **87**, 49–74.

Acar, W. and Aupperle, K. E. (1984) Bureaucracy as organizational pathology. *Systems Research,* **1**, 157–66.

Aggleton, P. and Chalmers, H (1986) *Nursing Models and the Nursing Process.* Macmillan, London.

Aguielera, D. C. (1967) Relationship between physical contact and verbal interaction between nurse and patients. *Journal of Psychiatric Nursing,* Jan/Feb, 13–17.

Ajzen, I. and Fishbein, M. (1980) *Understanding Attitudes and Predicting Social Behavior.* Prentice-Hall, Englewood Cliffs New Jersey.

Ajzen, I. and Madden, T. J. (1986) Prediction of goal-directed behavior: attitudes, intentions and perceived behavioral control. *Journal of Experimental Social Psychology,* **22**, 453–74.

Alagna, S. W. and Reddy, D. M. (1984) Predictors of proficient technique and successful lesion detection in breast self-examination. *Health Psychology,* **3**, 113–27.

Allen, V. L. and Levine, J. M. (1971) Social support and conformity: the role of independent assessment of reality. *Journal of Experimental Social Psychology,* **7**, 48–58.

Allport, G. W. (1954) *The Nature of Prejudice.* Addison-Welsey, Reading Mass.

Altschul, A. T. (1968) Measurement of patient–nurse interaction in relation to inpatient psychiatric treatment. M.Phil Thesis. *University of Edinburgh.*

Anderson, E. R. (1973) *The Role of the Nurse: Views of the Patient, Nurse, and Doctor in some General Hospitals in England.* Royal College of Nursing, London.

Archer, J. (1989) Childhood gender roles: structure and development. *The Psychologist: Bulletin of the British Psychological Society,* **9**, 367–70.

Argyle, M. (1972) *The Psychology of Interpersonal Behaviour.* Penguin, Harmondsworth.

Argyle, A., Furnham, A., and Graham, J. (1981). *Social Situations.* Cambridge University Press, Cambridge.

Argyle, M. (1988) *Bodily Communication.* Methuen. London.

Argyle, M., Alkema, K. and Gilmour, R. (1971) The communication of friendly and hostile attitudes by verbal and non-verbal signals. *European Journal of Social Psychology*, **1**, 385- 402.

Argyle, M., Henderson, M. and Furnham, A. (1985) The rules of social relationships. *The British Journal of Social Psychology*, **24**, 125–39.

Argyle, M., Salter, V., Nicholson, H., Williams, M., and Burgess, P. (1970). The communication of inferior and superior attitudes by verbal and non verbal signals. *British Journal of Social and Clinical Psychology*, **9**, 222–31.

Armstrong, D. (1983) The fabrication of nurse-patient relationships. *Social Science and Medicine*, **17**, 457–60.

Arvey, R. D. (1979) Unfair discrimination in the employment interview: legal and psychological aspects. *Psychological Bulletin*, **86**, 736–65.

Asch, S. E. (1946) Forming impressions of personality. *Journal of Abnormal and Social Psychology*, **69**, 258–90.

Asch, S. E. (1951) Effects of group pressure on the modification and distortion of judgements. In H. Guetzkow (ed.) *Groups, Leadership and Men*. Carnegie, Pittsburgh.

Asch, S. E. (1956) Studies of independence and conformity; a minority of one against a unanimous majority. *Psychological monographs* **70**, no. 9 (whole no. 416).

Ashworth, P. (1982) Change from what? A baseline descriptive study of clinical areas involved with the UK (Manchester) Collaborating Centre in research associated with WHO Medium Term Programme in Nursing/ Midwifery. Unpublished Report. Department of Nursing Studies, University of Manchester.

Ayllon, T. and Azrin, N. H. (1968) *The Token Economy: A Motivational System for Therapy and Rehabilitation*. Appleton-Century-Crofts, New York.

Ayllon, T. and Michael, J. (1989) The psychiatric nurse as a behavioural engineer. *Journal of Experimental Analysis of Behaviour*, **2**, 323–34.

Bales, R. F. and Slater, P. E. (1955) Role differentiation in small decision-making groups. In T. Parsons and R. F. Bales (eds) *Family Socialization and Interaction Processes*. The Free Press of Glencoe, Chicago, Ill.

Bandura, A. (1965) Influence of models' reinforcement contingencies on the acquisition of imitative responses. *Journal of Personality and Social Psychology*, **1**, 589–95.

Bandura, A. (1977a) *Social Learning Theory*, Prentice-Hall, Englewood Cliffs, New Jersey.

Bandura, A. (1977b) Self-efficacy: toward a unifying theory of behavior change. *Psychological Review*, **84**, 191–215.

Bandura, A. (1986) *Social Foundations of Thought and Action: A Social Cognitive Theory*. Prentice-Hall, Englewood Cliffs, New Jersey.

Bandura, A. (1989) Perceived-self efficacy in the exercise of personal agency. *The Psychologist: Bulletin of the British Psychological Society*, **10**, 411–24.

Barker, P. J. (1982) *Behaviour Therapy Nursing*. Croom Helm, London.

Barker, P., Baldwin, S. and Ulas, M. (1989) Medical expansionism: some implications for psychiatric nursing practice. *Nurse Education Today*, **9**, 192–202.

Barker, P., Docherty, P., Hird, J., and Hunter, M. H. (1978) Living and learning: a nurse-administered token economy programme involving mentally handicapped schoolboys. *International Journal of Nursing Studies*, **15**, 91–102.

Barker, P and Fraser, D. (1985) *The Nurse as Therapist: A Behavioural Model*. Croom Helm, London.

Barrera, M. Sandler, I. and Ramsay, T. (1981) Preliminary development of a scale of social support studies on college students. *Journal of Community Psychology August*, **9**, 435–47.

Barnett K. (1972) A Survey of the current utilisation of touch by health team personnel with hospitalised patients. *International Journal of Nursing Studies;* **9**, 195–209.

Barrett, E. (1988) A survey of why nurses remain in employment in Paddington and North Kensington. St Mary's Hospital Report.

Barton, E. S. (1975) Behaviour modification in the Hospital School for the severely subnormal. In Kiernan, C. C. and Woodford, F. P. (eds) Behaviour Modification with the Severely Retarded. Elsevier, Associated Scientific Publishers, Amsterdam.

Baston, C. D., Cochran, P. J., Biederman, M. F.

Blosser, J. L., Ryan, M. J. and Vogt, B. (1978) Failure to help when in a hurry: callousness or conflict. *Personality and Social Psychology Bulletin*, **4**, 97–101.

Beck, A. (1976) *Cognitive Therapy and Emotional Disorders*. International Universities Press, New York.

Becker, H. M., Hawfner, D. P., Kasl, S. V., Kirscht, J. P., Maiman, L. A. and Rosenstock, I. M. (1977) Selected psychosocial models and correlates of individual health-related behaviors. *Medical Care*, *15 (5, supplement)*, 27–46.

Becker, H. M., Drachman, R. H. and Kirscht, J. P. (1972) Predicting mother's compliance with medical regimens. *Journal of Pediatrics*, **81**, 843–54.

Beecher, H. K. (1956) Relationship of significance of wound to pain experienced. *Journal of the American Medical Association*, **161**, 1609–13.

Bem, S. L. (1974) The measurement of psychological androgyny. *Journal of Consulting and Clinical Psychology*, **42**, 155–62.

Bem, S. L. (1975) Sex-role adaptability: one consequence of psychological androgyny. *Journal of Personality and Social Psychology*, **31**, 634–43.

Benson, H. A. (1976) *The Relaxation Response*, Morrow, New York.

Bentler, P. M. and Speckart, G. (1981) Attitudes cause behaviours: structural equation analysis. *Journal of Personality and Social Psychology;* **40**, 228–38.

Berger, P. L. and Luckman, T. (1966) *The Social Construction of Reality: A Treatise in the Sociology of Knowledge*. Doubleday, New York.

Berkman, L. amd Syme, L. (1979) Social networks host resistance and mortality: a nine-year follow-up of Alemeda county residents. *American Journal of Epidemiology*, **109**, 186–204.

Berlo, D. K. (1960) *The Process of Communication: An Introduction to Theory and Practice*. Henry Holt, New York.

Berne, E. (1968) *Games People Play: The Psychology of Human Relationships*. Penguin, Harmondsworth.

Berry, D. S. and McArthur, L. Z. (1985a) Some components and consequences of a baby face. *Journal of Personality and Social Psychology*, **48**, 312–23

Berry, D. S. and McArthur, L. Z. (1985b) Perceiving characteristic in faces: the impact of age- related craniofacial changes on social perception. *Psychological Bulletin*, **100**, 3–18.

Berscheid, E. (1981) Interpersonal attraction. In Lindsey G. and Aronson E. (eds), *Handbook of Social Psychology,* 3rd edn. Addison-Wesley, New York.

Bierbrauer, G. (1979) Why did he do it? Attribution of obedience and the phenomenon of dispositional bias. *European Journal of Social Psychology*, **9**, 67–84.

Billig, M. and Tajfel, H. (1973) Social categorization and similarity in intergroup behavior. *European Journal of Social Psychology*, **3**, 27–52.

Birch, J.(1979) The anxious learner. *Nursing Mirror*, 8 Feb, 17–22

Blaxter, M. (1979) Concepts of causality: lay and medical models. In D. T. Oborne, M. M. Gruneberg and J. R. Eiser (eds) *Research in Psychology and Medicine: Vol. 2, Social Aspects: Attitudes Communication Care and Training*. Academic Press, London.

Bond, S. (1983) Nurses' communication with cancer patients. In J. Wilson-Barnett (ed.) Nursing Research: *Ten Studies in Patient Care*. Wiley. Chichester.

Boore, J. P. R. (1978) *Prescription for Recovery*. Royal College of Nursing Research Series, Churchill Livingstone, Edinburgh.

Bordieri, J. E., Soldoky M. L. and Mikos N. A. (1984) Physical attractiveness and nurses' perceptions of pediatric patients. *Nursing Research*, **34**, 24–26.

Bordow, S. and Porritt, D. (1979) An experimental evaluation of crisis intervention. *Social Science and Medicine*, **13A**, 251–56.

Boyle, C. M. (1970) Difference between patients' and doctors' interpretation of some common medical terms. *British Medical Journal*, **71**, 268–89.

Bradley, C. (1985) Psychological aspects of diabetes. *The Diabetes Annual*, **1**, 374–87.

Bradley, C., Brewin, C.R., Gamsu, D. S. and Moses, J. L. (1984) Development of scales to measure perceived control of diabetes mellitus and diabetes-related health beliefs. *Diabetic Medicine*, **1**, 213–18.

Brechin, A., Liddiard, P. and Swain, J. (eds) (1981) *Handicap in a Social World*. Hodder and Stoughton, London.

Brehm, J. W. (1966) *A Theory of Psychological Reactance*. Academic Press, New York.

Brewin, C. R. (1984) Perceived controllability of life events and willingness to prescribe psychotropic drugs. *British Journal of Social Psychology*, **23**, 285–87.

Briggs, A. (1972) Report of the Committee on Nursing. HMSO, London.

British Medical Journal (1897) The nursing of the sick under Queen Victoria. Vol. 1 (19 June, p. 1645). Cited in S. C. Davis (1980) *Rewriting Nursing History* (p. 45), Croom Helm, London.

Broadhead, W. F, Kaplan, B. H., James. S., Wagner. E., Schoenbach. V., Grimson, R., Heyden, S., Tibblin, G. and Gehlbach, S. H. (1983) The epidemiological evidence for a relationship between social support and health. *American Journal of Epidemiology*, **117**, 521–36.

Bronowski, J. (1973) *The Ascent of Man*. British Broadcasting Corporation, London.

Brophy, J. E. and Good, T. L. (1970) Teachers communication of differential expectations for children's classroom performance. *Journal of Educational psychology*, **61**, 365–74.

Broverman, I. K., Broverman, D. M.,Clarkson, F. E., Rosenkrantz, P and Vogel, S. R. (1970) Sex role stereotypes and clinical judgements of mental health. *Journal of Consulting and Clinical Psychology*, **34**, 1–7.

Brown, G. W., Birley, J. and Wing, A. (1972) The influence of family life on the course of schizophrenic disorders: a replication. *British Journal of Psychiatry*, **121**, 241–58.

Brown, G. W. and Harris, T. (1979) *The Social Origins of Depression*. Tavistock, London.

Brown, R. G. S. and Stones, R. W. H. (1973) *The Male Nurse*. Bell, London.

Brown, R. J. (1978) Divided we fall; an analysis of relations between sections of a factory work force. In H. Tajfel (ed.) *Differentiation Between Social Groups: Studies in the Social Psychology of Intergroup Relations*. Academic Press, London.

Brown, R. J. and Turner, (1981) Interpersonal and intergroup behavior. In J. C. Turner and H. Giles (eds) *Intergroup Behavior*. Blackwell, Oxford.

Brunson, B. and Matthews, K. A. (1981) The type A coronary-prone behavior pattern and reactions to uncontrollable stress: an analysis of performance strategies, affect and attributions during failure. *Journal of Personality and Social Psychology*, **14**, 564–78.

Bruner, J. S. and Tagiuri, R. (1954) The Perception of People. In G. Lindzey (ed.) *Handbook of Social Psychology*.Vol. 1. Addison-Wesley, Cambridge, Mass.

Bryant, B. M., Trower, P. E., Yardley, K., Urbieta, H. and Letmendia, F. (1976). A survey of social adequacy among psychiatric outpatients. *Psychological Medicine;* **6**: 101–12.

Bucher, R. and Stelling, J. (1969) Characteristics of professional Organizations.*Journal of Health and Social Behaviour*, **10**, 2–13.

Buhrmester, D. and Furman, W. (1983) Sex-role differences in socio-emotional adjustment to college. Unpublished manuscript, University of Denver, Denver, Colo.

Burns, T. and Stalker, G. M. (1961) *The Management of Innovation.* Tavistock, London.

Butterworth, C. A. and Skidmore, D. (1981) *Caring for the Mentally Ill in the Community.* Croom Helm, London.

Byrne, D. (1961a) The influence of propinquity and opportunities for interaction on classroom relationships. *Human Relations,* **14,** 63–69.

Byrne, D. (1961b) Interpersonal attraction and attitudinal similarity. *Journal of Abnormal and Social Psychology,* **62,** 713–15.

Byrne, D. (1971) *The Attraction Paradigm,* Academic Press, London.

Byrne, P. S. and Long, E. L. (1976) *Doctors Talking to Patients; A Study of the Verbal Behavior of General practitioners Consulting in their Surgeries.* HMSO, London.

Canter, D. (1984) The environmental context of nursing: looking beyond the ward. In S. Skevington (ed.) *Understanding Nurses: The Social Psychology of Nursing.* Wiley, Chichester.

Cantor, N. and Mischel, W. (1977) Traits as prototypes: effects on recognition memory. *Journal of Personality and Social Psychology,* **35,** 38–48.

Cantor, N. and Mischel, W. (1979) Prototypes in Person Perception. In L. Berkowitz (ed.) *Advances in Experimental Social Psychology,* **12,** Academic Press, New York.

Caplaw, T. and Forman, R. (1950) Neighbourhood interaction in a homogenous community. *American Sociological Review,* **15,** 357–66.

Carlson, R. E. (1971) Effect of interview information in altering valid impressions. *Journal of Applied Psychology,* **55,** 443–48.

Cartwright, D. and Zander, A. (1968) Leadership and Performance of Group Functions. In D Cartwright and A Zander (eds) *Group Dynamics; Theory and Research (3rd edn).* Tavistock, London.

Carver, C. S. and Humphries, C. (1982) Social Psychology of the type A Coronary-Prone Behavior Pattern. In G. S. Sanders and J. Suls (eds) *Social Psychology of Health and Illness.* Lawrence Erlbaum, Hillsdale, New Jersey.

Carver, C. S. and Scheier, M. F. (1981) The self- attention-induced feedback loop and social facilitation. *Journal of Experimental Social Psychology,* **17,** 545–68.

Central Statistical Office (1985) *Social Trends 15.* HMSO London.

Chalmers, A. F. (1978) *What is this thing called Science.* Open University Press, Milton Keynes.

Chapman, C. R., Casey, L. K. Dubner, R., Florey, K. M., Gracely, R. H. and Reading, A. E. (1985) Pain measurement: An Overview. *Pain,* **22,** 1–31.

Chemers, M. M., Hays R. B., Rhodeawlt, F. and Wysocki, J. (1985) A person-environment analysis of job stress; a contingency model explanation. *Journal of personality and Social Psychology,* **49,** 628–35.

Cheyne, W. M. (1970) Stereotyped reactions of speakers with Scottish and English regional accents. *British Journal of Social and Clinical Psychology,* **9,** 77–9.

Chomsky, N. (1959) Review of B. F. Skinner's verbal behaviour. *Language,* **35,** 26–58.

Choon, G. L. and Skevington, S. M. (1984) How do women and men in nursing perceive each other? In S. Skevington (ed.) *Understanding nurses: The Social Psychology of Nursing.* Wiley, Chichester.

Christie, M. J. and Mellett, P. G. (eds) (1986) *The Psychosomatic Approach: Contemporary Practice of Whole Person Care.* Wiley, Chichester.

Clark, R. D. III and Ward, L. E. (1972) Why don't bystanders help? Becaue of ambiguity? *Journal of Personality and Social Psychology;* **24,** 392–400.

Clegg, F. (1988) Bereavement. In S. Fisher and J. Reason (eds) *Handbook of Life Stress, Cognition and Health.* Wiley, Chichester.

Cohen, J. and Syme, S. L. (1985) Issues in the study and application of social support. In J. Cohen and S. L. Syme (eds)*Social Support and Health*. Academic Press, New York.

Cohen, S. and Hoberman, H. M. (1983) Positive events and social support as buffers of life change stress. *Journal of Applied psychology*, **13**, 99–125.

Condry, J. and Condry S. (1976) Sex differences: a study in the eye of the beholder.*Child Development*, **47**, 812–19.

Cooley, C. H. (1956)*Human Nature and the Social Order*. The Free Press of Glencoe, New York.

Cooper, D. (1967) *Psychiatry and Anti-psychiatry*. Tavistock, London.

Corbett, J. (1989) The quality of life in the independence curriculum. *Disability, Handicap and Society*. **4**, 145–65.

Cormack, D. (1975) *Psychiatric Nursing Observed*. Royal College of Nursing, London.

Coser, L. (1962) *Life on the Ward*. Michigan State University Press, East Lansin, Michigan

Cottingham, M. (1987) Putting men in the picture. *Nursing Times*, **83**, May, 28–9.

Cronin-Stubbs, D. and Brophy, E. B. (1985) Burnout: Can social support save the psychiatric nurse. *Journal of Psychosocial and Nursing Mental Health Service*, **23**, 8–13.

Cummings, K. M., Becker, M. H., and Maile, M. C. (1980) Bringing the models together; an empirical approach to combining variables used to explain health actions. *Journal of Behavioural Medicine*, **3**, 123–45.

Cunningham, C. C. (1975) Parents as Therapists and Educators. In Kiernan, C. C. and Woodford, F. P. (eds) *Behaviour Modification with the Severely Retarded*. Elsevier, Associated Scientific Publishers, Amsterdam.

Damrosch, S. P. (1982) More than skin deep: relationships between perceived physical attractiveness and nursing students assessments. *Western Journal of Nursing Research*, **4**, 423–33.

Darley, J. M. and Latane, B. (1968) Bystander intervention in emergencies: diffusion of responsibility.*Journal of Personality and Social Psychology*, **8**, 377–83.

Davies, B. (1981) Social skills in nursing. In M. Argyle (ed.) *Social Skills and Mental Health*.Methuen, London.

Davies, F. (1975) Professional socialisation as subjective experience: the process of doctrinal conversion among student nurses. In C. Cox and A. Mead (eds) *A Sociology of Medical Practice*. Collier-Macmillan, London.

Davis, M. S. (1968) Physiologic, psychological and demographic factors in patient compliance with doctors' orders. *Medical Care*, **5**, 115–22.

Dawkins, J. E., Depp, F. C. and Selzer, N. E. (1985) Stress and the psychiatric nurse.*Journal of Psychosocial Nursing*, **23**, 9–15.

Dean, P. G. (1986) Expanding our sights to include social networks. *Nursing and Health Care*, December. 545–50.

Deaux, K. (1985) Sex and gender, *Annual Review of Psychology*, **36**, 49–81.

Deci, E. L. (1975) *Intrinsic Motivation*. Plenum, New York.

Department of Health and Social Security DHSS (1976) *Prevention and Health: Everybody's Business, A Reassessment of Personal and Public Health*. HMSO, London.

Department of Health (1989) *Working for Patients*. Cm 555, HMSO, London.

Deutsch, M. and Gerard, H. B. (1955) A study of normative and informational influence on individual judgement.*Journal of Abnormal and Social Psychology*, **51**, 629–36

Dewe, P. V. (1989) Stressor frequency, tension, tiredness and coping. Some measurement issues and a comparison across nursing groups. *Journal of Advanced Nursing*, **14**, 308–20.

DeWever, M. K. (1977) Nursing home patients' perception of nurses' affective touching. *Journal of Psychology*, **96**, 163–71.

DiMatteo, M. R., Friedman, H. S. and Taranta, A. (1979). Sensitivity to bodily non-verbal communication as a factor in practitioner–patient rapport. *Journal of Non-Verbal Behaviour;* **4**, 18–26.

DiMatteo, M. R., Hays, R. D. and Prince L. M. (1986) Relationship of Non-Verbal communication skill to patient satisfaction: appointment non-compliance and physician workload. *Health Psychology;* **5**, 581–94.

Dingwall, R (1977) The place of men in nursing. In M. College and D. Jones (eds) *Reader in Nursing.* Edinburgh, Churchill Livingstone.

Dion, K. Berscheid, E. and Walster, E. (1972) What is beautiful is good. *Journal of Personality and Social Psychology,* **245**, 285–90

Dittes, J. E. and Kelley, H. H. (1956) Effects of different conditions of acceptance on conformity to group norms. *Journal of Abnormal and Social Psychology,* **59**, 204–9.

Dodd, H. (1988) Realistic thinking, *Nursing Times,* **84**, 35–7.

Dornbusch S. M., Hastorf, A. H., Richardson, S. A., Muzzy, R. E., and Vreeland, R. S. (1965) The perceiver and the perceived: their relative influence on the categories of interpersonal cognition. *Journal of Personality and Social Psychology.* **1**, 434–40.

Doyal, L. and Pennell, I. (1979) *The Political Economy of Health.* Pluto Press, London.

Dracup, K., Meieis, A. and Edlefsen, P. (1984) Family-focused cardiac rehabilitation: a role supplementation program for cardiac patients and spouses. *Nursing Clinics of North America,* **19**, 113–24.

Duck, S. (1975) Attitude similarities and interpersonal attraction: right answers and wrong reasons.*British Journal of Social and Clinical Psychology,* **14**, 311–12.

Duck, S. (1977) *The Study of Acquaintance.* Saxon House, Farnborough.

Duncan, B. L. (1976) Differential social perception and attribution of intergroup violence: testing the lower limits of stereotyping of Blacks, *Journal of Personality and Social Psychology,* **34**, 508–8.

Dunkell-Schetter, C. (1982) Social support and coping with cancer. Unpublished PhD Dissertation. Northwestern University, Evanston.

Dunkell-Schetter, C. and Wortman, C. (1982) The interpersonal dynamics of cancer. Problems in social relatonships and their impact on the patient. In H. S. Freedman and M. R. DiMatteo (eds) *Interpersonal Issues in Health Care.* Academic Press. New York

Durkheim, E. (1951) *Suicide.* Free Press. New York.

Dweck, C. S. and Licht, B. G. (1980) Learned helplessness and intellectual achievement. In J. Garber and M. E. P. Seligman (eds) *Human Helplessness: Theory and Applications.*Academic Press, London.

Ebbesen, E. B., Kjos, G. L. and Konecini, V. L. (1976) Spatial ecology: its effects on the choice of friends and enemies.*Journal of Experimental Social Psychology,* **12**, 505–18

Egan, G. (1990) *The Skilled Helper; A Systematic Approach to Effective Helping* (4th edn.). Brooks/Cole California.

Eagly, A. H. (1989) Gender stereotypes and attitudes toward men and women. *Personality and Social Psychology Bulletin,* **14**, 543–58.

Egbert, L. D., Battit, G. E., Welch, C. E., and Bartlett, M. K. (1964) Reduction of post operative pain by encouragement and instruction of patients, *New England Journal of Medicine,* **270r, 825–7.**

Eiser, C. and Patterson, D. (1983) Slugs and snails and puppy dog tails – children's ideas about the inside of their bodies. *Child: Care, Health and Development,* **9**, 233–40.

Eiser, R. (1982) Addiction as Attribution: Cognitive Processes in Giving up Smoking. In R. Eiser (ed.) *Social Psychology and Behavioral Medicine.* Wiley, Chichester.

Elliot, T. S. (1974) *Collected Poems, 1909–1962.*Faber and Faber, London.

Ellis, A. (1962) *Reason and emotion in psychotherapy*. Lyle Stuart, New York.

Ellis, A. (1976 Rational-emotive therapy. In Binder, V., Binder, A. and Rimland, B. (eds) *Modern Therapies*, Prentice-Hall, Englewood Cliffs New Jersey.

Emerson, J. (1970) Behaviour in private places: sustaining definitions of reality in Gynaecological examinations. In H. P. Dreitzel (ed.) *Recent Sociology* No. 2. Macmillan, London.

Emrick, C. D., Lassen, C. L. and Edwards, M. T. (1977) Nonprofessional peers as therapeutic agents.In A. S. Gurman and A. M. Razin (eds) *Effective Psychotherapy: A Handbook of Research*. Pergamon Press, Oxford.

Engel, G. L. (1977) The need for a new medical model: a challenge for biomedicine. *Science*, **196**, 129–36.

Fabrikant, B. (1974) The psychotherapist and the female patient: perceptions and change. In V. Franks and V.Burtle (eds) *Women in Therapy*. Bruner-Mazel, New York.

Faris, R. and Dunham, H. W. (1939) *Mental Disorders in Urban Areas*. University of Chicago Press, Chicago, Ill.

Faulkner, A. (1979) Monitoring nurse-patient conversations in a ward. *Nursing Times*, **75**, Supplement, 95–96.

Faulkner, A. (1980) Communication and the nurse. *Nursing Times*, Occasional Papers 76, **21**, 93–5.

Faulkner, A. (1985) The organizational context of interpersonal skills in nursing. In C. Kagan (ed.) *Interpersonal Skills In Nursing*. Croom Helm, London.

Faulkner, A. (1985b) *Nursing: A Creative Approach*. Bailliere Tindell, Eastbourne UK.

Faukner, A., McLeod-Clark, J., Bridges, W. (1983) *Teaching Communication in Schools of Nursing*. Royal College of Nursing Conference, Brighton, England.

Fawcett, J. (1984) *Analysis and Evaluation of Conceptual Models of Nursing*. Davis, Philadelphia, Pa.

Feilder, F. E. (1967) *A Theory of Leadership Effectiveness McGraw-Hill, New York*.

Festinger, L. (1954) A theory of social comparison processes. *Human Relations*, **7**, 117–40.

Festinger, L. (1957) *A Theory of Cognitive Dissonance*. Stanforn University Press, Stanford.

Feuerstein, M., Labbe, E. E. and Kuczmierczyk, A. R. (1986) *Health Psychology: A Psychobiological Perspective*. Plenum Press, New York.

Fielding, R. G. and Llewelyn, P. M. (1987) Communication training in nursing may damage your health and enthusiasm: some warnings. *Journal of Advanced Nursing*, **12**, 281–90.

Flor, H., Kerns, R. D., and Turk, D. C. (1987) The role of spouse reinforcement, perceived pain and activity levels of chronic pain patients. *Journal of Psychosomatic Research*, **31**, 251–9.

Flowers, M. L. (1977) A laboratory test of some implications of Janis' groupthink hypothesis. *Journal of Personality and Social Psychology*, **35**, 888–86.

Fodor, J. A. (1976) *The Language of Thought*. Harvester Press, Hassocks.

Fontana, D. (1989) *Managing Stress*. British Psychological Society and Routledge, Leicester.

Fordyce, W. (1976) *Behavioural Methods for Chronic Pain and Illness*. Mosby, St Louis.

Franks, C. M. (1966) Conditioning and conditioned aversion therapies in the treatment of the alcoholic. *International Journal of the Addictions*, **1**, 61–98.

Fraser, C. (1984) Communication in interaction. In H. Tajfel and C. Fraser (1984) *Introducing Social Psychology*. Penguin, Harmondsworth.

French, P. (1983) *Social Skills for Nursing Practice*. Croom Helm, London.

Friedman, M. and Rosenman, R. H. (1974) *Type A Behavior and Your Heart*. Fawcett Books, New York.

Frunkel, M. and Wilson D. (1985) I want to know what's in my file. *Report for the*

Campaign for Freedom of Information. London.

Gamarnikov, E. (1978) Sexual division of labour: the case of nursing. In A. Kuhn and A. M. Wolpe (eds) *Feminism and Materialism.* Routledge and Kegan Paul, London.

Gaze, H. (1987) Men in nursing. *Nursing Times*, **83**, May, 25–27.

Geitgey, D. A. (1966) A study of some effects of sensitivity training on the performance of students in associate degree programs of nursing education. Dissertion Abstracts 27B: 2000–1.

Gekas, V. and Schwalbe, M. L.(1983) Beyond the looking-glass self. Social structure and efficacy-based self esteem. *Social Psychology Quarterly*, **46**, 77–88.

Gergen, K. J. (1973) Social psychology as history. *Journal of Personality and Social Psychology*, **26**, 309–20.

Ghiselli, E. E. (1973) The validity of aptitude tests in personnel selection. *Personnel Psychology*, **26**, 461–77.

Gibb, C. A. (1954) Leadership. In G. Lindzey (ed.) *Handbook of Social Psychology*, vol. 2. Addison-Wesley, Cambridge, Mass.

Giles, H. and Powesland, P. F. (1975) *Speech Style and Social Evaluation.* Academic Press, London.

Gilligan, C. (1982) *In a Different Voice; Psychological Theory and Women's Development.* Harvard University Press, Harvard, Mass.

Glass, D. C. (1977) *Behavior Patterns, Stress and Coronary Heart Disease.* Lawrence Erlbaum, Hillsdale, New Jersey.

Glass, D. C. and Singer, J. E. (1972) *Urban Stress: Experiments on Noise and Social Stressors.* Academic Press, New York.

Goebel, B. L. (1984) Age stereotype held by student nurses. *Journal of Psychology*, **116**, 249–54.

Goldberg, P. (1968) Are women prejudiced against women? *Transaction*, **5**, 28–30.

Goffman, E. (1955) On face-work: an analysis of the ritual elements in social interaction. psychiatry. *Journal for the Study of Interpersonal Processes*, **12**, 213–31.

Goffman, E. (1961) Encounters: two studies in the sociology of interaction. The Bobbs-Merrill Company Inc., Indianapolis.

Goffman, E. (1969) *The Presentation of Self in Everyday Life.* Penguin, Harmondsworth.

Goffman, E. (1972a) *Relations in Public: Microstudies of the Public Order.* Penguin, Harmondsworth.

Goffman, E. (1972b) *Encounters: Two Studies in the Sociology of Interaction.* Allen Lane, Harmondsworth.

Goffman, E. (1974) *Frame Analysis.* Penguin, Harmondsworth.

Gordon Pugh, W. T. (1969) *Practical Nursing, 21st edn.* Allen Lane. London.

Gore, S. (1978) The effect of support in moderating the consequences of unemployment. *Journal of Health and Social Behaviour*, **19**, 157–64.

Graham, R. J. (1981) Understanding the benefits of poor communication. *Interface*, **11**, 80–82.

Gruen, W. (1975) Effects of brief psychotherapy during the hospitalisation period of the recovery process in health attacks. *Journal of Consulting and Clinical Psychology*, **43**, 223–32.

Gray-Toft, P. A. and Anderson, J. G. (1981) Stress among hospital nursing staff: its causes and effects. *Social Science and Medicine*, **15A**, 639–47.

Gray-Toft, P. A. and Anderson, J. G. (1985) Organisational stress in the hospital. Development of a model for diagnosis and prediction. *Health Service Research*, **19**, 753–74.

Greene, J. and D'Oliveria, M. (1982) *Learning to use Statistical Tests in Psychology: A Student's Guide.* Open University Press, Milton Keynes.

Greenspoon, J. (1955) The reinforcing effects of two spoken sounds on the frequency of two responses. *American Journal of Psychology*, **68**, 409–16.

Gregory, R. L. (1977) *Eye and Brain*. (3rd edn.) McGraw-Hill, New York.

Guardian, The (1984) Police catcall costs £100. *The Guardian*, 17 November.

Hackett, G. and Betz, N. E. (1981) A self-efficacy approach to the career development of women. *Journal of Vocational Behaviour*, **18**, 326–39.

Haefner, D. P. and Kirscht, J. P. (1970) Motivational and behavioral effects of modifying health beliefs. *Public Health Reports*, **85**, 478–84.

Hall, D. J. (1977) *Social Relations and innovation: Changing the State of Play in Hospitals*. Routledge and Kegan Paul, London.

Hamner, W. C. and Organ, D. W. (1978) *Organisational Behaviour; An Applied Psychological Approach*, Dallas Business Publications, Dallas, Texas.

Haney, C., Banks, C. and Zimbardo, P. (1973) Interpersonal dynamics in a simulated prison. *Journal of Criminology and Penology*, **1**, 69–97.

Hargreaves, D. H. (1980) Common-sense models of action. In A. J. Chapman and D. M. Jones (eds) *Models of Man*. The British Psychological Society, Leicester.

Harré, R. (1979) *Social Being*. Blackwell, Oxford.

Harré, R. (1983) *Personal Being*. Blackwell, Oxford.

Harris, P. R. (1985) Asch's data and the Asch effect: a critical note. *British Journal of Social Psychology*, **24**, 229–30.

Hastings, G. B. and Scott, A. C. (1987) Aids publicity: pointers to development. *Health Education Journal*, **46** (2), 58–9.

Hawkins, L., Cooper, C., Harris, P. (1982) Smoking stress and nurses. *Nursing Mirror*, **155** (15), 18–22.

Hawkins, L. (1987) An ergonomic approach to stress. *International Journal of Nursing Studies*, **24**, 307–18.

Hauser, S.T. (1981) Physician–Patient Relationships. In Mishler, E. G., Amaraingham, L. R., Osherson, S. D. Hauser, S. T., Waxler, N. E. and Liem, R. (eds) *Social Contexts of Health, Illness and Patient Care*. Cambridge University Press, Cambridge.

Hayward, J. (1975) Information – a prescription against pain. *The Study of Nursing Care Project Reports*, Series 2, No. 5, Royal College of Nursing, London.

Heider, F. (1958) The Psychology of Interpersonal Relations, Wiley, New York.

Helfer, R. E. (1970) An objective comparison of the pediatric interviewing skills of freshman and senior medical students. *Pediatrics*, **45**, 623–7.

Henderson, D. and Gillespie, R. (1964) *Textbook of Psychiatry*. Oxford University Press, London.

Henley, N. M. (1977) *Body Politics: Power, Sex and Non-verbal Communication. Prentice-Hall, Englewood Cliffs, New Jersey*.

Henry, C. and Tuxill, A. C. (1987) Persons and Humans. *Journal of Advanced Nursing*, **12**, 383–8.

Hersey, P. and Blanchard, K. (1982) Organizational Behaviour; Utilizing Human Resources, (4th edn.). Prentice-Hall, Englewood Cliffs, New Jersey.

Hingley, P. and Cooper, C. L. (1986) *Stress and the Nurse Manager*. Wiley, New York.

Hinshaw, A. S., Smeltzer, C. H. and Atwood, J. R. (1987) Innovative retention strategies for nursing staff. *Journal of Nursing Administration*, **17**, 8–16

Hofling, C. K., Brotzman, E., Dalrymple, S., Graves, N. and Pierce, C. M. (1966) An experimental study in nurse-physician relationships. *Journal of Nervous and Mental Diseases*, **143**, 171–80.

Holmes, T. H. and Rahe, R.H. (1967) The social readjustment rating scale. *Journal of Psychosomatic Research*, **11**, 213–18.

Hollinger, L. M. (1980) Perception of touch in the elderly. *Journal of Gerontological Nursing*, **6**, 741–46.

Hollingshead, A. B. and Redlich, F. C. (1958) *Social Class and Mental Illness*. Wiley, New York.

Holroyd, K. A., Penzien, D. B., Hursey, K. G., Tobin, D. L., Rogers, L. Holm, J. E., Mercille, P. J., Hall, J. R., Chila, A. G. (1984) Change mechanisms in EMG biofeedback training: cognitive changes underlying improvements in tension headache. *Journal of Cosulting and Clinical Psychology*, **52**, 1039–53.

Horner, M. S. (1972) Towards an understanding of achievement-related conflicts in women. *Journal of Social Issues*, **28**, 157–75.

House, R. J. and Rizzo, J. R. (1972) Role conflict and ambiguity as critical variables in a model of organizational behaviour. *Organizational Behaviour and Human Performance*, **7**, 467–05.

Hovland. C. I., Janis, I. L. and Kelley, H. H. (1953) *Communication and Persuasion*. Yale University Press, New Haven, Conn.

Huckabay, L. M. D. and Jagla, B. (1979) Nurses' stress factors in the intensive care unit. *Journal of Nursing Administration*, **2**, 21–6.

Hughes, D. (1983) Consultation length and outcome in two general practices, *Journal of the Royal College of General practitioners*, **33**, 143–7.

Huston, T. L., Ruggiero, M., Conner, R., Geiss, G.

(1981) Bystander intervention into crime: a study based on naturally-occurring episodes. *Social Psychology Quarterly*, **44**, 14–23.

Ingleby, D. (1981) *Critical Psychiatry: The Politics of Mental Health*. Penguin, Harmondsworth.

Inglis, B. (1983) *The Diseases of Civilization*. Granada, London.

Insko, C. A. Drenan, S. Solomon M. R. and Wade, T. J. (1983) Conformity as a function of the consistency of positive self-evaluation with being liked and being right. *Journal of Experimental Social psychology*, **19**, 341–58.

Jahoda, M. (1982) *Employment and Unemployment: A Social Psychological Analysis*. Cambridge University Press, Cambridge.

James, W. (1890) *The Principles of Psychology*. Holt Rinehart and Winston, New York.

Janis, I. L. (1972) *Victims of Groupthink*. Houghton Mifflin, Boston.

Janz, N. K. and Becker, H. M. (1984) The health belief model: a decade later. *Health Education Quarterly*, **11**, 1–47.

Jaspers, J.M.F. (1978) The Nature and Measurement of Attitudes. In H. Tajfel and C. Fraser (eds) *Introducing Social Psychology*. Penguin, Harmondsworth.

Jay Report (1979) Report of the Committee of Enquiry into mental Handicap Nursing and Care. HMSO, London.

Jenkins, C. D. (1966) Group differences in perception: a study of community beliefs and feelings about tuberculosis. *American Journal of Sociology*, **71**, 417–25.

Jenkins, C. D. (1979) An approach to the diagnosis and treatment of health related behavior. *International Journal of Health Education*, **22**, 1–24.

Johnson, D. (1980) The behavioural system model for nursing, In Riehl, J. P. and Roy C. (eds) *Conceptual Models for Nursing Practice*. Appleton-Century-Crofts, Norwalk.

Johnston, M. (1976) Communication of patients' feelings in hospital. In A. E. Bennet (ed.) *Communications Between Doctors and Patients*. Nuffield Provincial Hospitals Trust, London.

Johnston, M. (1980) Anxiety in surgical patients, *Psychological Medicine*, **10**, 145–52.

Johnston, M. (1982) Recognition of patients' worries by nurses and other patients. *British Journal of Clinical Psychology*, **21**, 255–61.

Johnston, M. (1987) Emotional and cognitive aspects of anxiety in surgical patients. *Communication and Cognition* **20**, 261–76.

Jones, A. (1989) Bereavement counselling: applying ten principles. *Geriatic Medicine*, September, 55–8.

Jones, E. E. and Harris, V. A. (1967) The attribution of attitudes. *Journal of Experimental Social Psychology*, **3**, 1–24

Jones, E. E. and Nisbett, R. E. (1972) The actor and the observer; divergent perceptions of the causes of behavior. In E. E. Jones, D. E. Kenrose, H. H. Kelley, R. E. Nisbett, S. Valins, and B. Weiner (eds) *Attribution: Perceiving the Causes of Behavior*. General Learning Press, Morristown.

Jones, E. E. and Pittman, T. S. (1982) Towards a general theory of strategic self-presentation. In J. Suns (ed.) Psychological Perspectives on the Self. Erlbaum, Hillsdale, New Jersey.

Jones, J. G., Janman, K., Payne, R. L. and Rick, J. T. (1987) Some determinants of stress in psychiatric nurses. *International Journal of Nursing Studies*, **24**, 129–44.

Jones, M. (1953) *The Therapeutic Community*, Basic Books, New York.

Jones, M. C. (1924) The elimination of children's fears. *Journal of Experimental Psychology*, **7**, 382–90.

Jones, R. A. (1982) Expectations and illness. In H. S. Friedman and M. R. DiMatteo (eds) *Interpersonal Issues in Health Care*. Academic Press, New York.

Jorgensen, B. W. and Cervone, J. C. (1978) Affect enhancement in the pseudorecognition task. *Personality and Social Psychology Bulletin*, **4**, 285–8.

Jorgensen, S. R. and Sonstegard, J. S. (1984) Predicting adolescent sexual and contraceptive behavior: an application and test of the Fishbein model. *Journal of Marriage and the Family*, **46**, 43–55.

Jourard, S. M. (1966) An exploratory study of body accessibility. *The British Journal of Social and Clinical Psychology*, **5**, 221–31.

Kaplan, G. D. and Cowles, A. (1978) Health locus of control and health value in prediction of smoking reduction. *Health Education Monographs*, **6**, 129–37.

Kaplan, R. M., Atkins, C. J., and Reinsch, S. (1984) Specific efficacy expectations mediate exercise compliance in patients with COPD. *Health Psychology*, **3**, 223–42.

Karlins, M., Coffman, T.L. and Walters, G. (1969) On the fading of social stereotypes; studies in three generations of college students. *Journal of Personality and Social Psychology*, **13**, 1–6

Katz, A. (1970) Self help organizations and volunteer participation in social welfare. *Social Work*, **15**, 551–60.

Kayser, J. S. and Minnigerode, F. A. (1975) Increasing nursing students' interest in working with aged patients. *Nursing Research*, **24**, 23–6.

Kelley, H. H. (1967) Attribution theory in social psychology. In, D. Levine (ed.) *Nebraska Symposium on Motivation* (vol. 15), University of Nebraska Press, Lincoln, Nebraska.

Kelley, H. H. (1972) Attribution in interaction. In E. E. Jones, D. E. Kenrose, H. H. Kelley, R. E. Nisbett, S. Valins, and B. Weiner (eds) *Attribution: Perceiving the Causes of Behavior*. General Learning Press, Morristown, New Jersey.

Kelly, E. L. and Fiske, D. W. (1951) *The Prediction of Performance in Clinical Psychology*. University of Michigan Press, Michigan.

Kelly, G. A. (1955) *The Psychology of Personal Constructs*. Norton, New York.

Kelly, M. P. and May, D. (1982) Good and bad patients: a review of the literature and a theoretical critique. *Journal of Advanced Nursing*, **7**, 147–56.

Kelly, P. M. (1986) The subjective experience of chronic disease: some implications for the management of ulcerative colitis. *Journal of Chronic Diseases*, **39**, 653–6.

Kerckhoff, A. C. and Davis K. E. (1962) Value consensus and need complementarity in mate selection. *American Sociological Review*, **27**, 293–303.

Kessler, R. C. and McLeod, J. B. (1985) Social support and mental health in community samples. In S. Cohen and S. L. Syme (eds) *Social Support and Health*. Academic Press. New York.

Kilham, W. and Mann, L (1974) Level of destructive obedience as a function of transmitter and excutant roles in the Milgram obedience paradigm. *Journal of*

Personality and Social Psychology, **29**, 696–702.

Killilea, M. (1976) Mutual help organizations: interpretations in the literature. In G. Caplan and Killilea (eds) *Support Systems and Mutual Help; Multidisciplinary Explorations*. Grune and Stratton, New York.

King, J (1983) Attribution theory and the health belief model. In, M. Hewstone (ed.) *Attribution Theory: Social an Functional extensions*. Blackwell, Oxford.

King, J. (1984) Psychology in nursing 2: the health belief model. *Nursing Times*, **80**, (Oct. 24): 53–5.

Knox, R. E. and Stafford, K. L. (1976) Group caution at the race track. *Journal of Experimental Social Psychology*, **12**, 317–24.

Kolb, D. A., Winter, S. K., and Berlew, D. E. (1968) Self-directed change: two studies, *Journal of Applied Behavioural Science*, **4**, 453–72.

Koos, E. (1954) *The Health of Regionsville: What the People Thought and Did About It.* Columbia University Press, New York.

Korman, A. (1967) 'Consideration', initiating structure; and organizational criteria, *Personnel Psychology*, **18**, 349–60.

Korsch, B. M., Gozzi, E. K. and Francis, V. (1968) Gaps in doctor–patient communication: 1. Doctor–patient interaction and patient satisfaction. *Pediatrics*, **42**, 855–71.

Kulik, J. A. and Mahler, H. I. M. (1989) Social support and recovery from surgery. *Health Psychology*, **8**, 221–38.

Labov, W. (1973) The logic of nonstandard English. In N. Keddie (ed.) *Tinker, Tailor... The myth of Cultural Deprivation*. Penguin, Harmondsworth.

Laing, R. D. (1959) *The Divided Self.* Tavistock, London.

Laing, R. D. (1967) *The Politics of Experience and the Birds of Paradise*. Penguin, Harmondsworth.

Laing, R. D. and Esterson, A. (1970) *Sanity Madness and the Family*. Tavistock, London.

Lamm, H. and Myers, D. G. (1978) Group-induced polarization of attitudes and behaviour. In L. Berkowitz (ed.) *Advances in Experimental Social Psychology*, Vol, 11. Academic Press, New York.

Langer, E. J. and Abelson, R. P. (1972) The semantics of asking a favour. How to succeed in getting help without really dying. *Journal of Personality and Social Psychology*, **24**, 26–32.

Langer, E. J., Blank, A. and Chanowitz, B. (1978) The mindlessness of ostensibly thoughtful action: the role of 'placebic' information in interpersonal interaction. *Journal of Personality and Social Psychology*, **36**, 635–42.

LaPiere, R. T. (1934) Attitudes versus actions. *Social Forces*, **13**, 230–37.

Larson, P. A. (1977) Influence of patient status and health condition on nurse perceptons of patient characteristics. *Nursing Research*, **26**, 416–21.

Larson, P. J. (1984) Important nurse caring behaviours perceived by patients with cancer. *Oncology Nursing Forum*, **11**, 46–50.

Latané, B. and Darley, J. M. (1970) *The Unresponsive Bystander; Why Doesn't He Help.* Appleton-Century-Crofts, New York.

Latané, B. and Nida, S. (1981) Ten years of research on group size and helping. *Psychological Bulletin*, **89**, 308–24.

Latané, B. and Rodin, J. (1969) A lady in distress: inhibiting effects and strangers on bystander intervention. *Journal of Experimental Social Psychology*, **5**, 189–202.

Lazarus A. A. (1976) Multimodal Assessment, In A. A. Lazarus (ed.) *Multimodal Behavior Therapy*, Springer, New York.

Lazarus, R. S. (1966) *Psychological Stress and Coping Process*. McGraw-Hill, New York.

Lebet, J. M. and Levinson, P. M. (1973) Concepts of social skills with special reference to the behaviour of depressed persons. *Journal of Consulting and Clinical*

Psychology, **40**, 304–12.

Lees, S. an Ellis, W. (1990) The design of a stress management programme for nursing personnel. *Journal of Advanced Nursing*, **15**, 946–61

Leiberman, M. (1982) The effects of social supports on responses to stress. In L. Goldberg L. and S. Breznitz (eds) *Handbook of Stress*. The Free Press, New York.

Lepper, M. R., Greene, D. and Nisbett, R. E. (1973) Undermining children's interest with extrinsic reward: a test of the overjustification hypothesis, *Journal of Personality and Social Psychology* , **28**, 129–37.

Lerner, M. J. (1980) *The Belief in a Just world: A Fundamental Delusion*. Plenum, New York.

Levenson, H. (1974) Activism and powerful others: distinctions within the concept of internal–external control. *Journal of Personality Assessment*, **38**, 377–83.

Leventhal, H. (1970) Findings and theory in the study of fear communications. In L. Berkowitz (ed.) *Advances in Experimental psychology*, Vol. 5. Academic Press, New York.

Lever, J. (1976) Sex differences in games children play, *Social Problems*, **23**, 478–87.

Levy, L. (l976) Self-help groups; types and psychological processes. *Applied Behavioural Research*, **12**, 310–22.

Ley, P. (1977) Communicating with the patient. In J. C. Coleman (ed.) *Introductory Psychology: A Text Book for Health Students*. Routledge and Kegan Paul, London.

Ley, P. (1979a) The psychology of compliance. In D. T. Oborne, M. M. Gruneberg and J. R. Eiser (eds) *Research in Psychology and Medicine: Vol. 2, Social Aspects; Attitudes Communication Care and Training*. Academic Press, London.

Ley, P. (1979b) Improving clinical communication: effects of altering doctor behavior. In D.T. Oborne, M. M. Gruneberg and J. R. Eiser (eds) *Research in Psychology and Medicine: Vol 2, Social Aspects; Attitudes Communication Care and Training*. Academic Press, London.

Ley, P. (1982) Satisfaction, compliance and communication. *British Journal of Clinical Psychology*, **21**, 241–54.

Ley, P. (1988) *Communicating with Patients: Improving Communication, Satisfaction and Compliance*. Croom Helm, London.

Lewin, K. (1948) *Resolving social conflicts: selected papers on group dynamics*. Harper and Row, New York.

Lieberman, M. A., Yalom, I. D. and Miles, M. B. (1973) *Encounter Groups: First Facts*. Basic Books, New York.

Lierman, L. M., Young, H. M., Kasprzyk, D. and Benoliel, J. Q. (1990) Predicting breast self- examination using the theory of reasoned action, *Nursing Research*, **39**, 97–101.

Litt, M. D. (1988) Self-efficacy and perceived control: cognitive mediators of pain tolerance. *Journal of Personality and Social Psychology*, **54**, 149–60.

London, M. and Hakel, M. D. (1974) Effects of applicant stereotypes, order and information on interview impressions. *Journal of Applied Psychology*, **59**, 157–62.

Lopez, J. L. R. (1990) Work organizations as social activity. In R. Bhaskar (ed.) *Harre and his Critics: Essays in Honour of Rom Harre with his commentary on them*. Blackwell, Oxford.

Lorensen, M. (1983) Effects of touch in parients during a crisis situation in hospital. In J. Wilson-Barnett (ed.) *Nursing Research: Vol. 10, Studies in Patient Care*, Wiley, Chichester.

Luchins, A. S. (1957) Primary-recency in impression formation. In C. I. Hoveland (ed.) *The Order of Presentation in Persuasion*. Yale University Press, New Haven, Conn.

Luke, R. A. (1972) The internal normative structure of sensitivity training groups. *Journal of Applied Behavioural Science*, **8**, 421–37.

Luria, A. R. (1981) *Language and Cognition*. Winston, Washington, DC.

Maccoby, E. E. and Jacklin, C. N. (1974) *The Psychology of Sex Differences.* Stanford University Press, Stanford, Calif.

Macleod Clark, J. (1981) Communication in nursing. *Nursing Times,* 1 January, 12–18.

Macleod Clark, J. (1984) Verbal communication in nursing. In A. Faulkner (ed.) *Recent Advances in Nursing 7: Communication.* Churchill Livingstone, Edinburgh.

MacPhillamy, D. J. and Lewinsohn, P. M. (1982) The pleasant events schedule: studies on reliability, validity and scale intercorrelation. *Journal of Consulting and Clinical Psychology,* **50**, 363–80.

McCorkle, R. (1974) Effects of touch on seriously ill patients. *Nursing Research* **23**, 125–32.

McDowell, J. R. S. (1989) For the love of the job. Unpublished Mental Nursing dissertation. University of Glasgow.

McGrath, A., Reid, N. and Boore, J. (1989) Occupational stress in nursing. *International Journal of Nursing Studies,* **26**, 343–58.

McGuire, W. J. (1969) The nature of attitudes and attitude change. In G. Lindzey and E. Aronson (eds) *Handbook of Social Psychology,* Vol 3, 2nd edn. Addison-Welsey, Reading, Mass.

McGuire, W. J. (1985) Atitudes and attitude change. In G. Lindzey and E. Aronson (eds) *Handbook of Social Psychology,* Vol. 2, 3rd edn. Random House, London.

McGuire, P. (1979) Teaching essential interviewing skills to medical students. In D. J. Oborne, M. M. Gruneberg and J. R. Eiser (eds) *Research in Psychology and Medicine II, Social Aspects: Atitudes Communication, Care and Training.* Academic Press, London.

McKinley, J. (1972) Social networks, lay consultation and help seeking behaviour. *Social Forces,* **51**, 275–81.

McWhinney, I. (1989) The need for a transformed clinical method. In M. Stewart and D. Roter (eds) *Communicating With Medical Patients.* Sage, New York.

Magee, B. (1973) *Popper.* Fontana, London.

Maggs, C (1984) A new history of nursing 2, *Nursing Times,* 19 September, 31–4.

Marsh, A. (1985) Smokers and illness: what smokers really believe. *Health Trends,* **17**, 7–12.

Marsh, A. and Matheson, J. (1983) *Smoking Attitudes and Behavior: an enquiry carried out on behalf of the Department of Health and Social Security.* HMSO, London.

Mathews, A. and Ridgeway, V. (1984) Psychological preparation for surgery. In A. Mathews and A. Steptoe (eds) *Health care and Human Behaviour.* Academic Press, London.

Mathews, S. M. (1988) Nothing to fear but fear, *Nursing Times,* **84**, (July 13) 35–7.

Mayer, D. K. (1987) Oncology Nurses' versus cancer patients' perceptions of nurse caring behaviours: a replication study. *Oncology Nursing Forum,* **14**, 48–52.

Mayfield, E. C. (1964) The selection interview: a reevaluation of published research. *Personnel Psychology,* **17**, 239–60.

Mayo, C. and La France, M. (1973) *Gase Direction in interracial dydadic communication.* Presented at the meeting of the Eastern Psychological Association, Washington, D.C.

Mauksch, H. O. (1966) Organizational context of nursing practice. In F. Davies (ed.) *The Nursing Profession.* Wiley, New York.

Mead, G. H. (1934) *Mind, Self and Society. Chicago University Press, Chicago, Ill.*

Meeus, W. H. J. and Raaijmakers, Q. A. W. (1986) Administrative obedience: carrying out orders to use psychological-administrative violence. *European Journal of Social Psychology,* **16**, 311–24.

Mechanic, D. (1978) *Medical Sociology* (2nd edn). Collier-Macmillan, London.

Meichenbaum, D. (1977) *Cognitive Behavior Modification: An Integrative Approach.* Plenum Press, New York.

Meichenbaum, D. and Turk D. (1977) The cognitive-behavioural management of anxiety, anger and pain. In P. O. Davidson (ed.) *The Behavioural Management of Anxiety, Depression and Pain*. Brunner Mazel, New York.

Melia, K. (1981) Student nurses account of their work and training. Unpublished PhD Thesis. University of Edinburgh, Edinburgh.

Melzack, R. (1975) The McGill Pain Questionnaire; major properties and scoring methods, *Pain*, **1**, 277–99.

Melzack, R. and Wall, P (1965) Pain mechanisms; a new theory, *Science*, **150**, 971–9.

Melzack, R. and Wall, P (1988) *The Challenge of Pain*, (2nd edn). Penguin, Harmondsworth.

Menzies, E. P. (1970) *The Functioning of Social Systems as a Defence Against Anxiety*. Tavistock, London.

Merton, K. (1957) The role set: problems in sociological theory. *British Journal of Sociology*, **8**, 106–20.

Meyerowitz, B. E. and Chaiken. S. (1987) The effect of message framing on breast self-examination attitudes, intentions and behavior. *Journal of Personality and Social Psychology*, **52**, 500–10.

Milgram, S. (1970) The experience of living in cities, *Science*, **167**, 1461–68.

Milgram, S. (1974) *Obedience to Authority*. Tavistock, London.

Mill, J. S. (1872) *A System of Logic*. Reprinted by Toronto University Press, 1973, Toronto.

Miller, A. (1985) Nurse/patient dependency – is it iatrogenic. *Journal of Advanced Nursing*, **10**, 63–9.

Miller, M. (1978) *The Body in Question*. Cape, London.

Miller, N., Maruyama, G.,Beaber, R. J. and Valone, K. (1976) Speed of speech and persuasion. *Journal of Personality and Social Psychology*, **34**, 615–24.

Millett, K. (1977) *Sexual Politics*. Virago, London.

Mills, C. W. (1940) Situated actions and vocabularies of motive. *American Sociological Review*, **5**, 904–13.

Mixon, D. (1972) Instead of deception. *Journal for the Theory of Social Behaviour*, **2**, 145–78.

Money, J. (1974) Prenatal hormones and postnatal socialization in gender identity differentiation. In J. K. Cole and A. Dienstbier (eds) *Nebraska Symposium on Motivation 1973*. University of Nebraska Press, Lincoln, Nebraska.

Money, J. and Ehrhardt, A. (1972) *Man, Women, Boy, Girl*. Johns Hopkins University Press, Baltimore, Md.

Morgan, B. S. (1985) A sementic differential measure of attitudes towards black American patients. *Research in Nursing and Health*, **7**, 155–62.

Morgan, M., Calnan, M. and Manning, N. (1986) *Sociological Approaches to Health and Medicine*. Routledge, London.

Morimoto, F. R. (1955) Favoritism in personnel – patient interaction. *Nursing Research;* **3**, 109–12.

Moscovici, S. (1961) *La Psychanalyse: Son Image et Son Public*. Presses Universitaires de France, Paris.

Moscovici, S. (1968) On social representation. In J. Forgas (ed.) *Social Cognition Perspectives on Everyday Understanding*. Academic Press, London.

Moscovici, S. (1976) *Social Influence and Social Change*. Academic Press, London.

Moscovici, S. (1980) Toward a theory of conversion behaviour. In L. Berkowitz (ed.) *Advances in Experimental Social Psychology*, Vol. 13. Academic Press, New York.

Moscovici, S. Lage, E. and Naffrechoux, M (1969) Influence of a consistant minority on the responses of a majority in a colour perception task. *Sociometry*, **32**, 365–80.

Moscovici, S. and Personnaz, B. (1980) Studies in social influence. V: Minority influence and conversion behaviour in a perceptual task. *Journal of Experimental Social Psychology,* **16**, 270–82.

Moscovici, S. and Zavalloni, M. (1969) The group as a polarizer of attitudes. *Journal of Personality and Social Psychology,* **12**, 125–35.

Moss, H. A. (1970) Sex, age and state as determinants of mother-infant interaction. In K Danziger (ed.) *Readings in Child Socialization.* Pergamon Press.

Muhlenkamp, A. F. and Sayles, J. A. (1968) Self esteem, social support and positive health practices. *Nursing Research,* **35**, 334–38.

Mumford, E., Schlesinger, H. J. and Glass, G. V. (1982) The effects of psychological intervention on recovery from surgery and heart attacks. An analysis of the literature, *American Journal of Public Health,* **72**, 141–51.

Murstein, B. I. (1977) The Stimulus-Value-Role (SVR) theory of dyadic relationships. In S. W. Duck (ed.) *Theory and Practice in Interpersonal Attraction.* Academic Press, London.

Murstein, B. I. MacDonald, M. G. and Cerreto, M. (1977) A theory and investigation of the effects of exchange-orientation on marriage and friendship. *Journal of Marriage and the Family,* **39**, 543–48.

Nahemow, L. and Lawton, M. P. (1975) Similarity and propinquity in friendship formation. *Journal of Personality & Social Psychology,* **32**, 205–13.

Naismith, L. D., Robinson, J. D., Shaw, G. B. and Macintyre, M. M. (1979) Psychological rehabilitation after myocardial in farction, *British Medical Journal,* **1**, 439–41.

National Development Group (1978) *Helping Mentally Handicapped People in Hospital.* National Development Group, Manchester.

National Health Service and Community Care Act (1990) *Care in the Community,* HMSO, London.

Nelson-Jones, R. (1990) *Counselling and Helping Skills.* Holt, Rinehart and Winston, London.

Neuman, B (1982) The Neuman health care system: a total approach to client care. In B. Neuman (ed.) The Neuman System Model. Appleton-Century-Crofts, New York.

Newcomb, T. (1961) *The Acquaintance Process.* Holt Rinehart, New York.

Newnes, C. (1981) Black stockings and frilly caps? *Nursing Mirror, 28 October,* 28–30.

Nichols, K. A. (1984) *Psychological Care in Physical Illness.* Croom Helm, London.

Nicholson, N., Steven G. C. and Rocklin, T. (1985) Conformity in the Asch situation: A comparison between contemporary British and US university students. *British Journal of Social Psychology,* **24**, 59–63.

Novaco, R. W. (1978) Anger and coping with stress: cognitive behavioural interventions. In J. P. Foreyt and D. P. Rathjen (eds) *Cognitive Behaviour Therapy: Research and Application.* Plenum, New York.

'Nursing': Survey Report on Nursing Ethics (1974) *Nursing,* September, 35–44.

Oakley, A. (1972) *Sex, Gender and Society.* Temple-Smith, London.

Oakley, A. (1974) *The Sociology of Housework.* Martin Robertson, London

Oakley, A. (1984) The importance of being a nurse. *Nursing Times,* 12 December, 24–7.

Oatley, K. (1980) Theories of personal learning in groups. In P. B. Smith (ed.) *Small Groups and Personal Change.* Methuen, London.

Oatley, K. (1988) Life events, social cognition and depression In S. Fisher and J. Reason (eds) *Handbook of Life Stress, Cognition and Health.* Wiley, Chichester.

O'Brien, C. P., Chaddock, B., Woody, G., and Greenstein, R. (1974) Systematic extinction of narcotic drug use using narcotic antagonists *Psychosomatic Medicine,* **36**, 458.

O'Brien, M. E. (1980) Effective social environment and haemodialysis adoptation; a panel analysis. *Journal of Health and Social Behaviour*, **21**, 360–70.

O'Dell, S. (1974) Training parents in behaviour modification. *Psychological Bulletin*, **81**, 418–33.

Ogier, M. (1984) How do ward sisters influence learning by nurses in the wards. In S. Skevington (ed.) *Understanding nurses: The Social Psychology of Nursing*. Wiley, Chichester.

Oppenheim, A. N. (1955) *The Function and Training of Mental Nurses*. Chapman and Hall, London.

Orbell, S., Hopkins, N. and Gillies, B. (1991) *A Survey of People Providing Care to an Elderly Person in Dundee*. Department of Epidemiology and Public Health, University of Dundee, Dundee.

Orem, D. (1985) *Nursing: Concepts of Practice, (2nd edn)*. McGraw Hill, New York.

Orton, H. D. (1981) *Ward Learning Climate*. Royal College of Nursing, London.

Orton, H. D. (1984) Learning on the ward - how important is climate? In S Skevington (ed.) *Understanding nurses: The Social Psychology of Nursing*. Wiley, Chichester.

Osgood, C. E. (1962) Studies in the generality of affective meaning systems, *American Psychologist*, **17**, 10–28.

Oswin, M. (1978) *Children Living in Long Stay Hospitals*. Spastics International Medical Publication, Heinemann, London.

Pahl, J. (1979) Refuges for battered women: social provision or social movement. *Journal of Voluntary Action Research*, **8**, 25–35.

Parkes, C. M. (1972) *Bereavement: Studies of grief in Adult Life*. Tavistock, London.

Parkes, C. M. and Weiss , R. S. (1983) *Recovery from Bereavement*. Basic Books, New York.

Parkes, K. R. (1982) Occupational stress among student nurses: a natural experiment, *Journal of Applied Psychology*, **67**, 784–96.

Parsons, T. (1951) *The Social System*. The Free Press of Glencoe, New York.

Patterson, C. H. (1985) *The Therapeutic Relationship; Foundations for an Eclectic Psychotherapy*. Brooks/Cole California.

Pavlov, I. P. (1927) *Conditioned Reflexes: An Investigation of the Physiological Activity of the Cerebral Cortex*. Dover, New York.

Peat Marwick McLintock (1989) *Review of the United Kingdom Central Council and the Four National boards for Nursing, Midwifery and Health Visiting*. Peat Marwick McLintock, London.

Perrow, C. (1972) *Complex Organizations: A Critical Essay*. Scott, Foresman, Glenview, Ill.

Peters-Golden, H. (1982) Breast cancer: varied perceptions of social support in the illness experience. *Social Science and Medicine*, **16**, 483–91.

Peters, R. S. (1958) *The Concept of Motivation*. Routledge and Kegan Paul, London.

Pietroni, P. (1976) Non-verbal communication in the general practice surgery. In B. Tanner (ed.) *Language and Communication in General Practice*. Hodder and Stoughton, London.

Piliavin, J. A. and Piliavin I. M. (1972) Effects of blood on reactions to a victim. *Journal of Personality and Social Psychology*, **23**, 353–61.

Piliavin, I. M. Rodin, J. and Piliavin, J. A. (1969) Good samaritanism: an underground phenomenon. *Journal of Personality and Social Psychology*, **13**, 389–99.

Pollak, S. and Gilligan, C. (1982) Images of violence in Thematic and perception test stories. *Journal of Personality and Social Psychology*, **42**, 159–67.

Popper, K. (1959) *The Logic of Scientific Discovery*. Hutchinson, London.

Potter, J. and Wetherell, M. (1987) *Discourse Analysis and Social Psychology*. Sage, London.

Powell, D. R. (1981) Creating and sustaining parent groups: critical program process dimensions. Presented to Society for Research in Child Development. Boston, Mass.

Powell, L. H. and Friedman, M. (1986) Alteration of Type A Behavior in Coronary Patients. In M. J. Christie and P. G. Mellett (eds) *The Psychosomatic Approach: Contemporary Practice of Whole Person Care.* Wiley, Chichester.

Price Waterhouse (1988) *Nurses Retention and Recruitment.* Price Waterhouse, London.

Project 2000 (1986) *A New Preparation for Practice.* United Kingdom Central Council for Nurses, Midwives and Health Visitors, London.

Raines, G. N. and Rohrer, J. H. (1955) The operational matrix of psychiatric practice: consistency and variability in interview impressions of different psychiatrists. *American Journal of Psychiatry,* **111**, 721–33.

Rank, S. G. and Jacobson, C. K. (1977) Hospital nurses compliance with medication overdose orders: a failure to replicate. *Journal of Health and Social Behaviour,* **18**, 188–93.

Rapoport, R. N. (1960) *Community as Doctor,* Tavistock, London.

Raps, C. S., Peterson, C., Jonas, M., Seligman, M. E. P. (1982) *Journal of Personality and Social Psychology,* **42**, 1036–41.

Raven, B. H., Freeman, H. E. and Haley, R. W. (1982) Social science perspectives in hospital infection control. In A. W. Johnson, O. Grusky and B. H. Raven (eds) *Contemporary Health Services: Social Science Perspectives,* Auburn House, Boston.

Raven, B. H. and Haley, R. W. (1980) Social influence in a medical context: Hospital- acquired infections as aproblem in medical social psychology. In L. Bickman (ed.) *Applied Social Psychology Annual,* Vol. 1. Sage, Beverly Hills, Calif.

Reicher, S. D. (1984) Social influence in the crowd: Attitudinal and behavioural effects of deindividuation in conditions of high and low group salience. *British Journal of Social Psychology,* **23**, 341–51.

Reiss, H. T., Wheeler, L., Spiegel, N., Kernis, M. H., Nezlek, J., and Perri, M. (1982) Physical attractiveness in social interaction 2: Why does appearance affect social experience? *Journal of Personality and Social Psychology,* **43**, 979–96.

Report of the Committee of Nursing (1972) (The Briggs Report). HMSO, London.

Rescorla, R. A. (1968) Probability of schock in the presence or absence of CS in fear conditioning. *Journal of Comparative and Physiological Psychology,* **66**, 1–5.

Reverby, S. (1987a) *Ordered to Care: The Dilemma of American Nursing.* Cambridge University Press, New York.

Reverby, S. (1987b) A caring dilemma: womenhood and nursing in historical perspective. *Nursing Research,* **36**, 5–11.

Rheingold, H. L. and Cook, K. U. (1975) The contents of boy's and girl's rooms as an index of parents' behaviour. *Child Development,* **46**, 459–63.

Richman, N., Douglas, J., Hunt, H., Lansdown, R., Levere, R. (1985) Behavioural methods in the treatment of sleep disorders – a pilot study, *Journal of Child Psychology and Psychiatry,* **26**, 581–90.

Riehl, J. P. (1980) The Riehl interaction model. In Riehl, J. P. and Roy C. (eds) *Conceptual Models for Nursing Practice.* Appleton-Century- Crofts, New York.

Rivicki, D. A. and May, H. J. (1989) Organizational characteristics: occupational stress and mental health in nurses. *Behaviour and Medicine,* **15**, 30–6.

Robbins, L. (1974) *The Viet Nam Drug User Returns.* McGraw-Hill, New York.

Robinson, D. (1980) Self-help health groups. In P. B. Smith (ed.) *Small Groups and Personal Change.* Methuen, London.

Robinson, D. and Robinson Y. (1979) *From Self-Help to Health.* Concord Books, London.

Rogers, C. R. (1957) The necessary and sufficient conditions of therapeutic personality change. *Journal of Counselling Psychology,* **21**, 95–103.

Rogers, M. E. (1980). Nursing: A science of unitary man. In Riehel, J. P. and

Ray, C. (eds). *Conceptual Models for Nursing Practice.* Appleton-Century-Crofts, New York.

Rosenfeld, H. M. (1967) Non-verbal reciprocation of approval: an experimental analysis. *Journal of Experimental Psychology,* **3**, 102–111.

Rosenkrantz, P., Vogel, S., Bee, H., Broverman, I. K., Broverman, D. M. (1968) Sex role sterotypes and self-concepts in college students. *Journal of Consulting and Clinical Psychology,* **32**, 287-95.

Rosenman, R. H. Friedman, M. and Strauss, R. (1966) CHD in the Western Collaborative Group Study. *Journal of the American Medical Association,* **195**, 86–92.

Rosenstock, I. M. (1960) What research in motivation suggests for public health. *American Journal of Public Health,* **50**, 295–302.

Rosenstock, I. M. (1966) Why people use health services. *Milbank Memorial Fund Quarterly,* **44**, 94–127.

Rosenstock, I. M. (1974) The health belief model and preventive health behavior. *Health Education Monographs,* **2**, 354–86.

Rosenthal, R. and Jacobson, L. (1968) *Pygmalion in the Classroom.* Holt, Rinehart and Winston, New York.

Rotter, D. (1989) What facets of communication have strong effects on outcome – a meta-analysis. In M. Stewart and D. Rotter (eds) *Communicating with Medical Patients.* Sage, London.

Rotter, J. B. (1966) General expectancies for internal versus external control of reinforcement. *Psychological Monographs,* **80** (whole part).

Rowland, A. J. and Cooper, P. (1983) *Environment and Health.* Edward Arnold, London.

Roy, C. (1984) *Introduction to Nursing: An Adaption Model.* Prentice-Hall, Englewood Cliffs, New Jersey.

Ruano, B. J. (1971) This I believe. . . about nurses innovating change. *Nursing Outlook,* 19 June, 416–8.

Rush, A. J. and Giles, D. E. (1982) Cognitive therapy; theory and research. In A. J. Rush (ed.) *Short-Term Psychotherapies for Depression.* Wiley, Chichester.

Saegel, D., Bloom, J.R. and Yalom, I. (1981) Group support for patient with metastatic cancer. A randomized prospective outcome study. *Archive of General Psychiatry,* **38**, 527–33.

Sanger, S., Weir, K. and Churchill, E. (1981) Treatment of sleep problems: the use of behaviour modification techniques by health visitors. *Health Visitor,* **54**, 421–24.

Sarah, E., Scott, M. and Spender, D. (1980) The education of feminists: the case for single sex schools. In D. Spender and E. Sarah (eds) *Learning to Lose: Sexism and Education. The Women's Press, London.*

Schank, R,. and Abelson, R. (1977) *Scripts, Plans, Goals and Understanding: An Inquiry into Human Knowledge Structures.* Lawrence Erlbaum, Hillsdale, New Jersey.

Schmidt, F. L. and Hunter, J. E. (1981) Employment testing: old theories and new research findings. *American Psychologist,* **36**, 1128–37.

Schmidt, N. (1976) Social and situational determinants of interview decisions: implications for the employment interview. *Personnel Psychology,* **29**, 79–102.

Schneider, J. and Conrad, P. (1981) Medical and sociological typologies: the case of epilepsy. *Social Science and Medicine,* **15**, 211–19.

Schutz, A. (1953) Commonsense and scientific interpretation of human action. *Philosophy and Phenomenological Research,* **14**, 1–37.

Schutz, A. (1967) *Collected Papers.* Martinus Nijhoff, The Hague.

Schwartz, S. H. and Howard, J. A. (1981) A normative decision-making model of altruism. In J. P. Rushton and R. M. Sorrentino (eds) *Altruism and Helping Behaviour.* Erlbaum, Hillsdale, New Jersey.

Schwarzer, R. and Leppin, A. (1989) Social support and health: a meta-analysis.

Psychology and Health, **3**, 1–15.

Scott, M. (1980) Teach her a lesson: sexist curriculum in patriarchial education. In D. Spender and E. Sarah (eds) *Learning to Lose: Sexism and Education*. The Women's Press, London.

Scott, M. and Lyman, S. (1968) Accounts, *American Sociological review*, **33**, 46–62.

Secord, P.F. and Backman, C. W. (1974) *Social Psychology, (2nd edn)*. McGraw-Hill International, London.

Seligman, M. E. P. (1975) *Helplessness*. Freeman, San Francisco.

Seligman, M. E. P., Abrahamson, L. Y., Semmel, A. and von Baeyer, C.(1979) Depressive attribution style. *Journal of Abnormal Psychology*, **88**, 242–7.

Selye H (1974) *Stress Without Distress*. Lippincott, Philadelphia, Pa.

Shaffer, , D. R. and Graziano, W. G. (1983) Effects of positive and negative moods on helping tasks having pleasant or unpleasant consequences. *Motivation and Emotion*, **7**, 269–78.

Shanley, E. (1984) *Evaluation of Mental Nurses by their Patients and Charge Nurses.* Unpublished PhD Thesis, University of Edinburgh, Edinburgh.

Shanley, E. and Murray, I. (1986). *A proposal for change in RMN training*. PNAS Publishers, Dundee.

Shanley, E. and Murray, I. (1991) *Preparation for Mental Health Nursing Practice*. Psychiatric Nurses' Association Publication, Edinburgh.

Shatz, M. and Gelmen, R. (1973) The development of communication skills: modifications in the speech of young children as a function of listener, Monographs of the Society for *Research in Child Development*, **38** (5), (whole no. 152).

Sherif, M. (1935) A study of some factors in perception. *Archives of psychology*, **27**, no. 187.

Shotland, R. L. and Heinold, W. D. (1985) Bystander response to arterial bleeding: helping skills, the decision-making process and differentiating the helping response. *Journal of Personality and Social Psychology*, **49**, 347–56.

Shotter, J. (1974) What is it to be human? In N. Armistead (ed.) *Reconstructing Social Psychology*. Penguin, Harmondsworth.

Shotter, J. (1980) Men the magicians: the duality of social being and the structure of moral worlds. In A. J. Chapman and D. M. Jones (eds) *Models of Man*. The British Psychological Society, Leicester.

Sidel, V. W. and Sidel, R. (1976) Beyond coping. *Social Policy*, **7**, 67–9.

Simon, J. G. and Feather, N. T. (1973) Causal attributions for success and failure at university examinations. *Journal of Educational Psychology*, **64**, 46–56.

Simpson, I. H. (1973) Patterns of socialization into professions; the case of student nurses. In D.R. MacQueen (ed.) *Understanding Sociology through Research*. Addison-Wesley, London.

Skevington, S. (1981) Intergroup relations and nursing. *European Journal of Social Psychology*, **11**, 43–59

Skevington, S. (1984) How will nurses cope with radical changes in training? In S. Skevington (ed.) *Understanding Nurses: The Social: Psychology of Nursing*. Wiley, Chichester.

Skinner, B. F. (1938) *The Behaviour of Organisms*, Appleton-Century-Crofts, New York.

Skinner, B. F. (1957) *Verbal Behaviour*. Appleton- Century-Crofts, New York.

Smith, P. B. (1980a) Group Processes and personal Change. Harper and Row, London.

Smith, P. B. (1980b) Introduction. In P. B. Smith (ed.) *Small Groups and Personal Change*. Methuen, London.

Smith, P. B. (1980c) The outcome of sensitivity training and encounter groups. In P. B. Smith (ed.) *Small Groups and Personal Change*. Methuen, London.

Snell, B. (1960) *The Discovery of Mind: The Greek Origins of European Thought.* Harper and Row, London.

Snyder, M. (1979) Self-monitoring processes. In L. Berkowitz (ed.) *Advances in Experimental Social Psychology,* **12**, 85–128, Academic Press, New York.

Sorrentino, R. M. and Boutillier, R. G. (1975) The effect of quality and quantity of verbal interaction on rating of leadership ability. *Journal of Experimental and Social Psychology,* **11**, 403–11.

Sosa, R., Kennell, J., Klaus, M., Robertson, I. and Urrutia, J. (1980) The effect of a supportive companion on perinatel problems, length of labour and mother infact interaction. *New England Journal of Medicine,* **303**, 597–600.

Speedling, E. J. (1982) Heart attack; *The Family Response at Home and in Hospital.* Tavistock, London.

Spence, J. T. and Helmreich, R. L. (1978) *Masculinity and Feminity: Their Psychological Dimensions, Correlates and Antecedents.* Texas University Press, Austin, Texas.

Spender, D. and Sarah, E. (eds) (1980) *Learning to Lose: Sexism and Education.* The Women's Press, London

Spiegel, D., Bloom, J. C. and Yalom, I. (1981) Group support for patients with metastatic cancer. A randomised propective outcome study. *Archieve of General Psychiatry,* **38**, 527–33.

Stachnik, T. J. (1980) Priorities for psychology in medical education and health care delivery. *American Psychologist,* **35**, 8–15.

Stansfield, J. (1986). Verbal communication and non-verbal communication. In Stanley E. (ed.) *Mental Handicap: Handbook of Care.* Churchill-Livingston, Edinburgh.

Steffens (1980) Perception of stress. 1800 nurses tell their stories. In Claus, K. and Bailey, J. (eds). *Living with stress and promoting well-being: A handbook for nurses.* CV Maskey, St. Louis.

Stein, L. I. (1968) The doctor/nurse game. *American Journal of Nursing,* **68**, 1–5.

Sternbach, R. A. and Tursky, B. (1965) Ethnic differences among housewives in psychophysical and skin potential responses to electric shock. *Psychophysiology,* **1**, 241–6.

Stewart, J., de Wit, H. and Eikelboom, R. (1984) Role of unconditioned and conditioned drug effects in the self administration of opiates and stimulants. *Psychological Review,* **91**, 251-68.

Stimson, G. V. and Webb, B. (1975) *Going to see the Doctor: The Consultation Process in General Practice.* Routledge and Kegan Paul, London.

Stockwell, F. (1972) *The Unpopular patient: The Study of Nursing Care Project Reports,* Series 1, No. 2. Royal College of Nursing, London.

Stogdill, R. M. (1974) *Handbook of Leadership; A Survey of Theory and Research.* Free press, New York.

Stoner, J. A. F. (1961) A comparison of individual and group decisions involving risk. Unpublished master's thesis. School of Industrial Management, Massachusetts Institute of Technology.

Strauss, A., Schatzman, L., Ehrlich, D., Bucher, R. Sabshin, M. (1963) The Hospital and its Negotiated order. In E. Freidson (ed.) *The Hospital in Modern Society.* Free Press, New York.

Strickland, B. R. (1978) Internal-external expectancies and health-related behaviors. *Journal of Counselling and Clinical Psychology,* **46**, 1192–211.

Stroebe, W., Stroebe, M. S., Gergen, K. J. and Gergen, M. (1982) The effects of breavement on mortality: a social psychological analysis. In J. R. Eiser (ed.) *Social Psychology and Behavioural Medicine.* Wiley, London.

Sudnow, D. (1967) *Passing On: The Social Organization of Dying.* Prentice-Hall, London.

Szasz, T. S. (1961) *The Myth of Mental Illness.* Harper and Row, New York.

Szivos, S. E. and Travers, E. (1988) Consciousness raising among mentally handicapped people: a critique of the implications of normalization. *Human Relations*, **41**, 641–53.

Tagliacozzo, D. L. and Mauksch, H. O. (1972) The patient's view of the patient's role. In E. G. Jaco (ed.) *Patients, Psychiatrists, and Illness* (2nd edn). Free Press, New York.

Tajfel, H. (ed.) (1978) *Differentiation Between Social Groups: Studies in the Social Psychology of Intergroup Relations*. Academic Press, London.

Tajfel, H., Flament, C., Billig, M. G., Bundy, R. P. (1971) Social categorization and intergroup behavior. *European Journal of Social Psychology*, **1**, 149–78.

Tajfel, H. (1972). Experiments in a vacuum. In J. Israel and K. Tajfel (eds). *The context of Social Psychology*. Academic Press, London.

Tajfel, H. and Turner, J. C. (1979) An integrative theory of intergroup conflict. In W. C. Austin and S. Worchel (eds) *The Social Psychology of Intergroup Relations*. Brooks Cole, Monterey, Calif.

Tannenbaum, R and Schmidt, W. H. (1957) How to chose a leadership pattern, *Harvard Business Review*, March–April, 95–101.

Taylor, C. (1971). Interpretation and the sciences of man *Review of Metaphysics*, **25**, 1–51

Taylor, D. M. and McKirnan, D. J. (1984) A five stage model of intergroup relations. *British Journal of Social Psychology*, **23**, 291–301.

Taylor, S. E. (1979) Hospital patient behaviour: reactance, helplessness or control? *Journal of Social Issues*, **35**, 156–84.

Taylor, S. E. (1983) Adjustment to threatening events: a theory of cognitive adaption. *American Psychologist*, **38**, 1161–173.

Tedeschi, J. T. (1981) *Impression Management Theory and Social Psychological Research*. Academic Press, New York.

Thompson, J. O. (1989) Recruiting men. *Nursing Times*, **85**, December, 45.

Thorndike, E. L. (1911) *Animal Intelligence*. Macmillan, New York.

Toffler, A. (1971) *Future Shock*. Pan Books, London.

Tolman, E. C. (1925) Purpose and cognition: the determinants of animal learning. *Psychological Review*, **32**, 285–97.

Tolman, E. C. and Honzik, C. H. (1930) Introduction and removal of reward and maze learning in rats. *University of California Publications in Psychology*, **4**, 257–75.

Towell, D. (1975). *Understanding psychiatric Nursing*. Royal College of Nursing, London.

Travelbee, J. (1966) *Interpersonal Aspects of Nursing*. F. A. Davies, Philadelphia, Pa.

Triandis, H. C. (1972) *An Analysis of Subjective Culture*. Wiley, New York.

Trower, P., Bryant, B. and Argyle, M. (1978) *Social Skills and Mental Health*. Methuen, London.

Truax, C. B. and Mitchell, K. M. (1971) Research on certain therapist interpersonal skills in relation to process and outcome. In A. E. Bergin and S. L. Garfield (eds) *Handbook of Psychotherapy and Behaviour Change*. Wiley, New York.

Tuckman, B. W. (1965) Developmental sequences in small groups. *Psychological Bulletin;* **63**, 384–98.

Turk, D. C. and Flor, H. (1987) Pain behaviour: One utility and limitations of the pain behaviour construct. *Pain;* **31**, 277–95.

Turk, D. C. and Kerns, R. D. (1983) Conceptual issues in the assessment of clinical pain. *International Journal of Psychiatry in Medicine*, **13**, 57–68.

Turk, D. C., Meichenbaum, D. and Genest M. (1983a) *Pain and Behavioural Medicine: A Cognitive- Behavioural Perspective*. Guildford, New York.

Turk, D. C., Wack, J. T. and Kerns, R. D. (1985b) An empirical examination of the 'pain behaviour'" construct. *Journal of Behavioural medicine*, **8**, 119–30.

Turner, J. C. (1982) Towards a cognitive redefinition of the social group. In H.

Tajfel (ed.) *Social Identity and Intergroup Relations.* Cambridge University Press, Cambridge.

Ulrich, L. and Trumbo, D. (1965) The selection interview since 1949. *Psychological Bulletin,* **63,** 100–16.

van Knippenberg, A. and van Oers, H. (1984) Social identity and equity concernsin intergroup perceptions. *British Journal of Social Psychology,* **23,** 351–63.

Verplanck, W. S. (1955) The control of the content of conversation: reinforcement of statements of opinion. *Journal of Abnormal and Social Psychology,* **51,** 668–76.

Waite, R. and Hutt, R. (1987) Attitude, job and mobility of qualified nurses. A report for the Royal College of Nursing, Institute of Manpower Studies 130. University of Sussex.

Waitzkin, H. and Stoekle, J. (1972) The communication of information about illness. *Advanced Psychosomatic Medicine,* **8,** 108–215.

Walker, S. (1984) *Learning Theory and Behaviour Modification.* Methuen, London.

Wallston, K. A. and Wallston, B. S. (1982) Who is responsible for your health? The construct of locus of control. In G. S. Sanders and J. Suls (eds) *Social Psychology of Health and Illness.* Lawrence Erlbraum, Hillsdale, New Jersey.

Wallston, K. A., Wallston, B. S. and DeVellis, R. (1978) Development of the multidimensional locus of control (MHLC) scales. *Health Education Monographs,* **6,** 161–70.

Walsh, P. A. and Ashcroft, J. B. (1974) Nurses' uniforms – do they affect patient–staff interaction? *Nursing Times,* 7 March, 363.

Watson, D. (1982) The actor and the observer: how are their perceptions of causality different? *Psychological Bulletin,* **92,** 682–700.

Watson, J. B. (1913) Psychology as a behaviourist views it. *Psychological Review,* **20,** 158–77.

Watson, J. B. and Rayner, R. (1920) Conditioned emotional reactions. *Journal of Experimental Psychology,* **3,** 1–4.

Watson, O. M. (1970) *Proxemic Behaviour: A Cross Cultural Study.* Mouton, The Hague.

Watson, W. (1975) The meaning of touch in geriatric nursing. *Journal of Communication,* **25,** 104–12.

Webb, C. (1982) The men wear the trousers, *Nursing Mirror, 13 January, 29–31.*

Webb, C. (1984) Feminist methodology in nursing research. *Journal of Advanced Nursing,* **9,** 249–56.

Weber, M. (1947) *The Theory of Social and Economic Organizations.* (T. Parsons (ed.), A. M. Henderson and T. Parsons (trans.). Free Press, New York.

Weiner, B. (1974) *Achievement, Motivation and Attribution Theory.* General Learning Press. Morristown, New Jersey.

Weiner, B. (1980) A cognitive attributional emotion-action model of motivated behaviour : an analysis of judgements of helpgiving. *Journal of Personality and Social Psychology,* **39,** 186–200.

Weinberg, R. S., Gould, D. and Jackson, A. (1979) Expectations and performance: an empirical test of Bandura's self-efficacy theory, *Journal of Sport Psychology,* **1,** 320–31.

Weinman, J. and Johnston, M. (1988) Stressful medical procedures: an analysis of the effects of psychological interventions and the stressfulness of the procedures. In S. Maes, C. D. Spielberger, P. B. Defaras and I. G. Sarason (eds) *Topics in Health Psychology.* Wiley, Chichester.

Weisberg, P. (1963) Social and nonsocial conditioning of infant vocalization, *Child Development,* **34,** 377–88.

Wells, T. (1980) *Problems in Geriatric Nursing Care.* Churchill Livingstone, Edinburgh.

Wheeler, L., Reis, H. and Nezlek, J. (1983) Loneliness, social interaction and sex roles. *Journal of Personality and Social Psychology*, **45**, 943–53.

Whitcher, S. J. and Fisher, J. (1979) Multidimensional reaction to therapeutic touch in a hospital setting. *Journal of Personality and Social Psychology*, **37**, 87–96.

White, R and Lippit, R (1968) Leader behaviour and member reaction in three 'social climates'. In D. Cartwright and A Zander, A. (eds) *Group Dynamics: Theory and Research*. Tavistock, London.

Wicker, A. J. (1969) Attitudes versus actions: the relationship of verbal and overt behavioral responses to attitude objects. *Journal of Social Issues*, **25**, 41–78.

Wiedenfeld, S. A., O'leary, A., Bandura, A., Brown. S., Levine, S. and Raska, K. (1989) Impact of perceived self-efficacy in coping with stressors on components of the immune system. Cited in Bandura, A. (1989) Perceived self efficacy in the exercise of personal agency. *The psychologist: Bulletin of the British Psychological Society*, **10**, 411–24.

Wiener, M, Devoe, S, Rubinow, S. and Giller, J. (1972) Non-verbal behaviour and non-verbal communication. *Psychological Review*, **79**, 185–214.

Wilkinson, S. R. (1987) Germs: nursery school children's views on the causality of illness. *Clinical Pediatrics*, **26**, 465–69.

Williams, J. E. and Best, D. L. (1982) *Measuring Sex Stereotypes: A Thirty Nation Study*. Sage, Beverly Hills, Calif.

Williams, J. E. (1979) Psychological androgeny and mental health. In O. Hartnert, G. Boden and M. Fuller (eds) *Sex Role Sterotyping*. Tavistock, London.

Wills, T. A. (1981) Downward comparison principles in social psychology. *Psychological Bulletin*, **90**, 245–71.

Wills, T. A. (1985) Supportive function of interpersonal relationships. In S. Cohen and S. J. Symes (eds) *Social Support and Health*. Academic Press, Orlando.

Wilson-Barnett, J. (1980). Prevention and alleviation of stress in patients. *Nursing;* **10**, 432–36.

Wilson-Barnett, J. (1984) Interventions to alleviate patients' stress: a review. *Journal of Psychosomatic Research*, **28**, 63–72.

Wilson-Barnett, J. (1988) Patient teaching or patient counselling? *Journal of Advanced Nursing*, **13**, 215–22.

Wolfensberger, W. (1972) *The Principle of Normalization in Human Services*. National Institute on Mental Retardation, Toronto.

Wolfensberger, W. (1984) Social role valorization: A proposed new term for the principle of normalization. *Mental Retardation*, **34**, 234–39.

Wood, M. J. (1980) Implementing the Riehl interaction model in nursing administration. In Riehl, J. P. and Roy C. (eds) *Conceptual Models for Nursing Practice*. Appleton-Century-Crofts, New York.

Wolpe, J. (1958) *Psychotherapy by Reciprocal Inhibition*. Stanford University Press, Stanford, Calif.

Worden, J. W. (1982) *Grief Counselling and Grief Therapy*. Tavistock, London.

World Health Organisation (1956) Report of the Expert Committee on Psychiatric Nursing. First Report. *WHO Technical Series*, No. 105. WHO, Geneva.

Worsley, A. (1980) Exploration of student nurses' sterotypes of patients. *International Journal of Nursing Studies*, **17**, 163–74.

Wortman, C. B. and Conway, T. L. (1985) The role of social support in adaptation and recovery from physical illness. In S. Cohen and S. J. Symes (eds) *Social Support and Health*, Academic Press, Orlando, Florida.

Wortman, C. B. and Dunkell-Schetter, C. (1987) Conceptual and methodological issues in the study of social support. *Psychometrics*, **20**, 780–7.

Yandrell, B. and Insko, C. A. (1977) Attributions of attitudes to speakers and listeners under assigned- behaviour conditions: Does behaviour engulf the field. *Journal of Experimental Social Psychology*, **13**, 269–78.

Zajonc, R. B. (1965) Social facilitation. *Science*, **149**, 269–74.

Zander, A. (1979) The psychology of group processes, *Annual Review of Psychology*, **30**, 417–51.

Zborowski, M. (1952) Cultural components in response to pain. *Journal of Social Issues*, **8**, 16–30.

Zola, I. K. (1975) Culture and symptoms: an analysis of patients' presenting complaints. In, C. Cox, and A. Mead (eds) *Sociology of Medical Practice*. Collier-Macmillan, London.

INDEX